THE
SOUTH
BEACH
DIET
GLUTEN
SOLUTION

THE
SOUTH
BEACH
DIET
GLUTEN
SOLUTION

The Delicious, Doctor-Designed, Gluten-Aware Plan for Losing Weight and Feeling Great—FAST!

ARTHUR AGATSTON, MD
WITH NATALIE GEARY, MD

RODALE.

© 2013 by Arthur Agatston, MD
The South Beach Diet® is a Registered Trademark of the SBD Holdings Group Corp.

Rodale books may be purchased for business or promotional use or for special sales.
For information, please write to:
Special Markets Department, Rodale Inc., 733 Third Avenue, New York, NY 10017.

Printed in the United States of America
Rodale Inc. makes every effort to use acid-free ♾, recycled paper ♺.

Book design by Amy King

Cartoon on page 3 © Alex Gregory/The New Yorker Collection/www.cartoonbank.com

Illustrations by Enid Hatton

Library of Congress Cataloging-in-Publication Data is on file with the publisher.

ISBN-13: 978-1-62336-045-0 hardcover

Distributed to the trade by Macmillan

2   4   6   8   10   9   7   5   3   1   hardcover

TO MY UNCLE, ROBERT AGATSTON,
WHO FIRST MADE ME GLUTEN AWARE

AND, AS ALWAYS, TO MY WIFE, SARI,
AND SONS, EVAN AND ADAM

CONTENTS

PART III: REAL-LIFE GLUTEN SOLUTIONS

ACKNOWLEDGMENTS

THERE ARE SO MANY PEOPLE WHO HAVE HELPED ME PROGRESS ON MY gluten-aware journey, which began with my initial gluten revelations and moved on to a better understanding of the influence of celiac disease and gluten sensitivity on our collective health. First, I would like to thank Dr. Natalie Geary for her insights and contributions to this book in the area of pediatrics. As I delved into the research, the names of gluten gurus Alessio Fasano of the University of Maryland, Peter H. R. Green of Columbia University, and Joseph Murray of the Mayo Clinic kept coming up. These remarkable doctors have pioneered a new and important area of medicine and one that has not been as widely funded as other areas, and I have learned a great deal from their writings.

Dr. Martin Blaser, my medical school classmate, was the first to make me aware of our changing microbiota and its influence on our health. In the past year, I have read many of his papers, and his work has directly led to my understanding of the potential role of our gut flora, and the factors that affect it, on the digestion of gluten. Fellow cardiologist Dr. William Davis recently raised America's gluten consciousness in his book, *Wheat Belly*. I believe he has been instrumental in bringing the importance of gluten to the public square. I am also grateful to Jennifer Lapidus, an expert in artisanal baking, who opened my eyes to the important role of fermentation in bread baking and the possible dangers of its absence. And, as always, I thank Marie Almon, MS, RD, who counsels patients about gluten awareness and a healthy diet on a daily basis in our practice. Her help has been invaluable. I am also grateful to Dr. Holly Atkinson for keeping me abreast of the latest research.

My appreciation also goes to my publicists Sandi Mendelson and Cathy Gruhn of Hilsinger-Mendelson East and to my agents Mel Berger and Eric Zohn at William Morris Endeavor. I would also like to thank Kate Slate and

Sandra Rose Gluck for developing and testing the delicious gluten-free recipes for this book.

Thanks as well to Maria Rodale, for championing the South Beach Diet brand and for allowing me to expand its scope. Much appreciation also goes to executive editor Trisha Calvo for her editing expertise; Amy King, executive director of art and design, for the book design; and to senior production editor, Nancy Bailey, for shepherding the book to completion.

Finally, my deepest thanks to my two personal editors, my friend and colleague, Marya Dalrymple, and my wife, Sari. In addition to being constant advocates and sounding boards, they keep an eye on me, making sure I am truly gluten aware.

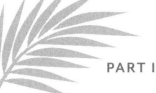

PART I

THE GLUTEN EFFECT

CHAPTER 1

THE ACCIDENTAL
GLUTEN DOCTOR

CONFUSED BY THE LATEST DIET CRAZE—GLUTEN FREE?

You're not alone.

The *New Yorker* cartoon below captures the current state of the nation when it comes to gluten. Many of us have heard about the phenomenon but really don't understand what gluten is or what, if anything, we should be doing about it. Yet millions of us are turning our lives upside down trying to avoid it.

Relax. We are here to help. You won't be confused about gluten after reading this book. And you won't be changing life as you know it. As a matter of fact, life is about to get a whole lot better.

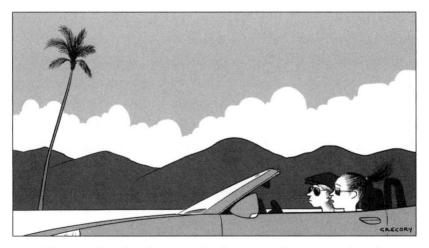

"I have no idea what gluten is, either, but I'm avoiding it, just to be safe."

3

The South Beach Diet Gluten Solution doesn't necessarily mean gluten free forever or that gluten is not a problem. What this program does do is teach you to become gluten *aware,* not gluten *phobic,* and how to make the changes in your diet that are right for you.

As you come to understand the real story about gluten, you may discover that you don't have to say good-bye for good to your favorite pasta dish or your grandma's homemade bread. You won't be walking around cranky and hungry. And yes, you will lose weight quickly and easily without feeling deprived.

On our program, you will be giving up gluten for 4 weeks, but it won't be hard. You'll eat a wide variety of foods, including lots of gluten-free whole grains and other good carbohydrates to satisfy your need for that slice of pizza or piece of rye toast. If it turns out that gluten is a problem for you, you are going to feel a lot better—*fast.* I know this because so many of my patients have seen positive results within days of starting the Gluten Solution Program. Not only do they have much more energy and fewer aches and pains, they no longer complain about bloat, digestive problems, or brain fog.

So what exactly is *gluten*?

Gluten is the major protein found in some grains. These include all forms of wheat (bulgur, durum, semolina, spelt, farro) as well as barley and rye and a wheat-rye cross called triticale. It's also a common additive in many pre-pared foods, cosmetics, and even medicines.

It can make some people very sick. But not everyone.

In fact, many people obsessed with avoiding gluten don't have anything to worry about. These are individuals who don't have to eliminate whole-wheat, barley, and rye products from their lives and who *should* enjoy them, because these whole grains are good sources of vitamins, minerals, and fiber.

At the same time, there are countless others who should be avoiding or at least limiting their intake of foods containing gluten. The vast majority of these people haven't the faintest idea that gluten is at the root of many of their health problems.

A STEALTH DISEASE

For some people—about 1 percent of the population—gluten can be a matter of life or death. These people have a condition known as celiac disease. True celiacs, as they are called, are so sensitive to gluten that even a small amount—really just a trace—can make them very sick. Because gluten damages the lining of the small intestine, it can lead to a host of health problems ranging from chronic fatigue and skin rashes to severe abdominal cramping and osteoporosis. And people with celiac disease are at higher risk for some cancers as well.

Until a decade ago, celiac disease was thought to be extremely rare, affecting 1 in 10,000 people in North America. But in 2003, Dr. Alessio Fasano, one of the world's leading researchers in the field, reported a surprising finding: The rate was actually 1 in 133. That's 100 times more common than was previously believed. Today, Dr. Fasano and other celiac experts suggest that this estimate is probably low and that the disease may be present in 1 in 100 people. To make matters worse, the great majority of these people don't realize they have it. These "silent celiacs" suffer symptoms, sometimes debilitating, without knowing why, and they continue to unwittingly eat gluten, making their condition worse.

But the real focus of this book is on a much more common disorder—the recently recognized problem of gluten sensitivity, a condition with symptoms often similar to celiac disease but that may not require giving up gluten entirely.

With the significant increase in our gluten intake over the past 50 years due to the ubiquity and overconsumption of products made with highly refined wheat flour—along with other surprising factors that I'll tell you about later—we are just beginning to appreciate gluten's impact on our health. As a society, we are in a state of "gluten overload," and millions of people of all ages and all walks of life are suffering as a result.

In my cardiology practice, I have been amazed at the number of patients who have gluten sensitivity and who have gone undiagnosed for many years. When they eat foods containing gluten, it triggers unpleasant symptoms—

stomach pains, diarrhea, heartburn, body aches, headache, skin rashes, fatigue, brain fog, and depression—and sometimes leads to or exacerbates chronic illnesses such as rheumatoid arthritis and fibromyalgia.

We now know that there is a relationship between this new epidemic of gluten sensitivity and the epidemics of obesity and diabetes, two related and reversible conditions that have been the principal focus of my earlier South Beach Diet books.

While there are specific diagnostic tests that can confirm celiac disease, this is not the case for gluten sensitivity. So, if you have symptoms and have tested negative for celiac disease, you may well be gluten sensitive. The only way you know whether gluten is a problem for you—and to what degree—is by observing whether your symptoms are relieved when gluten is sharply reduced or eliminated from your diet.

But I'm not advocating that we all become gluten phobic. My goal is to clear up the confusion and help you determine whether or not *you* are gluten sensitive—and if you are, just how sensitive. By following the South Beach Diet Gluten Solution Program in Part II, you will have the answers in just a few weeks.

The good news is that even if you are gluten sensitive, you don't have to give up *all* whole grains. There are many grains that do not contain gluten and that will not cause symptoms. And depending on your degree of sensitivity, you may be able to have some gluten-containing grains as well.

EAT WELL, FEEL WELL, STAY WELL

I am a history buff and find the evolution of the gluten story in this country and around the world fascinating. Wheat, and accordingly gluten, has been part of our diet for thousands of years. Throughout the book, I am going to touch on the pivotal changes that have made to the "staff of life" a problem for so many of us today.

But first let me tell you a bit about my own history and why I am so anxious to teach you about gluten—a topic that was barely covered when I attended medical school.

I am a preventive cardiologist. My entire career has been devoted to keeping people out of emergency rooms and coronary care units. I am best known in scientific circles for developing the Calcium Score (also known as the Agatston Score) along with my colleague Warren Janowitz. This is a method of screening for coronary atherosclerosis (hardening of the arteries) years before it leads to a heart attack or stroke. It is considered by most experts to be the single best predictor of heart disease, and it is used at medical centers throughout the world. I created the South Beach Diet to help my cardiac and diabetes patients lose weight and improve their blood chemistries in order to stop the progression of atherosclerosis and thus prevent heart attacks and strokes.

I never expected to write a best-selling diet book and thus have been referred to as an "accidental diet doctor." I was inadvertently pushed into the role when I noticed that the so-called heart healthy nationally recommended low-fat diet popular at that time was actually making my patients fatter and sicker. Once I switched my patients to our good fats, good carbs, lean protein, high-fiber strategy, I was amazed at how quickly their health improved and their waistlines shrank.

To apply these fundamentals easily to busy lives, we developed a three-phase approach that we still recommend today.

During Phase 1 of the South Beach Diet, which typically lasts for 2 weeks, all grains (including whole grains) and other starches, sugars (including fruits and fruit juices), and alcohol are excluded. This is the rapid but healthy weight-loss phase designed to eliminate cravings for sweet, sugary foods and refined starches. As a result, you gain control over what you eat and get quick, positive feedback from the many pounds shed. Phase 1 is tailored for people with greater than 10 pounds to lose and those who have difficulty controlling cravings. After 2 weeks most people move on to Phase 2.

People with fewer than 10 pounds to lose and who aren't bothered by cravings can begin the diet on Phase 2. In this phase, whole grains and other healthy starches, most fruits, and even alcohol are gradually reintroduced. Each individual learns which foods—and how much of those foods—he or

(continued on page 10)

MY NEW SECRET WEIGHT-LOSS WEAPON

I have written a great deal about the epidemics of diabetes and obesity and their well-established relationship to heart disease and to most other chronic diseases. I have laid the blame squarely on our sedentary lifestyle and our poor diet filled with empty-calorie, low-fiber, nonnutritious foods—especially in the form of refined carbohydrates.

Our addiction to highly processed starches has led us to consume more gluten than ever before. The irony here is that the more of these junk foods we eat, the more we crave them and the more we continue to eat them. It is a vicious cycle that leaves millions of people struggling with their weight, feeling exhausted and depressed, and suffering from a variety of health problems that are diminishing their quality of life.

I live in South Beach, so many of my patients have been happy to take my diet advice. While I was interested in making them healthier, their primary interest was in looking good. Whatever the motivation, weight was lost, blood chemistries improved, and success was achieved.

But some patients simply didn't care all that much about losing weight. The threat of diabetes and coronary artery disease sometime in the future was not "real" enough to induce them to make changes in the here and now. Interestingly, my new understanding of the Phase 1 gluten-free connection has led me to develop a different strategy for diagnosing and helping my patients. If these noncompliers have symptoms like joint pain, headaches, or difficulty concentrating that I think may be gluten related, I simply explain that relief may be at hand if they make some dietary changes and eliminate gluten for a few weeks. I stress the "feel better fast" part of the program to spark their enthusiasm and initial participation. Typically, if they only lose weight, *this* type of patient may fall off the wagon. But if they feel great and their troublesome symptoms disappear, they will remain faithful to our healthy eating principles for life.

Here's a real-life case in point:

I have followed my patient Tom, who is now 50 years old, for more than 20 years because of a problem with a heart valve. In the past few years, he has gained a middle-aged belly and developed an elevated hemoglobin A1C, which indicates high blood sugar and is a sign of prediabetes. He had never been compliant with my diet recommendations, and I didn't feel that scare tactics would work with him beyond the short term.

In addition to his prediabetes, Tom had a persistent complaint about ankle pain due to osteoarthritis from an old football injury. This actually bothered him more than the threat of future diabetes or heart attack. His ankle hurt—and it hurt now. He had tried all kinds of conventional and unconventional remedies to treat it. These included localized injections as well as "magic remedies" that he had seen on late-night infomercials. I told Tom that while I was certainly not sure, eliminating gluten for a month might improve his ankle pain, making it easier for him to exercise. I hoped that, like many of my other patients, he might feel so good limiting gluten (and by default so many refined carbohydrates) that he'd stick with the diet and that his belly fat would recede and his risk of diabetes would diminish along with his ankle pain.

I saw Tom a few months after he started the South Beach Diet Gluten Solution Program (he had been consulting with our nutritionist by phone in the meantime) and, as in so many other cases, his results exceeded my expectations. He reported that his ankle pain was much relieved after several weeks on the program. He had also lost 20 pounds, and the results of his bloodwork were better than they had been in years.

But even more impressive is that now, more than a year later, he remains committed to his gluten-aware diet (for him, this means eating some gluten-containing foods but not much and not often), not just because his ankle improved but because he "just feels so much better." He has trouble defining it more precisely than that. As a result, Tom has kept off the extra weight he was carrying, his waist circumference is down 2 inches, and his hemoglobin A1C is well below the diabetes zone. He also says that he has more energy now than ever—and this from a guy who didn't think he had a low energy level before.

And, by the way, his wife loves the new Tom.

she can eat without rekindling cravings. This slow and steady weight-loss phase is continued until you achieve your weight-loss goal.

Then a slimmer, healthier, and happier you moves on to Phase 3, the maintenance phase of the diet, where there are no absolute food prohibitions. You will have learned how to sustain a healthy weight, and the South Beach Diet will have become a lifestyle. Even those with no weight to lose should follow the South Beach Diet Phase 3 principles for optimal health.

Our South Beach Diet Gluten Solution Program, which is based on our time-tested principles, seamlessly incorporates a similar strategy that allows you to determine your personal gluten threshold while losing weight and getting healthy.

PHASE 1 FOREVER?

Now you would think that people following the "no grains, no fruits" dictum for the 2 weeks of Phase 1 would be eager to move on to Phase 2. We have found that this is often not the case. In fact, many South Beach dieters want to stay on the grain-free Phase 1 forever. Fifteen years ago, when I first recommended this diet to my patients, I was perplexed by the reaction of these "Phase 1 lovers." I attributed their euphoria to their rapid weight loss and stabilization of blood sugar. But as I saw patients with lifelong rheumatoid arthritis and psoriasis go into remission, I began to wonder if there might be something more to Phase 1 than met the eye. What I would eventually and unexpectedly discover is that it had to do with gluten.

FACT OR FAD?

Recently, there has been an explosion of articles, news stories, and publications about gluten. On store shelves, on menus, in sports arenas, in pizza joints, and around the office watercooler, "gluten free" is everywhere and it's the topic du jour. Many of your friends, acquaintances, family members, and business associates may be touting how much better they feel. Many of mine have told me the same thing. Is this all just a passing fad, or is there real science behind it? I am convinced it is very real and very important.

As new research emerges, the South Beach Diet always updates its recommendations for both diet and exercise. Now, new nutrition science—along with my own clinical experience and that of researchers in the field—is pointing to the fact that we should be gluten aware but not necessarily gluten free. In other words, we each need to determine our own level of sensitivity and enjoy the widest range of foods possible as long as they don't reactivate symptoms.

Becoming gluten aware may transform how you look and feel, increasing your energy level and mental focus. In some cases, it may literally cure conditions you have suffered from for many years. That was my experience. Simply curtailing my intake of whole-wheat bread and pasta, but not eliminating whole wheat entirely, has made a huge difference in how I feel—less morning stiffness and fewer muscle aches, not as much postnasal drip, and definitely more energy.

So from the accidental diet doctor, I have become the "accidental gluten doctor." Just as I never expected to write my original diet book, I never expected to be writing a book about gluten. But thanks to some revelations about Phase 1 (and a lot of digging into the medical literature), there's a new and exciting story to tell.

CHAPTER 2

MY JOURNEY TO GLUTEN AWARENESS

COINCIDENTALLY, AS I AM WRITING THIS CHAPTER, MY WIFE, SARI, and I are getting ready for a visit from my Uncle Robert, who first brought gluten to my attention. Uncle Robert is not your typical houseguest. Whenever he stays with us, we have to take great care at meals and in the kitchen. He can't have any gluten whatsoever, so there can be no slipups. If one of us spreads jam on our morning toast and puts that knife back into the jam jar, it can trigger a nasty reaction if Uncle Robert then uses the same jam.

Think Superman and kryptonite. That's Uncle Robert and gluten.

Along with my Phase 1 observations, Uncle Robert is the major reason why I became gluten aware. It all started about a decade ago, when he was diagnosed with celiac disease. Remember, celiac disease is the most severe of all gluten-related health problems. Although his diagnosis came late in life, Uncle Robert probably had latent celiac disease for many years before it was identified. There were telltale signs that were not recognized, mainly because their connection to celiac disease was not known by his physicians at the time.

For example, Uncle Robert was always on the skinny side as a teenager, struggling to maintain a normal weight although he ate ample amounts of food. This can be an indicator of celiac disease. Later, in his thirties, his doctor told him his blood sugar readings were on the high side. In retrospect, this was the beginning of type 1 diabetes, which, unlike the more common type 2 diabetes, is an autoimmune condition characterized by the inability of the pancreas to produce enough insulin. Like many autoimmune diseases, type 1 diabetes is associated with celiac disease, but nobody knew this when Uncle Robert was in his thirties. When he was in his seventies, Uncle Robert developed chronic diarrhea, a more obvious celiac-related symptom, and eventually he found a doctor who performed the appropriate diagnostic tests. Finally, he learned what had been responsible for his lifelong medical issues: He had celiac disease. Once he banned gluten from his diet, his diarrhea subsided and his blood sugar problems became easier to control.

Like so many people with celiac disease, Uncle Robert, a retired geologist, had to become a "gluten specialist" of sorts in order to manage his own problem. After adopting a strict gluten-free diet, he was mystified when he experienced a flare-up. He did a bit of digging online to see what could have gone wrong. His detective work led him to the discovery that there was a small amount of gluten in the capsule of a new medication he was taking. That minuscule amount was enough to make him sick.

The lesson here is that celiac disease is serious business—there can be no "I'll eat a bite of birthday cake just this once." Celiac patients have to avoid gluten like the plague and need to be well educated about its many hidden sources. As little as 50 milligrams of gluten per day (the amount in a few crumbs of bread) can set in motion an inflammatory reaction that causes further damage to the small intestine. If you have celiac disease, even adding a little soy sauce— yes, many brands of soy sauce contain wheat—to flavor your plain grilled chicken could make you sick. And because gluten is found in other unexpected places—imitation seafood, flavored yogurt, self-basting poultry—and inadvertently ingested, celiac patients must be advised by a knowledgeable nutritionist and regularly monitored by a gastroenterologist.

I learned a great deal from Uncle Robert's experience. It seemed tragic to me that the Uncle Roberts of the world can suffer so much discomfort for so many years before they finally find a doctor who makes the correct diagnosis. What's even sadder is that this is a disease that can be quickly and simply resolved by adhering to a strict gluten-free diet.

After several years of living gluten-free and reading everything he could on the subject, Uncle Robert put one other important piece of information in my head. He said that he had read somewhere that gluten problems were much more common than was generally appreciated and that nonceliac patients might also be sensitive to gluten.

THE REVELATION

I kept thinking about what Uncle Robert had told me—that gluten problems might be much more pervasive than anyone realized. At the same time, I continued to hear my patients rave about how much better they felt on Phase 1 of the South Beach Diet. I also observed and heard about some remarkable improvements in conditions ranging from depression and colitis to chronic skin problems and migraines. At this point, I put two and two together.

My revelation came when I realized that Phase 1, while *intentionally* grain free, was *unintentionally* gluten free.

A case I observed firsthand was so dramatic that it reinforced to my current obsession with all things gluten.

Jane, a new South Beach Diet editor, had long suffered from severe psoriasis, an autoimmune disorder. She had recently met with her dermatologist, who recommended that she consider starting Enbrel, a drug that dampens the immune response and carries a risk of serious side effects. While mulling over this decision, Jane began Phase 1 of the South Beach Diet, not to lose weight—she was slim to begin with—but to enhance her understanding of the eating plan.

To her delight, over the 2 weeks on Phase 1, her psoriasis significantly improved and the difficult decision regarding whether to take Enbrel became moot. Her dermatologist was amazed at the change in her skin.

Jane has been nearly psoriasis free for more than 5 years, except for occasional flares when she overdoes it on wheat products (wheat is America's number-one source of gluten) or when she gets a viral or bacterial infection, two known triggers. Jane tested negative for celiac disease, yet there can be no doubt that her skin erupts when she consumes grains containing gluten.

Thanks to Jane, I experienced an "aha moment," realizing that Phase 1 of the South Beach Diet had reversed Jane's psoriasis. This led me to further investigate the brave new and expanding world of gluten medical literature. What I learned began to explain other observations that our South Beach Diet team had made when following patients on Phase 1.

DÉJÀ VU ALL OVER AGAIN

Coming to terms with the gluten phenomenon is eerily reminiscent of my experience with the low-fat versus low-carb debate back in the late 1980s and 1990s. That's what led to the first South Beach Diet book in 2003. The expert guidelines at the time recommended a low-fat, high-carb diet. Both physicians and patients were quite frustrated with these recommendations, because they were hard to follow, and any health or weight-loss results were short lived at best. At the same time, the public was experimenting with, and losing weight on, low-carbohydrate diets, some of which were not particularly healthy.

The South Beach Diet emphasized that it was the *quality* of fats, carbohydrates, and protein that was important—and we were right. Millions of Americans embraced the South Beach Diet's good fats, good carbs philosophy, and its principles have become the basis of our national nutrition guidelines today. This acceptance led me to conclude that the diet debates were over.

But apparently, the diet debates are not over. Today the controversy is all about gluten—whether we've become gluten phobic for no reason, whether we should be paying more attention to it than we do, and whether gluten sensitivity even exists at all. Whatever the answers, the public's interest is clear. The gluten revolution is sweeping the country to the tune of an estimated $4 billion to $7 billion annually in sales of gluten-free products. And, again, just as the public's interest pushed the medical establishment to rethink the way we look at fats and carbohydrates, our current obsession with everything gluten free is compelling the medical and academic communities to take a good hard look at the way gluten may be affecting our health.

It's my hope that *The South Beach Diet Gluten Solution* will clear up the confusion about gluten in the same way *The South Beach Diet* cleared up the low-fat versus low-carb controversy more than a decade ago.

GLUTEN AWARE FOREVER

Jane's surprising remission confirmed my suspicions that there was more to Phase 1 than just weight loss and improved blood chemistries. Many of our Phase 1 dieters continued to report not only significant weight loss but also more energy, better sleep, better concentration, and the resolution of heartburn, headaches, rashes, and other ailments. When they reintroduced gluten-containing grains on Phase 2, however, their unpleasant symptoms sometimes returned along with a decrease in energy and an increase in brain fog. They just didn't feel as good as they felt on Phase 1. When I tested such patients for celiac disease, they were almost always negative, but their symptoms still suggested a gluten-related problem.

It's important to note that although Phase 1 of our original South Beach Diet eliminated all grains, it didn't entirely eliminate all forms of gluten. We didn't, for example, ban soy sauce, in which wheat is often a major ingredient. So even if people were following Phase 1 religiously, odds are that they were not gluten free to the degree required for a celiac patient. Yet since so many of them were feeling so much better, I realized that if someone is not a true celiac, being *absolutely* gluten free might not be necessary and in fact could be an unnecessary hardship.

The slow and deliberate addition of grains in Phase 2 allowed me to make another discovery: My patients had various reactions to the reintroduction of gluten grains. The same people who had reported relief from symptoms on Phase 1, and the return of symptoms on Phase 2, noted the change at different *stages* of Phase 2. Some patients began to feel the return of headaches, stomach discomfort, and other symptoms as soon as they added one serving of whole-wheat bread or cereal, while others felt just fine until they increased their servings. I found that some people, like myself, can eat a handful of whole-wheat crackers or occasionally indulge in an empty-calorie pastry and stay symptom free. Others may have a relapse after just one bite of a bagel. The threshold was decidedly different, depending on the degree of gluten sensitivity.

It became very clear to me that individuals without celiac disease can have varying degrees of gluten sensitivity. These people achieved good results by simply becoming gluten aware. It was at this point that I adapted Phase 2 for those people who appeared to be gluten sensitive, eliminating wheat, barley, rye, and other obvious sources of gluten for 4 weeks but allowing nongluten-containing whole grains instead of *all* the whole grains that would normally have been allowed on Phase 2. I called this Gluten Solution Phase 2, or GS Phase 2. For those patients with suggestive symptoms but no weight to lose, I created a modified version of GS Phase 2 that allowed them to eat healthfully—and gluten free—without losing weight.

GLUTEN FREE OR GLUTEN AWARE?

"What does 'gluten free' mean?" "How is 'gluten free' different from 'gluten aware'?" "Which one is right for me?" These are critical questions, because it can be very difficult to follow a totally gluten-free diet. If you have celiac disease, you have no choice.

The generally accepted definition of gluten free means that a food must contain less than 20 parts per million (ppm) of gluten, though labeling laws are yet to be passed (see page 158, "Be Aware: Gluten Is Everywhere"). That's the amount in about $\frac{1}{48}$ of a slice of bread: just a tiny sliver. In addition, grain products—cereals, baked goods, and other products—are not truly gluten free unless they are made in their own gluten-free facilities to prevent cross-contamination from wheat, rye, or barley products. For example, if an oatmeal cereal is made in a factory that makes cream of wheat, although the oatmeal is made from oats and nothing else, cross-contamination with traces of wheat picked up from the same machines that processed the wheat can bring the oatmeal above the 20 ppm threshold.

For people with celiac disease, gluten must be completely avoided to prevent continuing damage to the small intestine, which can lead to serious complications. And it's not just a matter of avoiding gluten-containing grains. Celiacs have to be gluten sleuths, alert to hidden sources of gluten in such divergent products as toothpaste and vitamin supplements. And they also need to recognize that gluten is an additive in many commercial food and nonfood products. Complications with celiac patients often arise when their symptoms, such as diarrhea, respond to a less severe restriction of gluten. They allow a little gluten back into their diet because they feel better physically, but in actuality their small intestine is suffering further assault, and this can lead to a host of other health problems.

For those who don't have celiac disease, simply understanding that gluten could be the cause of their symptoms is the first step to gluten awareness. Next is learning whether you feel better eliminating it. Finally, gluten-containing foods are slowly reintroduced in small quantities so you can discern how much you can tolerate without triggering symptoms.

Once you have determined that you are gluten sensitive, you will likely adopt a diet like most of my gluten-sensitive patients. You'll end up avoiding wheat-based breads, cereals, baked goods, and pasta (and barley- and rye-based products as well) most of the time, and you won't have to worry too much about the hidden sources of gluten. You'll have learned just how much of a problem gluten is for you and how concerned about gluten you need to be. This is my definition of being gluten aware.

My observations were only strengthened as I put more patients on the Gluten Solution Program. Recently, a patient who had done very well without gluten announced when she showed up for an exam that she felt "irritable, anxious, and tired" and she didn't know why. After some friendly interrogation, she remembered that on the way home the night before, she had grabbed a quick fast-food grilled chicken sandwich and had eaten half the bun. Mystery solved. She was in a hurry and thought she could get away with a half a bun. Some can; she couldn't.

Today, our nutritionist, Marie Almon, spends a lot of time at patients' first visits teaching those who appear to be gluten sensitive how to be gluten aware. In part, this means understanding where gluten can be found and also knowing how to look for gluten-containing ingredients on a food label—both important lessons for success on our program. We don't want patients to become paranoid about gluten; we're just teaching them to be gluten smart.

MORE POSTGRADUATE EDUCATION

My gluten education continued both in and out of the office. I did more research and began talking to other physicians about their own experiences. In doing so, I had the good fortune to meet Dr. Natalie Geary, who had a busy pediatric practice in New York City. For the previous 10 years, she had been treating kids with allergies and other symptoms with a gluten-free diet and was seeing incredible results. It was fascinating to meet a brilliant physician with so much clinical experience in helping children with gluten sensitivities who could corroborate my own observations.

One of the problems Dr. Geary encountered in her practice was the remarkable number of children suffering with recurrent ear infections. I had often wondered how problems like chronic ear infections, asthma, multiple allergies, and other ailments, so uncommon when I was growing up, could be so common in children today.

Dr. Geary provided insight into this phenomenon as well as some practical advice. She told me how she had successfully cured recurrent ear infections along with asthma, stomachaches, runny noses, rashes, behavior issues, and other conditions in many children by taking them off of wheat. When I (rather sheepishly) repeated our conversation to a well-known Ear Professor Emeritus, I was in for a surprise. Not only did he not discount Dr. Geary's experience, but he told me that during his training in the 1970s, an ear, nose, and throat allergist he worked with had advocated doing the same thing—because it worked. Even though avoiding gluten had apparently helped many patients, it was not widely reported.

Now there is evidence that kids sensitive to gluten do produce more mucus and, because of the angle of children's ear canals at a young age, this mucus finds its way into the middle ear much more easily than it does in adults. So less gluten, less mucus, fewer ear infections in kids; it makes sense.

Dr. Geary reaffirmed my own observations that many adults and children feel better after eliminating or cutting back on their gluten consumption. She also gave me a better understanding of the spectrum of gluten sensitivity and how widely the symptoms can vary.

On one end of the spectrum is the 1 percent of the population who has celiac disease and for whom reliable tests are available to make a precise diagnosis. The remaining 99 percent of Americans without celiac disease populate the rest of the spectrum—from highly gluten sensitive to no sensitivity at all. Because there are no reliable lab tests to confirm a diagnosis for the gluten sensitive, my program is primarily directed to them.

A major goal of mine is to help you understand that if you are part of the silent majority with a gluten-related problem and do not have celiac disease, then discovering where you are on the gluten spectrum and adjusting your diet accordingly may be your answer for better health.

CHAPTER 3

CELIAC DISEASE OR GLUTEN SENSITIVITY?

WHATEVER THE ANSWER TO THIS QUESTION, GLUTEN IS NOT your friend.

But not all gluten-related problems are created equal.

A key source of gluten confusion is the failure to distinguish between the two most common gluten-related disorders—celiac disease and gluten sensitivity. This is understandable, because much of what we know about celiac disease has only been learned in the last decade, and the recognition of gluten sensitivity as a separate disorder is only a few years old.

The distinction, however, is very important. For people with celiac disease, gluten must be treated as a potentially deadly enemy. All gluten must be banned. For the gluten sensitive, gluten is a troublemaker but not likely life threatening. Still, to experience relief from symptoms, these people must limit gluten or avoid it entirely depending on their degree of sensitivity.

Celiac disease is the most urgent and extreme form of gluten disorders, and it is what afflicted my Uncle Robert. Nonceliac gluten sensitivity is a similar but distinct condition that can have symptoms ranging from mild to fairly severe. (For the purposes of this book, we will continue to refer to nonceliac gluten sensitivity simply as gluten sensitivity.) Other gluten-related problems such as wheat allergy are more easily diagnosed and not so problematic for the general population. (See "What about Wheat Allergy?" on page 31.)

Most symptoms are similar in gluten-related disorders, making them hard to differentiate. Celiacs typically have GI symptoms like chronic diarrhea, bloating, and stomach pain, but so do many of those who are gluten sensitive. Individuals throughout the spectrum of gluten-related disorders can also have symptoms unrelated to the GI tract, sometimes called atypical symptoms, such as headaches, joint pain, canker sores, runny nose, and skin rashes or psoriasis. Celiacs may suffer with an autoimmune disease, and not uncommonly more than one (indeed, celiac disease is considered an autoimmune disease itself). But I have seen multiple symptoms, including autoimmune problems, in gluten-sensitive individuals as well. Some have terrible symptoms all the time, while others may have mild symptoms most of the time. Some have symptoms that go into remission for days or even years and then recur.

It can all be very confusing.

THE BATTLE INSIDE YOUR INSIDES

Whether you have celiac disease or gluten sensitivity, you have a problem with your small intestine.

The small intestine, which connects your stomach to your large intestine (colon), is unique in that it is the *only* part of the digestive tract where the nutrients from the food that fuels us are absorbed. These include "macronutrients," which we obtain from fats, carbohydrates, and protein, as well as "micronutrients," which include the vitamins and minerals necessary for good health.

The interior lining of this convoluted 20-foot-long tube is made up of tiny hairlike projections called villi and even smaller ones called microvilli. Both contain specialized cells that enable the absorption of nutrients into the bloodstream. If you were to look at a square inch of small intestine under a microscope and try to count the microvilli, you'd be at it for quite a while, because there are 10 billion in that square inch alone. You can imagine how these tiny villi create an enormous area in the small intestine to absorb our food and drink—about 4,000 square feet!

GLUTEN AND YOUR SMALL INTESTINE

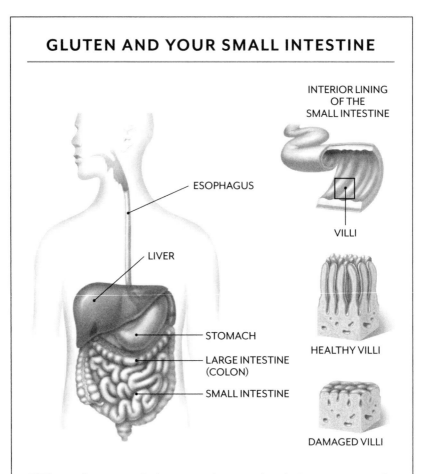

INTERIOR LINING
OF THE
SMALL INTESTINE

ESOPHAGUS

VILLI

LIVER

STOMACH

HEALTHY VILLI

LARGE INTESTINE
(COLON)

SMALL INTESTINE

DAMAGED VILLI

The small intestine, which connects the stomach to the large intestine, is the only part of the digestive tract where the nutrients from the foods we eat are absorbed into the bloodstream. The interior lining of the small intestine is made up of microscopic hairlike projections called *villi,* which contain specialized cells that enable the absorption of nutrients. Healthy villi stand up; in those with celiac disease, the villi are flattened in patches throughout the intestine (having been extensively damaged by the protein gluten) and are unable to absorb nutrients properly. The damaged intestinal cells ooze an enzyme, which stimulates an antibody response that can be measured in the blood. This is the first step in diagnosing celiac disease. Those with gluten sensitivity do not have extensive damage to the villi and do not leak the enzyme. Diagnosis of gluten sensitivity must therefore be made on the basis of symptoms and whether they are relieved by sharply reducing or removing gluten from the diet.

The small intestine has a big job. It must screen everything you eat and decide whether or not to grant admission into your bloodstream. You can actually think of the small intestine like a fine mesh strainer with very tiny openings that normally allow only individual food molecules through. Since a likely entryway for foreign proteins, including disease-causing proteins like bacteria and viruses, is through the food we eat, you can certainly understand why 80 percent of our immune system is located in the lining of the small intestine.

Once a threatening invader is recognized, it is the job of the immune system to activate a local inflammatory response to surround, wall off, and eat or expel the interloper. To combat these unfriendly proteins, the immune system recruits antibodies as well as specialized cells (T cells), which are designed to tag and remember the invader in case, once defeated, it returns. This allows the immune system to mount a more immediate and aggressive response the next time.

GLUTEN MAKES IT WORSE

When a protein is not a threat, our digestive system happily breaks it down into individual amino acid molecules for absorption through the wall of the small intestine and into the bloodstream (all proteins consist of a chain of amino acids connected like a string of beads). But gluten protein presents a much bigger challenge to the digestive process.

Unlike protein from the steak you ate for dinner last night, gluten protein contains particular amino acid molecules that have unusually strong attachments to their adjacent amino acid neighbors. These attachments make it very difficult for our digestive system to completely break down the chain into individual amino acids. That's why oftentimes gluten protein is only partially digested, resulting in smaller chains of amino acids, or fragments, called peptides, which are left behind in our small intestine.

In most people, these gluten-derived peptide strands continue down the small intestine and into the colon and are excreted without a problem. In those with celiac disease, however, some gluten peptides get trapped in the

IS GLUTEN THE CULPRIT?

By now you may be wondering if gluten sensitivity is at the root of your ailments and whether you need to adopt a gluten-aware lifestyle. Take the following short quiz to see if you have any of the common signs and symptoms of gluten sensitivity. We must point out that this is just a small sampling of symptoms. If you have ever been told that you have an autoimmune disorder, such as thyroiditis, type 1 diabetes, rheumatoid arthritis, psoriasis, fibromyalgia, or lupus, you should consider the possibility that gluten could be causing it or making it worse.

1.   **Do you often feel bloated after eating even a small amount of food?**
     ☐ Yes   ☐ No

2.   **Do you frequently suffer from constipation or diarrhea?**
     ☐ Yes   ☐ No

3.   **Do you often have abdominal pain or stomach cramps?**
     ☐ Yes   ☐ No

4.   **Do you often suffer from headaches?**
     ☐ Yes   ☐ No

5.   **Do you wake up with stiff joints?**
     ☐ Yes   ☐ No

6.   **Do you typically feel fatigued even after getting enough sleep?**
     ☐ Yes   ☐ No

7.   **Do you have excess mucus, postnasal drip, rhinitis, or sinus problems?**
     ☐ Yes   ☐ No

8.   **Do you have difficulty keeping your mental focus?**
     ☐ Yes   ☐ No

9.   **Do you have a problem with depression?**
     ☐ Yes   ☐ No

10. **Do you suffer from skin rashes?**
     ☐ Yes   ☐ No

If you answer yes to even one of these questions, you could be one of the millions of people with undiagnosed gluten sensitivity. If you undertake our South Beach Diet Gluten Solution Program and your symptoms diminish or disappear, it is likely you do have a problem with gluten.

villi and penetrate the protective lining of the small intestine, inciting an inflammatory response and immune reaction. In people with gluten sensitivity, the presence of these peptides also invokes an immune response, but the mechanism for how this happens is not yet well understood.

In those with celiac disease, the damage to the villi is quite extensive, and the villi are unable to carry out their normal function of bringing nutrients through the intestinal wall into the bloodstream. Furthermore, when these intestinal cells are injured, they ooze an enzyme called tissue transglutaminase (tTG), which stimulates an antibody response that can be measured in the blood as anti-tTG antibodies.

Therefore, a blood test is the first step in identifying celiac disease. A positive test for anti-tTG antibodies as well as for anti-endomysial antibodies is invariably associated with celiac disease and rarely associated with those who do not have the disease. Doctors can also request a genetic test to be run on the blood sample to check for the genes HLA-DQ2 and/or HLA-DQ8 that are almost always present in celiac patients.

In contrast, people with gluten sensitivity do not have significant damage to their small intestines and do not leak the tTG enzyme, which makes diagnosis that much harder. They also do not necessarily have the HLA-DQ2 or HLA-DQ8 genes.

Damage to the villi of the small intestine is usually "patchy," which means it can be scattered throughout the intestine. The extent and location of this damage can give rise to a wide spectrum of symptoms in both celiac suffers and the gluten sensitive, since each portion of the intestine is responsible for the absorption of different nutrients. Extensive damage produces the classic gluten-related symptoms of abdominal pain, bloating, and diarrhea. A more localized inflammatory reaction may cause more specific symptoms. For instance, if the area in the small intestine that absorbs iron is affected, the patient may have iron deficiency anemia but no abdominal complaints. A hunt for the source of iron loss, which usually occurs from blood loss due to bleeding from somewhere in the digestive tract, will be fruitless because the body is not losing iron, it's just not absorbing it in the first place.

CELIAC DISEASE: AN ANCIENT AILMENT

Imagine you're a parent living in AD 1st century Greece. You're understandably distraught because your child, who complains of stomach pain, is wasting away before your eyes, even though she is eating what you believe to be a perfectly adequate amount of food. You consult with the top physician of the day, Aretaeus of Cappadocia, to see if he can solve this mystery. The doctor explains that he has seen several other similar cases of children who complained of abdominal pain and who have been losing weight for no apparent reason. Unfortunately, this physician is as perplexed by the condition as you are, but he keeps track of these patients, many of whom die young.

Fast-forward to modern times. Today, Aretaeus of Cappadocia, who wrote several ancient medical texts, is credited with being the first physician to have documented celiac disease. In fact, the word *celiac* comes from the Greek *koiliakos*, meaning abdomen.

Greece was, of course, in the cradle of civilization where the first agricultural revolution began about 10,000 years ago. The agricultural revolution started with the discovery that the seeds of certain wild grasses, such as wheat, could be cultivated as fields of grain. This meant that much larger populations could be fed with much less time and effort than that required when procuring food from hunting and gathering alone. Spending most of their days finding food was how our hunter-gatherer ancestors managed to exist in small tribes for millennia. With agriculture, populations could feed themselves while having extra time to acquire and share the knowledge that has formed the basis for civilization and human progress ever since.

But the agricultural revolution was not *all* good for humankind. For one thing,

2.9 MILLION AND COUNTING

You would think that with all the attention focused on gluten and celiac disease in the media and the marketplace, combined with new simple screening tests, everyone with this problem would be getting diagnosed and treated. Unfortunately, just the opposite is true. Out of the nearly three million Americans estimated to have celiac disease, about 97 percent of them don't even know they have it! In fact, it typically takes up to *9 years* for a person with celiac disease to get an accurate diagnosis. And sometimes agricultural societies were often overdependent on a single source of nutrition rather than on the wide range of fruits and vegetables consumed by the tribes of hunter-gatherers. Consuming a variety helps ensure the intake of the nutrients we need for optimal health. Our DNA was designed to help us survive in the wild, hunting wild game and gathering fruits and vegetables—not eating grain—especially the grain that eventually became the staple of so many civilizations.

Remarkably, it was not until 1888 that British physician Samuel Gee described celiac disease as a chronic digestive disorder of young children and hypothesized that it might be related to diet. And it wasn't until after World War II that a Dutch pediatrician, Willem-Karel Dicke, discovered *what* in the diet was causing the disease. He observed that in the Netherlands, the war-related drop in bread intake led to a significant improvement in children with celiac disease. He also reported that when wheat products became more available after the war, the children's symptoms returned to prewar levels. Following Dicke's observations, other scientists finally determined that it was the gluten protein in wheat that was the culprit.

In the 1970s, the flexible endoscope made small bowel biopsies relatively easy to perform. With this procedure, damage to the small intestine could be detected, and more patients were diagnosed with celiac disease. It wasn't until new blood tests were developed over the past decade, however, that doctors could make a presumptive diagnosis of celiac disease without an invasive biopsy. With these blood tests, it became clear that many celiac patients had symptoms like fatigue and poor mental focus as well as autoimmune diseases such as thyroiditis and rheumatoid arthritis—none of which seem GI related. These diagnostic tools have led to the realization that celiac disease is far more common and manifests in a wider array of symptoms than previously believed.

much longer. That's right, there are 2.9 million people walking around with this disease, many suffering with multiple symptoms, who are totally unaware that their problems could be easily solved by eliminating gluten from their diet.

When you take into account that an estimated 50 percent of Americans have some degree of gluten sensitivity—and this includes children, too—you can understand why I am writing this book. The more we can educate both physicians and the public about gluten-related disorders, the more people can be spared from needless misery and the risk of potentially serious complications.

I was encouraged by the findings of a study in the *American Journal of Gastroenterology* highlighting how much better physicians could be at identifying and diagnosing celiac disease if they were provided with some simple information. All they need is a higher level of suspicion coupled with a few simple blood tests that are now readily available. In this study, 2,568 patients being treated by different primary-care physicians were preinterviewed by the researchers. If they had celiac disease risk factors, such as a family member with celiac, or they reported celiac-related symptoms, they were sent for a blood test to check for the telltale antibodies. If their antibody tests were positive, they were advised to get a small bowel biopsy to confirm damage to the small intestine. Through this aggressive screening, there were 43 times more patients diagnosed with celiac disease as compared to the number identified with the usual approach to diagnosis. Clearly, there is a great opportunity for physicians to do better. And the same holds true in detecting patients with gluten sensitivity. In the near future, however, I believe that only growing public awareness will make a significant dent in this problem.

MAKING A DIAGNOSIS JUST GOT EASIER

To create uniform, simple criteria for the diagnosis of celiac disease and gluten sensitivity, an expert consensus panel was convened not long ago, and their conclusions were published in 2012 in the journal *BMC Medicine*.

Celiac disease was defined as having four out of five of the following criteria:

1. You exhibit typical signs or symptoms of celiac disease, including but not limited to anemia, bloating, abdominal pain, weight loss, and diarrhea (symptoms may not necessarily involve the GI tract).

2. You have the genetic predisposition, which means that you have the HLA-DQ2 and/or the HLA-DQ8 gene. Ninety-five percent of individuals with celiac possess one or both of these genes. (At the

same time, these genes are present in 30 to 40 percent of the general population who *do not* have celiac disease.)

3. You show evidence of inflammation and damage to the cells lining the small intestine, which is manifested by specific antibodies present in your blood, as discussed above.

4. A biopsy of the small intestine documents characteristic damage to the intestine. The biopsy consists of collecting samples from the lining of the small intestine in a procedure called an upper endoscopy, during which a gastroenterologist passes a flexible instrument with a camera via your mouth through your esophagus and stomach into the first section of your small intestine, called the duodenum. The procedure is usually only mildly uncomfortable and is very safe. The samples are then reviewed under a microscope. If the results of the endoscopy show that your villi are damaged in a particular pattern, you will be diagnosed with celiac disease. In some cases, blood tests may be negative and the biopsy will still be performed when celiac disease is suspected due to family history and/or symptoms.

5. You show improvement in your symptoms (and a repeated blood test shows normal antibodies) when placed on a gluten-free diet.

CELIACS: DON'T BECOME COMPLACENT

I have already told you this, but it bears repeating: If you have been diagnosed with celiac disease, you must avoid *all* gluten *all* the time. Individuals with celiac disease may feel so much better after going on a gluten-free diet that they relax and become complacent about completely avoiding gluten in all its less-than-obvious places. Their symptoms, such as fatigue and bloating, may not recur, but damage to their small intestines nevertheless progresses even with very minimal gluten intake.

My patient Dr. Rogers illustrates this problem. For decades before I first saw him, Dr. Rogers had been suffering from diarrhea, bloating, and abdominal cramps, and yet surprisingly he was overweight. Having been given a copy of *The South Beach Diet* by a friend, he began the diet on his own to lose weight and to control a recent surge in his blood sugar. During Phase 1 of the diet, Dr. Rogers lost 12 pounds as expected, but to his amazement, his diarrhea resolved for the first time in more than 20 years.

Naturally wanting to discover what about the diet had cured his chronic stomach woes, Dr. Rogers began his own research. After a thorough review of the medical literature, he came to the conclusion that it was likely eliminating gluten grains that was responsible for his improvement. He concluded that he might have celiac disease, and he sought out a well-known celiac disease expert in New York City, where he lived. After blood tests and a small bowel biopsy, a diagnosis of celiac disease was indeed confirmed. He then sent his mother to the celiac specialist, since she had experienced lifelong undiagnosed stomach problems as well. She did in fact have celiac disease and later sadly developed small bowel lymphoma, a form of cancer associated with the disease.

Dr. Rogers continued to feel great on what he thought was his new gluten-free diet, but when he had a follow-up biopsy, his small bowel damage had actually progressed. The usual cause of this progression is either inconsistent compliance with a gluten-free diet or hidden sources of gluten being unknowingly consumed.

Since that biopsy, Dr. Rogers has realized that the gluten awareness he learned by happy accident while on Phase 1 of our diet, while adequate for preventing symptoms, was not adequate for preventing progression of intestinal damage. With celiac disease, he has had to learn to be strictly gluten free, not just gluten aware.

CELIAC DISEASE: WHO'S AT RISK?

Celiac disease is genetic. If any of your close relatives have had this disease, you should have a blood test done to see if you've inherited those genes. If you have, then further testing is warranted.

It's especially important for pediatricians to be aware of the diagnostic

WHAT ABOUT WHEAT ALLERGY?

Wheat allergy is also on the spectrum of gluten-related disorders, but its mechanism is different from that of celiac disease or gluten sensitivity.

An immune response to even a very small amount of wheat gluten is a fairly common food allergy, especially in children, who may outgrow it. Unlike some symptoms from other gluten-related disorders, which can strike at any time, even years after chronic exposure, symptoms of wheat allergy such as hives, an itchy rash, and nasal congestion occur within minutes to hours after exposure.

In some cases, a more severe "anaphylactic" reaction may occur, which presents as swelling or tightness of the throat, difficulty breathing due to an acute asthmatic reaction, and even dizziness or fainting. Anaphylactic reactions can be life threatening if an epinephrine injection is not quickly administered. Most people with severe wheat allergies carry an autoinjection pen for this purpose, but immediate medical attention may also be required.

Wheat allergies are diagnosed with skin and blood tests and respond well to avoiding the offending agent.

criteria. Celiac disease characteristically occurs in early childhood, often in infants after their first exposure to wheat products. Celiac expert Dr. Alessio Fasano has described celiac disease as analogous to a giant iceberg. Most celiac disease goes undiagnosed (like the hidden part of an iceberg below the water's surface) for years or even for decades, just as it did in the cases of Uncle Robert and Dr. Rogers.

During the years prior to a diagnosis, damage to the small intestine can progress, leading to serious complications down the road, including some types of cancer and even premature death. Therefore, getting a correct diagnosis as early as possible is critical. That's why I encourage parents to point out symptoms like gastrointestinal issues, frequent ear and sinus problems, and fatigue that could be indicative of celiac disease or gluten sensitivity to their children's pediatrician. You'll learn more about these and other symptoms and how to control them in Chapter 8, "It Starts Early."

TROUBLE ON THE OTHER END OF THE SPECTRUM

If you have symptoms (like abdominal bloating or abdominal pain) or a condition (like thyroid disease or anemia) and tests for celiac disease are negative, you may well have gluten sensitivity. But because there are no standardized tests to confirm gluten sensitivity, the diagnosis must be made on the basis of symptoms and response to therapy.

As discussed earlier, only recently has gluten sensitivity been recognized as a problem distinct from celiac disease. The same group of experts who established the criteria for diagnosing celiac disease in the 2012 consensus statement noted, "It is now becoming apparent that reactions to gluten are not limited to CD [celiac disease], rather we now appreciate the existence of a spectrum of gluten-related disorders."

The panel advised that gluten sensitivity should be considered if someone is exhibiting symptoms consistent with gluten-related disorders but does not have the telltale antibodies or the abnormal biopsy found in celiacs. Remember, their criteria for diagnosing gluten sensitivity is *whether these symptoms resolve when gluten is eliminated from the diet and recur when gluten is reintroduced.*

Such criteria make it difficult to perform the usual types of population studies that are done for diseases with more specific diagnostic tests. Diet studies are generally much harder and more expensive to design, to get funded, and certainly to control. And since the treatment approach for gluten sensitivity is dietary, there has been little incentive for pharmaceutical companies to support gluten research or gluten education.

Another well-known difficulty with trying to conduct controlled diet studies is that in the real world, it is nearly impossible to "blind" study subjects to what they are eating in the same way you can blind people to a placebo versus the real medication being tested. Add to this the previously held belief that only a small percentage of the population is affected, and you can understand why gluten sensitivity has been so long neglected. This is a formula for continuing controversy and unanswered questions about a condition that experts now believe to be far more common than was previously thought. And this is why you must become knowledgeable and empowered to become your own health advocate when it comes to gluten.

This might not be so easy, since some health professionals advise against treating gluten sensitivity until more research is done and all the facts are in. I strongly disagree, since I have seen so many lives improve when sensitive patients eliminate or cut back on gluten. It may be many more years before we have specific diagnostic tests for gluten sensitivity and understand the exact mechanisms by which it causes so many problems. But the fact is, the risk/reward calculation of becoming gluten aware is already clear. There is no health risk to a trial off of gluten. In fact, because it means lessening your intake of processed, refined carbohydrates, it actually has clear health benefits—even if it turns out you are not gluten sensitive.

On the other hand, ignoring the problem because a precise diagnostic test is not yet available means that millions of people with gluten sensitivity will continue to suffer needlessly. The only risk to a diagnosis of gluten sensitivity is if celiac disease is not tested for first and excluded.

DAZED AND CONFUSED

The confusion in the medical community—even among gastroenterologists—was experienced by my patient Julie. She sought my help because she had a total cholesterol level of over 300, which put her at elevated risk for a future heart attack or stroke. Julie is tall and slender, so her high cholesterol was not due to any dietary indiscretions, and the only way to bring it down was to have her take a cholesterol-lowering statin drug. One of the reasons she had come to me was because every single statin drug she had tried seemed to cause muscle aches and pains.

Upon close questioning, it became clear that Julie had suffered from body aches long before she ever started on a statin. In addition, she was being followed by a GI specialist for irritable bowel syndrome (IBS) and reflux esophagitis. She was also anxious and depressed, two symptoms commonly associated with IBS and gluten-related disorders. As if this wasn't bad enough, Julie had also been followed by a rheumatologist for more than 10 years because of positive antibody tests for lupus, rheumatoid arthritis, and generalized inflammation. To top it off, she had been documented with low vitamin D and B_{12} levels—indications of possible malabsorption of these nutrients in her small intestine.

I was pretty sure that Julie had a classic gluten-related problem, so I ordered antibody and genetic testing for celiac disease. The tests came back negative. Given her symptoms and the negative tests for celiac, the next step was following a gluten-free diet for 4 weeks. It was definitely worth a try.

When Julie returned to my office for a follow-up exam, I was amazed to hear how good she felt. Her GI and other symptoms had disappeared for the first time since she could remember, just days into her gluten-free diet. Her anxiety and depression had lifted, and she felt just great—that is, until she went back to see her gastroenterologist, Dr. Jones, for a routine follow-up of her irritable bowel syndrome and reflux. When she told him that her symptoms had vanished after Dr. Agatston had taken her off gluten, Dr. Jones replied rather haughtily, "You do not have celiac disease, and Arthur should stick to cardiology." (And I thought he was my friend!)

A DOUBTING DOCTOR

Dr. Jones then repeated the same celiac tests I had already performed, along with a small bowel biopsy. And again, all were negative. He announced that Julie could eat all the bread and baked goods she desired.

After being given a license to eat anything, Julie traveled to Vermont to visit her daughter and, with Dr. Jones' approval, indulged in a couple of slices of some freshly baked whole-wheat bread from a famous local bakery. Shortly afterward, she proceeded to demonstrate a characteristic response that occurs when gluten-sensitive individuals reintroduce gluten. She quickly experienced horrible bloating and abdominal cramps and realized almost immediately that gluten was the culprit. She again cut gluten out of her diet. From that moment on, her symptoms were gone.

Like so many others with gluten issues, Julie also noticed that her mental focus improved once she went gluten free. In particular, she realized that the "brain fog" that had been bothering her for years, and that she had dismissed as a normal part of aging, had vanished.

While "brain fog" is obviously not a precise medical diagnosis, my colleagues and I have been impressed at how common a complaint it is and how often it gets better when a patient cuts out or limits gluten. One year later, Julie is still feeling fabulous. In fact, a recent visit to her rheumatologist surprised both Julie and her doctor when her blood tests for lupus, rheumatoid arthritis, and inflammation were all normal for the first time since she began seeing him.

The lesson here is that many doctors—even gastroenterologists and rheumatologists—are still unaware of the full spectrum of gluten-related disorders, and gluten sensitivity is only now being recognized as a distinct condition.

I learned my own important lesson from Julie. It's that many symptoms of gluten sensitivity, such as headaches and chronic fatigue, which are so often dismissed by physicians (as well as friends and family) as "psychological," are very much physical and treatable.

The fact is that far too many patients—and even doctors—go for years suffering from an easily curable condition. Don't let this happen to you. I am hoping this book will help raise awareness of this problem, not just among lay people but among physicians as well. Maybe even Dr. Jones will read it. Meanwhile, if you believe you have gluten sensitivity, you must make sure you are heard. Contact a local celiac disease support group for recommendations of gastroenterologists specializing in gluten-related disorders. Also check out the Resources on page 231 for top celiac centers around the country that can refer you to a knowledgeable physician in your area.

CHAPTER 4

WHY NOW?

WHEN I TELL MY PATIENTS ABOUT THE INCREASING FREQUENCY OF gluten-related disorders documented in the United States and the increase in cases I am seeing in my own practice, some rightly ask, "But hasn't gluten been around forever? Why is it suddenly causing problems now?"

A few of them even quote a line I often use from Michael Pollan's *In Defense of Food*: "Don't eat what your great-great-grandmother wouldn't recognize as food."

Then they ask, "Well, Dr. Agatston, wouldn't my great-great-grandmother recognize whole-wheat bread or a roll as food?"

These are great questions, and the answers to them speak volumes about what has gone so terribly wrong with our modern diet. Yes, it's true that gluten has been around since wheat was introduced into the human diet. But the way wheat is now cultivated and processed into flour, the way dough is prepared and leavened for baking, and the way bread is enriched, fortified, and preserved are very different from the time of my great-great-grandmother Sarah.

All of these factors influence the amount of gluten we ingest and the way gluten is handled by the body. So even though the wheat rolls on dinner tables today may resemble the wheat rolls that Sarah enjoyed, they are very different indeed.

A ROLL IS A ROLL IS A ROLL . . . OR NOT?

I'll concede to my skeptical patients that, like the rolls we eat today, Great-Great-Grandma Sarah's roll did contain gluten. All wheat-based products do.

When wheat flour is made into dough, gluten (as its name suggests) acts like "glue," giving stickiness, structure, elasticity, and strength to the dough so it's easier to manipulate and bakes up nicely. The greater the gluten content in the flour, the more body in the dough.

But unlike the typical roll of today, Grandma Sarah's roll was not made from wheat that was mercilessly ground down to an ultrafine powder, stripped of virtually all of its fiber and nutrients, mass-produced in a giant factory using fast-rising yeast, loaded with preservatives along with more gluten in the form of additives, and shipped hundreds—if not thousands—of miles on trucks, trains, or ships to be sold in supermarkets.

Sarah likely made her own bread and rolls from flour that was ground on old-fashioned millstones. It certainly wasn't as white and fine as today's flour, the product of steel roller mills, but it was a lot healthier. Furthermore, her dough was fermented for hours as it rose. This fermentation process broke down much of the gluten, making it more digestible and less likely to cause problems. (We describe this process in "Slow Bread, Fast Bread," page 40.) In 1910, 75 percent of bread making in the United States was done in the home. The first industrially made, sliced, and packaged Wonder Bread was shipped in the 1930s.

But perhaps the real difference between then and now is the way in which our modern wheat flour baked goods are digested, as compared to Grandma Sarah's bread and rolls. Interestingly, because of the way wheat is processed today, this digestive process begins before we take our first bite.

To better "digest" this vital piece of information, however, you need to know a bit about the wheat seed.

SEEDS OF CHANGE

Even if you've never seen a kernel of wheat up close, if you eat bread, rolls, muffins, cookies, cakes, cereal, or anything else made from wheat flour, you need to know the difference between whole wheat and refined wheat.

And that begins with the grain kernel, or seed.

There are three parts of the wheat seed. The outer layer is the protective coat known as the *bran*. It contains practically all of the grain's fiber—the insoluble, indigestible carbohydrate that moves through your digestive system virtually unchanged. The bran also contains niacin and other B vitamins, along with some trace minerals. Beneath the bran is the *germ*, which is the seed's embryonic sprouting section and the part containing the most nutrients. The germ contains B vitamins, vitamin E, iron, calcium, magnesium, and other nutrients, as well as polyunsaturated fat. The third and innermost part is the *endosperm*, which comprises about 83 percent of the seed's weight. The endosperm is made up of starchy carbohydrate (chains of sugar molecules) and the protein gluten. Almost all of the gluten in wheat is found in the endosperm. All grains have proteins, but not all have a protein with the unique viscous and elastic properties of gluten.

When wheat is milled to make refined white flour, the bran and germ are removed, leaving only the endosperm and thus concentrating the effect of the gluten and starch, the only remaining components.

Think of it this way: Conventional wheat processing removes the healthy nutrients but leaves the problematic ones untouched. The irony is that processed bread products are often "enriched," which means adding back some, but not all, of the natural vitamins, like thiamine, riboflavin, niacin, and folic acid, that were lost when the bran and germ were removed. Highly processed bread products may also be "fortified" with ingredients not even found in whole wheat, like vitamin D and iron.

The purpose of grinding or milling wheat has always been to make flour that will produce dough that is malleable so that it can be baked and eaten. The invention of the steel roller mill in the late 19th century allowed the wheat to be highly refined and processed quickly and efficiently. The removal of the bran and germ resulted in a fine, white flour and a tasty product with an extended shelf life (the germ contains oil that can go rancid).

Although there were some early naysayers warning about the refinement of wheat and the loss of its nutrients, health did not enter the equation in a significant way until very recently. That's why the South Beach Diet has always emphasized eating 100 percent whole-wheat and whole-grain products, in which the fiber and nutrients contained in the bran and germ are still present.

For people who are not gluten sensitive, enjoying these nutritious high-fiber foods contributes to a varied and healthy diet. For those who are sensitive to gluten, however, even whole grains that contain gluten can be problematic.

MORE GLUTEN, MORE TROUBLE

Over the past 50 years in the United States, there has been a sharp rise in the consumption of food in general and an even sharper rise in the consumption of refined carbohydrates—mostly made from wheat. (I feel compelled to remind you that there has been no corresponding increase in physical exertion; in fact, quite the opposite is true.) On top of that, our portion sizes have grown, especially in this "supersize" era, which means that most of us are unwittingly getting an even higher dose of gluten in our daily diet. There is little doubt that this increased intake of gluten has played an important role in the epidemic of gluten-related disorders—not to mention diabetes and obesity, which are caused in large part by our increased consumption of refined-wheat products.

In addition, changes in the wheat itself are another possible contributor to the gluten problem. From time immemorial, farmers have been cross-breeding all kinds of crops for improved characteristics. Over the past half century, tremendous strides have been made to create wheat that is high yielding and resistant to environmental factors, including disease and insects as well as drought and other damaging weather. Wheat has also been hybridized for improved nutrient content and improved bread-making qualities, which accordingly means some strains have more gluten. While there is more gluten in most strains of today's wheat than there was 100 years ago, its relative impact on gluten-related disorders is not yet clear. (Don't mistake hybridized with genetically modified. While hybridized wheat is widely used in our bread products today, to date there is no genetically modified wheat sold anywhere in the United States or the world.)

And there's more to the tale. Over the past 40 years or so, gluten has been liberally added to flour to improve the baking characteristics of commercially produced breads and other baked goods. And because gluten is less expensive

SLOW BREAD, FAST BREAD

I'm not a baker—but I'm thinking of becoming one after learning how important baking methods are to our health and how much they have changed over the years. This is yet another chapter in the fascinating story of how the unintended consequences of technology have impacted our lives.

My education in traditional versus modern methods of baking began unexpectedly when I met Jennifer Lapidus, a professional baker and director of the North Carolina Organic Bread Flour Project. Jennifer is known in baking circles for her expertise in baking bread "the old-fashioned way."

By old-fashioned, I mean that Jennifer is part of the slow-baking movement, a trend among artisanal bakers around the country to return to healthier ways of baking bread. Instead of using fast-rising commercial yeast that makes it possible to move very quickly from dough to baked loaf, Jennifer relies on an age-old slow method. Instead of yeast, she and other "slow bakers" use different types of non-yeast starters, which allow the dough to ferment and rise naturally over many hours as it reacts to the good bacteria in the starter. The whole process takes about 18 hours, but the time is put to good use. All the while, good bacteria are breaking down the gluten protein in the dough, so that the bread is easier for us to digest. In fact, Jennifer and other slow bakers contend that many gluten-sensitive individuals can tolerate their slow-fermented bread for this reason.

In contrast, the fast-rising yeast bread that most of us eat has not had the benefit of slow fermentation, placing more of a burden on our digestive system to break down the gluten.

Human beings and wheat have always had a complex relationship. That's because the protective coat of the seed—the hard bran layer that is made up mainly of fiber—wasn't digestible. And the wheat seed's inner nutrients could be accessed (and

than other protein additives, it has also been used to "fortify" breads and other products in order to increase their protein content.

But I'm still not finished.

Because of its excellent thickening properties, gluten is added to many nonbread products such as condensed canned soups, tomato and spaghetti sauces, salad dressings, marinades, and flavored prepackaged rice mixes to improve texture.

digested) only by going through a preparation stage first—something that humans did not figure out how to do for hundreds of thousands of years.

It was only at the start of the agricultural revolution 10,000 years ago that man discovered that wheat could be eaten if the seeds were ground into flour. I like to imagine that the discovery probably occurred when one of our starving ancestors searching for food desperately gathered a pile of wheat seeds and smashed them with a stone to see if there was something inside that was edible. Think of it as the first "stone-ground wheat." He might have decided to soak the mixture to soften it and make it palatable. And fermentation was born.

Fermentation occurs when moisture is added to a grain at the right temperature. This attracts microbes (bacteria and yeast) that begin to chow down on the sugar in the starch, turning it into alcohol and carbon dioxide gas, which in turn cause the dough to rise. As I said above, this process can be fast or slow. Until the second quarter of the 20th century, when fast-rising yeast and new baking technology gave rise to industrial bread making, bread was made using this slow-fermentation technique.

After talking with Jennifer, I searched the medical and wheat science literature. Sure enough, there is good reason why slowly fermented breads are so well tolerated. For instance, studies of sourdough bread fermentation using lactic acid bacteria (*Lactobacilli*) confirm that gluten is predigested by the bacteria during fermentation, making it easier for humans—even those who are sensitive to gluten—to complete the digestive process.

In the United States, it's clear that with our overconsumption of modern fast bread, we are dumping more difficult-to-digest gluten, as well as preservatives and other additives, into our intestines without considering the health implications. Some of us are overwhelming our digestive enzymes with food constituents our bodies simply can't handle in the quantities we're eating.

Jennifer Lapidus thinks so. And from my review of the relevant science, I agree.

And if the ubiquity of gluten isn't the nail in the coffin, unlike in Great-Great-Grandma Sarah's day, the gluten in our bread and rolls today is no longer "predigested" as it was during the slow-rising fermentation process she used to prepare her dough before baking.

To understand how all this affects our digestion—*and our ability to digest gluten in particular*—let's follow Great-Great-Grandma Sarah's roll on its journey from her breakfast plate into her bloodstream.

DON'T FORGET TO CHEW

Whether we are eating a plain roll, a sushi roll, or a lobster roll, the purpose of digestion is to nourish our bodies and feed and replenish our cells. It starts when we take fairly large chunks of food into our mouths and then continues as that food is gradually broken down into individual molecules that can move through the wall of the small intestine and into our bloodstream. (Indigestible fiber and very small amounts of undigested proteins, fats, and sugars continue on to the large intestine and are expelled as waste.) Once in the bloodstream, these small molecules may be immediately used for fuel, incorporated into our body's tissues, or stored for future use. If we don't completely digest our food by breaking it down into individual molecules, then the partially digested particles of food continue down the digestive tract, where they can cause a whole host of problems. Think "indigestion."

When I was growing up, we were told to chew each mouthful of food slowly to make sure that we digested it well. Hopefully moms are still reminding their kids to do the same today. This is important, because as we chew our food, in addition to breaking it down *mechanically*, we are bathing it in enzymes from our saliva that start a *chemical* breakdown process.

The processes of mechanical and chemical breakdown continue once Great-Great-Grandma Sarah swallows the roll, sending it down through her esophagus into her stomach. Here, thanks to gastric juices, it undergoes transformation into a liquid soup that later empties into the small intestine. It is in the small intestine that the final deconstruction of that roll takes place, aided by additional enzymes that further reduce this soup into individual molecules that move through the wall of the small intestine into the bloodstream to provide sustenance for the body.

Many of these digestive enzymes are manufactured in the wall of the small intestine itself. Others come from the pancreas via the common bile duct. Bile, which aids digestion, is stored in the gallbladder, and after we eat a meal (or a roll), the gallbladder contracts, emptying its contents into the small intestine. (And, yes, you can live comfortably without your gallbladder; the bile is delivered through another mechanism.)

We also recently discovered the importance of additional enzymes needed to break down our food, which are manufactured by friendly bacteria (gut flora) that reside in the small intestine.

During the digestion process, the starch from the roll—a chain of glucose (sugar) molecules—is chemically broken into individual glucose molecules that can move through the intestinal wall into the bloodstream. In the case of Great-Great-Grandma Sarah's whole-wheat roll, the nutritious contents of the germ, including its B vitamins, vitamin E, iron, calcium, magnesium, and other nutrients, is directly absorbed through various specialized areas of the small intestine. The bran fiber, which is not digested because humans do not have the enzymes to break it down, continues moving through the small intestine into the large intestine, where it gives bulk to the stool and helps prevent Sarah from getting constipated.

In any case, whenever Sarah eats food of any sort, if proteins, starches, or fats are not completely digested into their molecular components, or if damage to the intestine prevents their full absorption through the intestinal wall, problems well beyond indigestion can arise.

But when things are going right with the roll, its primary protein, *gluten,* is broken down into its individual amino acid molecules, which are then transported through the intestinal wall.

Good or bad, Great-Great-Grandma Sarah's roll is now officially digested. End of story? I'm afraid not.

UNFINISHED BUSINESS

So what's happened that's made eating today's roll so problematic?

You already have a handle on how overprocessing, overglutenizing, and lack of fermentation has made the content of our rolls so different from Grandma Sarah's, but what about the difference in the number of rolls (or their equivalent) currently going into our mouths? It's clear that we are now consuming refined wheat products, and food in general, in amounts that would have been thought impossible in Grandma Sarah's time.

These days, our digestive enzymes are being overwhelmed by the

MILK GOT YOU?

Many people with celiac disease have a problem tolerating lactose, the sugar in milk. That's because the inflammation and damage to the small intestine that occurs with celiac disease may destroy the intestinal wall's ability to produce lactase, the enzyme needed to break down lactose. This problem may also manifest itself in the gluten sensitive, if there is an inflammatory response and damage to the small intestine.

If lactose is not digested, it continues down the small intestine, where bacteria will ferment it, producing excess gas that causes bloating and cramps. Still undigested, the lactose then moves into the large intestine, where it can produce diarrhea. The degree of inflammation in the small intestine and your natural lactase production will determine the severity of lactose intolerance.

Just as there are degrees of nonceliac gluten sensitivity, there are degrees of lactose intolerance. A mildly gluten-sensitive person might be able to have a piece of toast without triggering symptoms; similarly, someone with mild lactose intolerance may be able to have milk in their coffee and feel okay. For others with a high degree of sensitivity, even a little bit of the offending agent is too much.

If you've been having trouble digesting milk and other dairy products, you may want to consider whether you might have a gluten-related disorder that's contributing to the problem.

sheer quantities of gluten-containing foods we are eating. And even if we're not overeating, some of us lack the necessary enzymes to adequately break down gluten protein into individual amino acids.

Whether our enzyme function is affected by overconsumption of wheat, the higher concentration of gluten in our food, or damage to the intestinal wall, some of the incompletely digested chains of gluten molecules (peptides) may not move through the digestive tract into the colon. Instead, they get trapped in the villi and then seep through the intestinal lining, initially causing inflammation and possibly abdominal pain. This insult allows even more peptides to seep into the lining, which can ultimately result in the wide range of symptoms associated with celiac disease and gluten sensitivity.

But what happens if your problems *don't* primarily result from your inability to completely digest gluten? What if they result from factors that have nothing to do with the roll at all?

Some celiac experts believe that injury to the small intestine from bacterial or viral infections (infectious gastroenteritis) may set off gluten-related symptoms by making the intestinal wall more porous, thus facilitating the penetration of incompletely digested gluten peptides. But infectious gastroenteritis is certainly not new. In fact, there is a good chance that Great-Great-Grandma Sarah and her children suffered through some episodes.

So what else could be contributing to our epidemic of gluten-related disorders?

NSAID AND ANTIBIOTIC OVERUSE

In recent decades, there has been an ever-increasing use of pain relievers, particularly nonsteroidal anti-inflammatory medications (NSAIDS), both over the counter and prescribed. These include aspirin (Bayer, Bufferin), naproxen (Aleve), and ibuprofen (Advil, Motrin). While most of us have heard that NSAIDs can damage our stomachs, what you may not know is that they are just as likely to damage your small intestine. When you consider that more than 30 billion doses of over-the-counter and prescription NSAIDs are taken in the United States each year, the impact on our collective small intestines must be substantial. In the same manner that gastroenteritis allows incompletely digested gluten peptides to leak through the intestinal lining and cause symptoms, so can NSAID damage. This was not an issue in Sarah's day.

One other medical breakthrough—antibiotics—may also be contributing to our gluten-related problems. Keep in mind that Sarah certainly would not have had access to these "wonder drugs," since they weren't discovered until the late 1920s and were not developed for clinical use until the 1940s. As with NSAIDs, overuse and overprescription of antibiotics is rampant in the United States today, beginning in childhood. It is estimated that doctors prescribe antibiotics to a child at one out of every five visits, often for viral respiratory ailments like bronchitis and flu that do not require them.

Is our promiscuous use of antibiotics killing off the friendly bacteria in our intestines that help us to digest gluten? Read on.

CHAPTER 5

FRIENDLY BACTERIA (YOUR NEW BFF)

MICHELLE, WHO HAS BEEN WORKING WITH ME FOR MORE THAN 20 years, is an upbeat, hardworking nurse practitioner. She has suffered with severe reflux esophagitis (heartburn) for about 10 years. It seems that almost everybody does these days. In fact, probably the most common cause of chest pain seen by cardiologists is not from the heart but from the esophagus. Many of my patients who complain of chest pain turn out to have heartburn.

Over the years, Michelle had regularly seen a gastroenterologist and had undergone several endoscopies, one of which included a biopsy of the small intestine to rule out celiac disease. Her biopsy was negative, but her pain persisted. For relief, she took high doses of antacids and acid blockers. But nothing seemed to quell the fire from within.

About 2 years ago, I could see from Michelle's pained expression that she was having a particularly bad day with her reflux. I knew that she had already tried every conceivable medication to control her discomfort, so I suggested that she experiment with a gluten-free approach.

This was on a Thursday. When I saw her again on Monday, she was a new woman.

"Dr. Agatston," she said, barely able to contain her delight, "it was like turning off a faucet. My heartburn is gone."

She told me that she was doing so well off gluten, even in this short time, that she hadn't needed to take any antacids over the weekend. In the months that followed, Michelle discovered that as long as she kept her gluten intake to a bare minimum (no more than a bite or two of a bagel every once in a while), she felt great.

Pretty exciting stuff.

SYMPTOMS COME AND GO

After witnessing Michelle's remarkable improvement, I was curious to find out whether she had experienced any symptoms of gluten sensitivity as a child. When I asked, I learned that she had had a sensitive stomach for as long as she could remember. But it had gotten much better in early adulthood. It wasn't until she was in her fifties that her reflux struck big time and then became persistent.

I've heard this story from many of my gluten-sensitive patients. A good number of them report having had sensitive stomachs during childhood and as teenagers. This is followed by a period of remission (as if they "outgrew" it), only to have the signs and symptoms recur several years to several decades later.

Why this happens only raises more questions about gluten-related disorders. Why is there such variability of signs and symptoms in both celiac and gluten-sensitive patients over time? Why do people like Michelle have childhood symptoms that disappear, only to resurface in their forties or fifties or even beyond? What factors bring symptoms to the surface or cause them to recede?

The answers lie in part in the amount of refined wheat products we may be consuming at any given time and any damage to our small intestine that might have resulted from nonsteroidal anti-inflammatory drug (NSAID) use or other factors. But the fact is, there are 100 trillion other possible answers that I can condense into one word: *bacteria*! Or, to be precise, friendly bacteria, because not all bacteria are the same. It is the study of these friendly bacteria that may eventually help us answer these questions and better understand the increase in gluten disorders seen in recent decades.

BACTERIA—FRIEND, FOE, OR BOTH?

Before I explain how bacteria and gluten sensitivity are connected, it's important to understand a little bit about bacteria, both good and bad. Our bodies, including our skin, all our orifices, and in particular our intestines, are home to about 100 trillion good bacteria, collectively called our microbiota, which have been with us forever and are essential for good health. Unfortunately, we have not always differentiated between good and bad bacteria.

Ever since Louis Pasteur came up with the germ theory of disease in the 1860s, bacteria have been regarded as Public Enemy #1, a dangerous threat that needs to be wiped, sponged, or mopped out of existence. We hunt down bacteria in our bathrooms, in our food, in our drinks, and on our bodies. Our weapons are a vast array of consumer goods, including household cleaners, mouthwashes, antibacterial soaps, hand sanitizers, and, oh yes, our big guns, antibiotics. This paranoia is understandable, since bacteria have been the source of so much human misery, including the epidemics of bubonic plague, typhoid, and tuberculosis—to name a few. These diseases have ravaged entire societies—as well as entire armies—often causing more casualties than combat. However, we've lost sight of the fact that all of these weapons can indiscriminately kill good bacteria along with the bad.

I too was raised with a negative view of bacteria, which was passed down from my parents, who emphasized the popular notion that cleanliness was next to godliness; from my teachers, who frequently reminded us to wash our hands; and from my medical school training. I maintained that low opinion of bacteria until recently, when I was transformed from a "bacteriaphobe" into a "bacteriaphile."

YOU CALL THIS "PROGRESS"?

My transformation began one evening several years ago when I was having dinner with a medical school classmate, Martin Blaser, a renowned infectious disease specialist and the chairman of the department of medicine at the NYU School of Medicine. I asked him what he was working on, and Dr. Blaser surprised me with some new insights into what might be causing the changing pattern of gastrointestinal disease in America. Specifically, he addressed a phenomenon that I had also observed in my practice—the extraordinary rise in reflux cases (like Michelle's) and the near disappearance of gastric ulcers other than those associated with the overuse of NSAIDs.

During our medical training in the 1970s, ulcers were much more prevalent than reflux as a significant medical condition that brought patients in to see their doctors. But what happened? It's as if ulcers went out of style and reflux is suddenly in! We all know that skirt lengths can rise and fall following the dictates of fashion, but how could the same be true for stomach disease?

It is interesting that disease trends, much like fashion trends, are rooted in human behavior. As Dr. Blaser pointed out, we have known since the 1980s that the bacteria *Heliobacter pylori* are the major cause of gastric and duodenal ulcers (the duodenum is the first section of the small intestine attached to the stomach). *H. pylori* start out as beneficial bacteria, helping to regulate and suppress the acidity of our stomach contents. But sometimes this normally protective bacteria can turn on us, penetrating and weakening the stomach's protective mucous lining and leaving it more susceptible to ulcers. We can now "cure" these ulcers with antibiotics that kill *H. pylori*. So far so good. But what often happens is that former ulcer patients develop a new problem—reflux.

As it turns out, the presence of *H. pylori* in the gut flora (the microbiota of the intestine) of people living in the industrialized world has been continuously diminishing. This has been particularly true over the last 20 years as antibiotic use has increased. Today, these diminished *H. pylori* have left millions of adults suffering from reflux. And so are many children. *H. pylori* bacteria have gone from being a universal presence in our intestines to now being found in only 10 percent of children. Dr. Blaser hypothesizes that it is the excessive prescribing of antibiotics in childhood and beyond that has destroyed much of our usually friendly *H. pylori*, thus explaining the decrease of peptic ulcer disease and the increase in reflux and possibly the increase in asthma, rhinitis, and eczema as well.

That certainly seems to have been a factor in Michelle's experience. She confirmed that every time she developed the sniffles as a child, her well-meaning parents encouraged the doctor to treat her with antibiotics. During treatment for her stomach woes, she did indeed test negative for *H. pylori*. It now appears that it was Michelle's *H. pylori* deficiency (along with other changes to her gut flora from the antibiotics) that may have caused or exacerbated her gluten sensitivity and contributed to her reflux.

OUR CHANGING MICROBIOTA

Since my dinner with Dr. Blaser, I have kept up with his work and that of others who have pioneered a whole new area of medical investigation: the study of microbiota. It turns out the cells of our microbiota outnumber our own cells by 10 to 1. Bacterial communities have lived with us for as long as humans have inhabited the earth, and for them to survive and thrive, they logically must help us survive and thrive. And indeed they do.

We are just beginning to understand the enormous roles that gut flora and other good bacteria play in our health. Recently, we have learned that these microorganisms produce enzymes that are instrumental in the digestion of food and the absorption of vitamins, minerals, and other nutrients. These good bacteria also produce substances like lactic acid, which make the environment in all of our orifices and on our skin inhospitable to bad bacteria.

Our close relationship with friendly bacteria begins during birth, when infants pass through the birth canal and swallow some of their mother's bacteria. And although good bacteria are also passed on through breast-feeding, babies who are born via C-section and who miss the opportunity for good bacteria acquisition in the birth canal can have imbalances in gut flora that persist for up to 6 months after birth.

Throughout childhood, and continuing throughout our lives, our friendly microbiota continue to change in response to our use of medications, our diets, and our lifestyles. Studies show that children who eat a high-fiber diet in rural Africa have different gut flora from Western children who eat a low-fiber meat-and-starch diet. The gut flora of African children is protective against diarrhea and inflammatory disease, while the gut flora of Western children from industrialized countries is associated with a higher incidence of Western diseases such as diabetes, allergies, inflammatory bowel disorders—and obesity. A meat-heavy diet is also a contributor because of the way animals are raised and fed.

In addition to feeding animals a corn- and grain-based diet to fatten them up quickly, meat and poultry producers in America have used antibiotics as fattening agents for cattle, pigs, and chickens, among other animals, since the 1950s. Originally used to prevent disease, antibiotics began to be routinely added to the animals' food when it was realized that these drugs increased their body weight. Today, the use of antibiotics in animals has grown to the point where we're using about the same amount *or more* in animals as we do in humans.

At the same time that we've been pumping ourselves and our livestock full of antibiotics, we've also been consuming greater quantities of processed foods that are loaded with preservatives. The purpose of preservatives is to prevent potentially harmful bacteria and other microorganisms from spoiling food and from making us sick if we eat it. This is great when the preservatives are targeting bacteria like *Clostridium botulinum* or *E. coli*, two potential deadly threats in the food supply. But what if they are also killing the friendly bacteria in our food and in our guts?

I realize that preserving the quality of food in storage has been an age-old endeavor important for man's survival. It was the inability to store food that caused our hunter-gatherer ancestors to risk life and limb to acquire fresh food daily. Still, when we are using chemical preservatives that have not been used historically by traditional societies, we may be exposing ourselves to unintended consequences. Clearly, the jury is still out on whether (and to what degree) modern preservatives are affecting our health. Other than specific allergic reactions to such preservatives, I have not seen that they do. But I can't help wondering whether the widespread use of preservatives in the food supply is yet another reason why our gut flora has changed so markedly.

I'll be glad to see what ongoing research turns up.

THE BACTERIA-GLUTEN CONNECTION

So does all this new information about good and bad bacteria help solve the "why now, why so variable" gluten sensitivity conundrum? I think it may.

We already know that as a result of our efforts to wipe out disease-causing bacteria, we have inadvertently killed off good bacteria as well.

Without sufficient good bacteria in our small intestine, we may not produce enough enzymes to help break down gluten protein, which in turn could result in gluten sensitivity. And we're now learning that we need to pay attention to this problem very early in life. It appears that the amount of gluten ingested during a child's first year, along with other feeding patterns, can affect a susceptible infant's microbiota and his or her susceptibility to developing celiac disease later in life.

This was suggested in a 2012 study led by Maria Sellitto of the University of Maryland, which followed 26 infants genetically predisposed to celiac disease from birth to age 2. The study concluded that these genetically predisposed infants may benefit from delaying exposure to gluten from 6 months of age to at least 12 months. While the exact mechanisms of the benefit are still unknown, it is thought to be related to immature microbiota in the intestines of these infants.

The study authors hypothesized that the introduction of gluten to an infant with immature microbiota might trigger or accelerate the development of autoimmunity. At 12 months, most nonceliac infants have mature microbiota similar to that of adults, but Dr. Sellitto's study found that this is not the case in infants at risk for celiac disease. Their microbiota at 12 months remained immature. This led her group to postulate that delaying gluten exposure would give the predisposed infants' microbiota further time to develop and, although not reaching the maturation level of nonceliac infants, potentially help them better tolerate gluten in the future.

Another study, published recently in *BMC Microbiology,* demonstrated that children with untreated celiac disease have different gut flora from those who have been on a gluten-free diet, and that both are different from the gut flora of kids without celiac disease. The study authors suggest that new therapeutic strategies aimed at restoring the intestinal ecosystem balance are warranted.

One thing both of these studies make clear is that our gut flora's connection to gluten-related disorders cannot be overstated. We know that gut flora changes with age, diet, and antibiotic use, among other factors; this may well explain the variability in symptoms for gluten-related disorders over time.

THE BACTERIA-WEIGHT CONNECTION

Changes in our microbiota may also be a factor in our obesity crisis. A 2009 study in *Nature* showed that the gut flora of overweight individuals is different from the gut flora of thin individuals, and in the overweight it produces enzymes that break down carbohydrates into sugars more efficiently. This is thought to lead to increased absorption of sugars from starches and therefore to the absorption of more calories from carbohydrates—and weight gain.

Another study analyzing the connection between microbiota and weight gain, by Ilseung Cho, Martin Blaser, and colleagues, was published in the same journal in 2012. It showed how widespread antibiotic use is affecting our gut flora and possibly making us fat. The study looked at the effects of penicillin and other common antibiotics on just-weaned mice, using doses comparable to the amounts used by farmers to fatten their livestock. The results indicated that the drugs altered gut flora, causing metabolic changes— possibly affecting the metabolism of fatty acids and the increase of energy (calorie) extraction from the intestines—that led the treated mice to gain 10 to 15 percent more fat after 7 weeks than the untreated mice.

Another recent study of more than 11,000 English children, which was reported in the *International Journal of Obesity,* postulated that microbes in our intestines may play a critical role in how we absorb calories from food, and that exposure to antibiotics, especially early in life, may kill off healthy bacteria that influence the absorption of nutrients. This study found that giving babies antibiotics before the age of 6 months increased their chance of being overweight by age 3 *by 22 percent.*

While more research is clearly needed, these studies support an emerging body of evidence that links gut bacteria, and the effect of antibiotics on gut bacteria, with the development of obesity. These kinds of results cannot be ignored.

TO THE RESCUE: PROBIOTICS?

Assuming our modern diet and excessive use of antibiotics and preservatives are killing off our good bacteria, is there anything we can do to restore the proper balance of good and bad bacteria within our bodies? Maybe. There's a promising area of microbiota research that is shedding new light on recolonizing the bacteria in our intestines with probiotics (the word literally means "beneficial to life").

You've likely heard of probiotics. These good bacteria (which already reside in our intestines) have populated or have been added to a vast number of products ranging from yogurt to green drinks and other supplements for years. But despite some good rationale behind effficacy claims, we are still waiting for more evidence before probiotics can be established as an important component in achieving better health. That's in part because the various foods and supplements for oral delivery of probiotics don't necessarily spare these friendly bacteria from being destroyed by our stomach acid.

One use of probiotics that has been found to be beneficial, however, is in the treatment of the bacterial overgrowth of *Clostridium difficile*, a decidedly unfriendly enemy that attacks our intestinal linings, causing inflammation, abdominal pain, and diarrhea. It often occurs when friendly bacteria are killed by antibiotics during the treatment of pneumonia or other infections. Ironically, it takes a strong blast of another antibiotic to kill *C. difficile* and up to 3 months for good bacteria to repopulate the intestines following treatment. But there may be a faster way. First, the *C. difficile* bacteria are killed by a targeted antibiotic. Then a "stool transplant" from a normal person's colon is performed (in a non-icky way), quickly restoring the good bacteria in the afflicted person's colon. This gets around the oral-delivery problem I just mentioned.

Another use of probiotics may be in helping children fight common ailments. A well-designed, double-blind placebo-controlled study from Finland, a country with a documented and growing gluten problem, tested the value of lactobacillus (good probiotic bacteria) fortified milk in preventing illness in young kids attending daycare. While this study was performed in 2001 and the researchers were not considering gluten issues at the time, they found that those children drinking the fortified milk versus milk without lactobacillus had fewer days absent because of upper respiratory problems, ear infections, and stomach ailments. Could these results have been impacted by the probiotic bacteria helping digest gluten? Interesting question.

So while more studies are clearly needed before I can make a blanket recommendation of probiotics to you or my patients, I do think this is a promising area of investigation that could turn out to have a surprising health impact. Consult with your doctor before taking probiotics if you're interested. Hopefully these microorganisms will yield positive results for you.

CHAPTER 6

GLUTEN-RELATED DISORDERS: THE GREAT IMITATORS

THE DESIGNATION "GREAT IMITATOR" IS CLASSIC IN THE HISTORY OF medicine. It refers to a disease that is particularly difficult to diagnose because its symptoms, involving multiple organs or tissues, can mimic many other diseases. Consequently, the correct diagnosis is commonly delayed.

I would definitely include both celiac disease and gluten sensitivity—distinct but related ailments—among the great imitators. And I am not the first to consider this. Celiac disease has been called a "clinical chameleon" because it can affect any organ or tissue in the body and in nonspecific ways.

I have seen patients who have endured what turned out to be a gluten-related condition for 20, 40, even 50 years before the diagnosis was made. It's not uncommon for these people to a share a long, sad history of going from one specialist to another, often being told that their problems must be psychological. They present to the neurologist as numbness in an extremity, to the rheumatologist as joint pain, to the endocrinologist as a thyroid problem, to the dermatologist as a rash, to the obstetrician as infertility, to the internist as fatigue and depression, to the gastroenterologist as heartburn, and to the cardiologist as chest pain.

It is unlikely that a physician who hasn't spent time learning about gluten would immediately think "Gluten sensitivity!" when a patient comes in with an array of complaints like these. That's because gluten sensitivity, though common, was recognized as a condition distinct from celiac disease only very recently, and the nongastrointestinal features of celiac disease have been documented only over the past 10 years or so. For the most part, physicians were taught that celiac disease is an intestinal problem presenting primarily with diarrhea, bloating, and abdominal pain. And in this era of subspecialization, doctors may not appreciate the whole picture or recognize the confusing assortment of complaints as being gluten related. Most physicians are simply unaware of the non-GI symptoms associated with gluten sensitivity. And so they have trouble identifying the root cause of a mix of signs and symptoms that are giving so many people so much discomfort.

But with the growing awareness of gluten-related disorders and the associated symptoms, I hope that more doctors will naturally become "accidental gluten doctors."

THE "GLUTEN TRIFECTA"

As a physician who has recently become gluten aware, I marvel at the many different ways that gluten-related problems surface in patients and at how many are not classic intestinal complaints. We now know enough about our bodies' reactions to gluten to understand why the manifestations are so varied and confusing. I have already covered some of the potential problems that arise during gluten digestion, but now I want to show you how incompletely digested gluten protein can impact every cell and every system in your body.

There are three primary ways that gluten can negatively affect your health. I call them the "Gluten Trifecta": inflammation, diminished nutrient absorption, and autoimmune response. All are induced by incompletely digested gluten proteins and our immune system's reaction to them. Some gluten symptoms can be linked to more than one element of the trifecta; other symptoms result from mechanisms yet to be figured out.

1. INFLAMMATION—AND PAIN

As discussed in Chapter 3, inflammation is initiated when gluten proteins (long chains of amino acids) are incompletely digested, resulting in peptides (short chains of amino acids) that breach the inner lining of the small intestine and cause a local inflammatory response. In the case of celiac disease, the inflammation destroys the fine architecture of the intestinal villi. But in the case of the gluten-sensitive patient, although local inflammation is present, the villi in the lining of the small intestine are not damaged.

Whether due to celiac disease or gluten sensitivity, intestinal inflammation can trigger symptoms such as bloating, diarrhea, and reflux and can also cause systemwide reactions ranging from skin rashes and migraines to fatigue and muscles aches. You know how your body hurts all over when you have a respiratory flu or pneumonia. Those aches and pains you feel away from the site of the infection are due to the release of cytokines, which are produced by inflammatory cells and act as messengers to regulate our immune response. Cytokines can cause symptoms locally (such as pain from a cut on your hand or pneumonia in your chest), or they can provoke symptoms in regions far from the site of inflammation. You may have experienced the latter situation when you had a viral infection and an old football injury or chronic arthritic knee pain suddenly felt worse. This is the systemic, or bodywide, action of cytokines.

There is a gray area of gluten-related disorders in which the mechanism causing symptoms is not clear. For example, morning stiffness is a very common yet nonspecific early sign of many different types of arthritis, including degenerative osteoarthritis and the much less common autoimmune condition rheumatoid arthritis. They are both associated with local inflammation of the affected joint.

I have seen morning stiffness frequently respond to a reduction in gluten. In fact, I have seen it in myself. It used to be that when I hit the tennis court or the golf course on cool weekend mornings in Miami Beach (they do occur occasionally), I felt stiffness in my fingers that improved as I warmed up. Since I have become gluten aware, however, my morning stiffness has disappeared. Now I think that my stiffness was probably due to mild osteoarthritis exacerbated by the effects of cytokines arising from gluten-induced inflammation. Avoiding gluten or taking an anti-inflammatory medication relieved the stiffness, but I much prefer avoiding gluten.

Migraine headache is another common ailment that can sometimes be linked to gluten sensitivity and celiac disease. I believe that's the case with one of my patients, a 60-year-old physician. He initially went on the South Beach Diet to lose weight, and he dropped more than 20 pounds. He felt so good eliminating all grains, including wheat, for the 2 weeks of Phase 1 that he has kept his wheat intake to a minimum even after introducing grains. He recently reminded me that he had experienced severe migraines until he went on the South Beach Diet and that he has not experienced one since. (Interestingly, it has been postulated that cytokines associated with inflammation may be a trigger for migraines.) I considered trying to convince him to reintroduce wheat to see if the migraines would recur but have not yet mustered the courage.

2. GLUTEN OVERLOAD, NUTRIENT UNDERLOAD

Long before my "gluten obsession," I had often pointed out that too many Americans, while overfed, are undernourished because of the predominantly empty calories that they consume. All too often, these calories come in the form of highly processed fast foods containing sugar, refined starches, and bad fats with minimal nutritive value. It was only recently that I realized that poor absorption of nutrients due to gluten-related problems might also be contributing to this overfed/undernourished phenomenon. In the first place, refined, overly processed carbohydrates are hurting us by causing swings in blood sugar, resulting in cravings, and by not providing enough nutrients; in the second place, we're ingesting too much gluten by eating too many of these bad carbs. This gluten overload causes inflammation in susceptible individuals and, in turn, may block the absorption of nutrients from other, more wholesome foods.

Poor absorption of nutrients prevents us from getting the full complement of all the vitamins and minerals in food, which can lead to various nutrient deficiencies and their corresponding health problems. It would take several pages to list them all, but they run the gamut from anemia and hormone imbalances to mood disorders and neurological issues.

In fact, it may surprise you (and perhaps even your doctor) to learn that gluten sensitivity can contribute to osteoporosis, a progressive bone-thinning disease that increases the risk of fractures. About 55 percent of Americans over the age of 50 either have osteoporosis or are at high risk for developing it. I have always wondered why osteoporosis is so common in the industrialized world, despite our intake of calcium, magnesium, vitamin D, and other nutrients important for bone formation and strength. Interestingly, osteoporosis has traditionally been treated with calcium supplements, but their impact on stopping or reversing this disease has been minimal at best.

We know that with celiac disease, nutrient deficiencies resulting from a damaged small intestine stunt the growth of children and, indeed, prevent children from getting enough of these vital nutrients during their bone-building years. It seems likely that the osteoporosis that occurs later in life could be due to decades of poor absorption of the nutrients that were available from food but never got into the bloodstream and tissues.

Surprisingly, even with supplementation and exposure to sunlight, vitamin D deficiency, in particular, is still common today. In addition to its being a factor in osteoporosis development (vitamin D is needed to increase the intestinal absorption of calcium), the latest research indicates that this deficiency is linked to heart disease and several types of cancer. I believe that in some cases, it is also a marker for gluten disorders. If you have been told that you have a low vitamin D level, you should be tested for celiac disease, since damaged villi cannot adequately absorb this fat-soluble vitamin. Even if the results are negative, you should follow our Gluten Solution Program, monitor your response, and have your vitamin D rechecked after being off gluten. Conversely, if you find you are gluten sensitive after you've done our program, ask your doctor to test your vitamin D level and your levels other nutrients as well. You may need supplementation under your doctor's guidance.

3. AUTOIMMUNE RESPONSE TO GLUTEN

This is perhaps the most serious component of the Gluten Trifecta. Autoimmune diseases occur when our immune cells get involved in a case of "mistaken identity" and attack our own healthy cells and tissues. This may sound like a crazy thing for the body to do to itself, but in fact the immune system thinks that it is protecting us.

As explained earlier, with celiac disease, those incompletely digested strands of gluten protein—the peptides—penetrate the intestinal lining and are identified as foreign invaders by immune cells (also known as T cells) guarding this critical border from the outside world. Then these "first responder" immune cells call for backup, attracting a reserve army of more immune cells. Some of these reservists produce antibodies, so that if the invader shows up again, they will quickly recognize the uninvited guest and attack.

As if this isn't bad enough, sometimes these gluten peptides can look very much like parts of proteins that make up *all* of our body's tissues.

For example, if part of a gluten-derived peptide closely resembles part of a protein found in one of our joints, then our reserve army of immune cells might attack that joint, mistaking its protein for the targeted gluten protein. This destructive process, called molecular mimicry, can lead to a severe form of arthritis called rheumatoid arthritis (RA), which is just one fairly common autoimmune disease that is associated with celiac disease. RA can result in joint pain, joint deformity, and dysfunction. Unlike osteoarthritis, where joint damage is mainly the result of wear and tear due to gradual injury or to a more severe traumatic injury (such as an ankle fracture), in rheumatoid arthritis the immune system attacks the joints directly. Joint pain can be a symptom of other autoimmune conditions as well, such as lupus and fibromyalgia, which also have been associated with gluten-related disorders.

Another such case of mistaken identity occurs when an offending peptide, such as a gluten peptide, resembles protein from insulin-producing cells in the pancreas. The body ends up attacking its own pancreatic cells, interfering with insulin production and consequently with the body's ability to move glucose (blood sugar) from the bloodstream into the tissues. If the pancreas does not produce enough insulin, glucose accumulates in the blood, which is recognized when doctors detect high blood sugar levels. This type of autoimmune reaction is thought to be the major cause of type 1 diabetes, and, as you may remember, it is what happened to my Uncle Robert years before his diagnosis of celiac disease. It can also occur very early in life: A substantial number of children with type 1 diabetes have celiac disease—often undiagnosed. And, yes, a gluten-free diet has been shown to improve or even reverse type 1 diabetes in those children.

Unfortunately, our joints and our pancreas are not the only organs that may be in the crosshairs of our overzealous immune cells. The long list of these innocent bystanders includes our brain, our adrenal glands, our skin, and many more organs and tissues. Perhaps the most commonly attacked innocent bystander, however, is the thyroid. When it's under siege, it results in an inflammatory autoimmune condition called thyroiditis, which may show up as an overactive (hyperthyroidism) or underactive (hypothyroidism) thyroid.

In fact, there is practically no organ in the body that has been spared.

Because the mechanism of autoimmunity in gluten sensitivity is not as well understood as it is for celiac disease, its impact on those who are gluten sensitive remains ill defined. I have seen autoimmune issues in my own patients with nonceliac gluten sensitivity and await new research for a better understanding of how this happens.

At this time, the important message here is that if you have been diagnosed with one or more autoimmune conditions, be sure you get tested for celiac disease. If your tests are negative, then give the South Beach Diet Gluten Solution Program a try to determine your level of gluten sensitivity. You may be amazed by the results.

THE CHALLENGE AND THE OPPORTUNITY

It is not uncommon to have signs and symptoms from all three contributors to the Gluten Trifecta. A single patient might have abdominal cramps, bloating, and fatigue from small intestinal inflammation; iron deficiency anemia and osteoporosis from malabsorption; and psoriasis and type 1 diabetes from autoimmunity. Thus, gluten-related disorders not only mimic many ailments but actually cause a range of signs, symptoms, and conditions that are usually considered individually. But as in the case of my doctor friend, whom I discussed earlier, they may all be due to one problem—a reaction to gluten—and be cured with a gluten-free or gluten-aware diet.

There is no better case to illustrate the many disguises of gluten-related disorders and the full impact of the Gluten Trifecta on the body of an unsuspecting victim than the case of my patient Lisa. At 62 years old, Lisa had

A WORD ABOUT BLOATING

"I feel bloated" is one of the more common complaints doctors hear from patients, as well as from family, friends, and acquaintances. Add to that list abdominal pain, flatulence, diarrhea, and constipation. These problems have been traditionally lumped together and classified as irritable bowel syndrome (IBS). There has been a great deal of speculation as to possible causes of IBS, but the truth is, up until now, no one has had a good answer.

IBS symptoms also constitute the classic presentation of both celiac disease and gluten sensitivity, and here we have a much better understanding of what's going on. Remember, both celiac patients and gluten-sensitive patients have problems digesting gluten, and this is indeed a form of indigestion. The incompletely digested strands of gluten proteins proceed down the intestinal tract, dragging water with them that otherwise would have been absorbed into the bloodstream. This excess fluid can cause abdominal distension—in other words, bloating—as well as pain and loose, watery stools (diarrhea).

A second contributor to IBS-type symptoms in these patients is associated with intolerance to lactose—the sugar found in milk—and intolerance to other carbohydrates resulting from an insufficiency of enzymes needed to completely break down these chains of sugar molecules. (I discuss lactose intolerance in "Milk Got You?" on page 44.) This occurs because the injured intestinal lining can no longer produce certain enzymes in adequate amounts. In either case, the incompletely digested carbohydrates, just like the incompletely digested proteins, move down the intestine. In the case of the carbohydrates, when they meet up with additional bacteria, they undergo fermentation, generating a great deal of gas. This gas in turn produces bloating, cramps, and flatulence.

If you suffer from these kinds of intestinal complaints, changes in your diet—specifically reducing or eliminating both gluten and dairy—may relieve your symptoms.

pretty much given up hope of ever feeling well. With a medical record nearly as thick as a phone book, Lisa could barely remember all the specialists she had seen over time. Despite some improvement after treating her isolated conditions, she continued to feel drained, exhausted, and in pain. Her husband, who was a heart patient of mine, had frequently told me about her travails. After years of being just as perplexed as her doctors, I finally suggested she come see me because I suspected her ailments might be gluten related and I thought I might be able to help.

While in her early thirties, Lisa had developed a skin rash and was told she had lupus, a potentially serious autoimmune disease that can affect the skin and joints and lead to damage of major organs. In her forties, she was diagnosed with iron deficiency anemia. In her fifties, that diagnosis was upgraded to pernicious anemia, which occurs from an autoimmune defect that prevents the absorption of vitamin B_{12}. Her B_{12} levels were still low when she came to my office, as was her level of vitamin D.

Did I mention that this poor woman also had osteoporosis and debilitating migraines?

Unfortunately, I'm not finished. Lisa was taking thyroid hormone replacement for thyroiditis and had been diagnosed with hypopituitarism, a rare autoimmune hormone disorder. The endocrinologist who diagnosed that problem had actually tested her for celiac disease, but the results were negative.

Considering her vast array of symptoms, along with her classic digestive issues, I, too, had Lisa tested for celiac disease. Although the tests still came back negative, I believed that these seemingly unrelated symptoms and ailments might be traced back to gluten sensitivity. I suggested that Lisa become gluten free for at least a month and possibly longer.

A month later, when she came back to see me for a follow-up visit, Lisa was transformed. Not only did she have a great deal more energy and stamina after eliminating gluten from her life, but she had finally found relief from the chronic aches and pains that had been a problem since childhood. And so far, no more migraines! I congratulated her, had her see our nutritionist for some extra counseling, and told her to just keep doing what she had been doing.

Lisa has continued to do well for nearly 3 years—a very gratifying case.

With the advantage of 20/20 hindsight, it now seems obvious that many of Lisa's problems were rooted in, if not aggravated by, the Gluten Trifecta—inflammation, poor absorption of nutrients, and autoimmunity. The point is, if Lisa had been diagnosed with gluten sensitivity at a young age—and had been put on a gluten-free diet—she could have been spared many, if not all, of her maladies much earlier.

ONE OF HISTORY'S MYSTERIES: DID JFK HAVE CELIAC DISEASE?

There may be no better illustration of the disastrous consequences of failing to identify a gluten-related disorder than that of one of our most popular presidents. John Fitzgerald Kennedy (JFK), our second-youngest president, was perceived to be the vision of health and vigor (*viga* in Bostonese), but he was actually weak and sickly during much of his tragically short life. I have come to believe that celiac disease was probably the primary cause of his lifelong suffering. When his debilitating health history and his stoicism in the face of pain are fully appreciated, his accomplishments appear that much more courageous.

I had read some brief accounts of President Kennedy's health issues, but my real discovery of JFK's medical trials and tribulations began when I read the last volume of Robert Caro's highly acclaimed biography of former president Lyndon Johnson, *The Passage of Power.* It includes the fascinating story of the lead-up to the 1960 election, when Kennedy won the presidency, and then proceeds to cover Johnson's role as vice president and the passage of power after the tragic assassination of President Kennedy. Caro also gives a detailed account of JFK's medical problems, which started in childhood.

As I read about Kennedy's lifetime of struggle from an undiagnosed intestinal illness associated with many other seemingly unrelated problems, I kept thinking "celiac disease." Although the possibility of celiac disease was not mentioned in Caro's book, I looked to see if anyone else had come to this conclusion. I found further, earlier descriptions of Kennedy's health problems when White House health records were released in 2002 to historian Robert Dallek. He summarized the information in an article that year in the *Atlantic Monthly* titled "The Medical Ordeals of JFK." I also discovered that I was not the only one to postulate that Kennedy's problems originated from celiac disease. On the basis of the new information described by Dallek, celiac disease specialist Dr. Peter H.R. Green argued in an article published in 2004 on George Mason University's History News Network that JFK's underlying condition may well have been celiac disease. Interestingly, celiac disease is more common in those of Irish ancestry (and, of course, JFK was Irish). Possibly the long history of an almost gluten-free diet in Ireland, with its dependence on potatoes and corn as staples, has left the Irish with a limited ability to digest gluten.

In 2008, Dr. Lee R. Mandel had the opportunity to review Kennedy's health

(*continued*)

ONE OF HISTORY'S MYSTERIES:
DID JFK HAVE CELIAC DISEASE?—*CONTINUED*

records and, in 2009, he described Kennedy's medical problems and his thoughts about them in a history of medicine article in the prestigious *Annals of Internal Medicine*. He concluded that Kennedy had a syndrome that included autoimmune adrenal insufficiency and autoimmune thyroid disease. He also suggested that these autoimmune conditions, along with Kennedy's lifelong gastrointestinal symptoms, were consistent with a diagnosis of celiac disease.

JFK was in fact a sickly child due mainly to intestinal problems that continued throughout his life and that were never precisely diagnosed. He seemed always to be falling ill, and he endured many prolonged hospitalizations as a child for both treatment and uncomfortable testing in an ultimately vain attempt to make a diagnosis.

Kennedy suffered from chronic fatigue and was always very thin. At his boarding school, Choate, he spent a great deal of time in the infirmary, primarily with abdominal complaints, and at times was hospitalized. But his doctors never figured out what was wrong. He spent 4 months at the Mayo Clinic during his boarding school years and had to leave college during his freshman year, spending another 2 months in the hospital, this time at the Peter Bent Brigham Harvard-affiliated hospital in Boston. These sick days and hospitalizations were all due to stomach-related complaints—pain, nausea and vomiting, cramps, and diarrhea. Severe fatigue and collapse were associated with his worst episodes. Diagnoses of ulcers, colitis, spastic colitis, irritable bowel syndrome, and food allergies were all listed in his medical records. When he entered the navy in 1941, he was 6 feet tall but weighed only 150 pounds and could not have passed the military physical, getting in only through the influence of his powerful father.

After leaving the navy as a war hero, Kennedy ran for Congress and then the Senate, but his career was marked again by recurrent illnesses and hospital stays. When he fell ill on a visit to London in 1947, he was first given a diagnosis of Addison's disease—a deficiency of cortisone, a hormone that is synthesized by the adrenal glands, which sit atop the kidneys. This was probably an autoimmune disease, though Kennedy's likely use of cortisone injections over many years in an attempt to treat his intestinal inflammation may have suppressed his adrenal glands and produced a similar picture. Cortisone was first used clinically in the late 1930s and 1940s and was often thought to be a cure for any undiagnosed illness. Doctors prescribed it liberally, because its long-term complications were not yet appreciated. With its anti-inflammatory properties, cortisone might have given Kennedy some temporary relief from his intestinal inflammation, but only with dangerous long-term consequences. Later, he developed what appeared to be autoimmune thyroiditis. Both autoimmune Addison's disease and thyroiditis can be associated with celiac disease.

Kennedy was also plagued by back pain from well before his navy days and underwent a total of three life-threatening, unsuccessful back surgeries. He was diagnosed with severe osteoporosis, which could have been due to celiac disease and/or his chronic cortisone therapy. In addition, JFK suffered from migraine headaches, another celiac-associated condition.

As Kennedy was running for president, his primary and general election opponents attempted to uncover and make public the true state of his health. The offices of at least two of his physicians were burglarized in unsuccessful attempts to expose his medical history. Had this been done successfully, it is unlikely that he would have been elected in what was a razor-thin victory. But the true state of Kennedy's health was adequately protected thanks to deft language in an important press release by his physicians.

As successful and tragic as JFK's shortened life was, it's a shame to think that a disease that could have been treated with diet alone could have caused so much discomfort. During most of the years JFK was suffering, the connection between wheat and celiac disease had yet to be discovered. Small bowel biopsies were not performed until the 1950s (in fact, they were not performed easily until upper endoscopy was introduced in the 1970s). Gluten was not even identified as the culprit in celiac disease until the 1950s, and the antibody screening tests and genetic testing for celiac were not available during his lifetime.

Kennedy wrote a famous book, *Profiles in Courage,* before he was elected president in 1960. After having read how he found the inner strength and courage to overcome so many debilitating health problems, I believe it could be the title for his own biography. Today, there is no reason for gluten-related disorders to go undiagnosed and for so many to needlessly suffer as he did.

CHAPTER 7

THE NOT-SO-PLACEBO EFFECT

"IT'S ALL IN YOUR HEAD." THAT'S WHAT MANY GLUTEN-SENSITIVE patients have heard from their doctors, who are often too quick to dismiss patients' confusing symptoms. I might have thought the same thing myself on occasion, but now that I know more about gluten, I rarely make such an assumption.

Recently, Tiffany, the 28-year-old daughter of old friends, told me about her own misdiagnosis. A bright and attractive young woman, Tiffany looks and feels great today—no thanks to her doctors.

For most of her teenage years and early twenties, she suffered from stomach issues such as abdominal cramps after large meals, occasional diarrhea, and a generally sensitive stomach. Soon after she graduated from college and was eager to begin a career, things got worse for Tiffany. Her stomachaches progressed to the point where she was eating very little, losing weight, and feeling weak. She had also begun to feel anxious and depressed, which she insisted was unusual for her and unrelated to any life situation she could pinpoint. She consulted a battery of specialists and underwent plenty of tests without finding a solution to her problem. Finally, she agreed to take an anti-anxiety medication and an antidepressant prescribed by a psychiatrist. But the drugs offered little relief.

Like many patients who don't feel comfortable with their diagnosis—or nondiagnosis—Tiffany began doing her own research on the Internet. (While this isn't always a good idea, if you aren't getting the answers you need from your doctor, and you consult reputable sources, it's not always a bad idea either.) Her online detective work led her to diagnosis herself with gluten

JUST GOOGLE "GLUTEN"

There's no question that when the public is interested in a disease, they "Google it." When physicians are interested in a disease, we commonly do a search in PubMed (ncbi.nlm.nih.gov/pubmed), which is an easy way to review the medical literature quickly. What's fascinating is that the ratio of Google searches to PubMed searches on a particular medical topic can tell a lot about the relative interest of the public versus the medical profession. For conditions such as breast cancer and lung cancer, for example, there is a pretty consistent balance of public and physician interest. For gluten-related conditions, however, the ratio is 10 times greater in favor of public interest. Certainly, not every popular craze is rooted in good science, but occasionally one is. And as is sometimes the case when a trend outpaces the science, it may be a while before the medical profession takes it seriously. So keep Googling gluten! We suggest some reliable sites to visit in the Resources section, starting on page 231.

sensitivity. As soon as she eliminated gluten from her diet, relief was prompt and dramatic. Practically overnight, the stomachaches, poor appetite, anxiety, and depression vanished. Today, I am happy to report that Tiffany is happy and healthy and off all medication—and has been for more than 2 years. Needless to say, she spends very little time in doctors' offices.

A SURPRISE ENDING

Some of you may think that these "miraculous" turnarounds in symptoms— and in some cases, outright cures—after eliminating gluten are nothing more than the so-called placebo effect. That is, the positive results are not actually due to the absence of gluten but rather to the power of self-suggestion. With the lack of precise diagnostic tests, and because its symptoms resemble so many other conditions, gluten sensitivity's very existence has occasionally been questioned.

I am convinced that the placebo effect, while sometimes present, is *not* a significant factor in gluten sensitivity. In fact, a 2012 study from Scandinavia showed that both celiac and nonceliac gluten-sensitive patients were not inclined to "somaticize." This means that although symptoms of gluten sensitivity may mimic stress-related complaints, psychological stress *did not* tend to manifest itself as physical complaints in these patients. While I would never say that stress does not affect physical well-being, in my experience the vast majority of patients suffering with symptoms of gluten sensitivity turn out to have a completely physical problem. It's simply a matter of knowing how to interpret the symptoms. When you take these patients off gluten, their symptoms disappear, and so do they—from my office.

Let me tell you about one of my new patients, Ken, who came to see me for a cardiac prevention evaluation. The first words out of his mouth were most unusual. "Dr. Agatston, first you have to help me with my wife, or I am going to end up divorced." He then told me that his 55-year-old wife, Mary, to whom he had been married for 35 years, was suffering from chronic symptoms that included nausea, fatigue, headaches, generalized aches and pains, and a variety of problems that sounded like a possible sensitivity to gluten. Again, it would be reasonable to question whether these symptoms could be due to psychological stress, but, as in Tiffany's case, Mary's overall history suggested otherwise.

I told Ken of my suspicion but insisted that Mary come in for a complete physical with our internist Dr. Woolf, who had recently joined me on my gluten-awareness journey. After meeting with Mary, he found that in addition to the complaints Ken had mentioned, she was taking medication for depression, complaining of insomnia, and battling adult-onset acne. Antidepressants had not helped her, just as they not helped Tiffany. Her screening tests for celiac disease were negative, but she did have a low vitamin B_{12} level and osteopenia, or bone loss, indicating possible malabsorption of vitamin D. When tested, her vitamin D level was in fact low. After her tests, Dr. Woolf had Mary eliminate gluten from her diet with the help of our nutritionist.

A few days later, while I was out of town, I received a text from Dr. Woolf: "Arthur, while I don't want to feed your gluten obsession, Mary just called to say that she is nausea free for the first time in 2 years and that her aches and pains have disappeared. She says that she now knows her problems are gluten related."

I saw Mary about 6 weeks later, and she reported that all of her symptoms were gone. She felt energized, she was sleeping well, and she was able to focus much better. Perhaps her greatest thrill of all was that she could really enjoy her grandchildren, even playing on the floor with them without pain or fatigue. A year later, she is still doing well and rarely visits our office. Needless to say, her husband is happy, too. Maybe I should go into marriage counseling.

Mary's story illustrates several characteristics that suggest her response was not placebo. First, as with so many gluten-sensitive patients, she had consulted many other physicians and was exposed to many therapies, including several medications. Clearly, she would already have responded, at least in the short term, if she was susceptible to the placebo effect. Second, she responded more quickly than was expected. Third, and perhaps most important, her improvement has lasted more than a year. Most placebo effects have durations of weeks to months, not years. Our experience has been that when gluten-sensitive patients respond, they respond forever—that is, if they remain gluten aware after figuring out how much, if any, gluten they can tolerate. Long remissions are simply not characteristic of the placebo effect.

YET MORE PROOF

Some would rightly argue that complaints such as fatigue and brain fog are highly subjective and difficult to measure. Therefore, you can never really tell whether going off gluten is effective as a treatment or is an example of the placebo effect. For the reasons outlined in Mary's case, and more, I am convinced that the relief of symptoms experienced by these patients was not primarily due to the placebo effect.

In the case of fatigue, for example, there is an excellent double-blind, randomized, placebo-controlled study that considered "tiredness" and other symptoms in nonceliac gluten-sensitive patients just like Mary. This type of study is the gold standard for excluding the placebo effect in research trials.

Researchers at Monash University in Victoria, Australia, recruited 34 patients with irritable bowel syndrome suspected to be due to gluten sensitivity who had been on a gluten-free diet for the 6 weeks prior to the study. At that point, the patients were randomly assigned to either eat one *gluten-rich* muffin and two pieces of *gluten-rich* bread or one *gluten-free* muffin and two pieces of *gluten-free* bread daily for 6 weeks. Neither the patients nor the investigators knew who was consuming the gluten-containing foods. The participants answered questions about their symptoms weekly for the 6 weeks of the study and for 3 weeks after they returned to their original gluten-free diet.

Just a week after the muffins and bread were introduced, at the first opportunity to report their symptoms, there was a dramatic decrease in energy and increase in gastrointestinal symptoms noted in the group given the gluten-containing foods, which held true throughout the study. The quick return of symptoms is characteristic of the response of gluten-sensitive patients when gluten is reintroduced into their diet.

And even though the response time for improvement in symptoms once gluten is eliminated was not tested in this trial, many physicians, myself included, have observed a rapid improvement in many symptoms upon the removal of gluten. This was never my expectation with my early patients, and therefore I never communicated it to them. And yet, like Mary, they often called me within days to tell me how much better they were feeling.

WHAT CRIME SHOWS TAUGHT ME

There is another important factor that has helped convince me that symptom improvements in gluten-sensitive patients are not the result of the placebo effect. It can perhaps be best explained by what I call the "homicide detective rule."

Those of us who watch detective shows on TV and follow real-life crime events are well aware that detectives do not publicly release all the evidence gathered from a crime scene. This way, they can keep secret certain information that only the perpetrator would know. Similarly, I never tell patients about *all* the symptoms that might improve when they avoid gluten. For one thing, I wouldn't be able to list all the possible symptoms, and for another, I would probably sound more like a snake oil salesman than a doctor. And, frankly, there is just no need to. To encourage compliance with a gluten-free trial, I communicate optimism regarding the major symptoms I think will improve, but I don't make promises I am not sure I can keep. I simply wait to see what the patients report. When they return to my office and excitedly tell me about relief from symptoms we never discussed, I can be fairly sure that their improvement is not due to the placebo effect.

Mary definitely proved this to be true. Remember that she told me she could focus better after going off gluten? Interestingly, she had never complained about lack of focus during her visit with Dr. Woolf, and neither he nor I had suggested to her that it might be a symptom associated with gluten sensitivity.

Which brings me to the story of Harry, a patient who provides another good illustration of these "unexpected benefits."

For years I had tried to get my patient Harry to adopt the South Beach Diet, including an exercise regimen, to lose weight and manage his type 2 diabetes. He was totally noncompliant with these lifestyle measures. One day, when Harry returned to my office for a regular visit and complained of fatigue and joint pain, I told him he just might feel a whole lot better without gluten. Secretly, I hoped that he would end up eating a substantially healthier diet if he thought it would relieve his aching joints and pep him up. When Harry returned for a follow-up visit 2 weeks later, I was surprised to hear that the major change he noticed after avoiding gluten (in addition to the 12 pounds he reported he'd lost on Phase 1 of our program) was that it was much easier for him to focus. He asked me whether I had seen this in other patients, and I told him I had. After sharing Mary's story with him, I also recalled that a young man had told me that after eliminating gluten, he was better able to focus on studying for his business school entrance exam, which, as it turned out, he aced.

Now that I've seen this kind of improvement several times, I recommend becoming gluten aware to family, friends, and the older children of patients who are studying for important exams. If you're not gluten sensitive, you may not experience any change in your ability to concentrate, but it's certainly worth a "test" before the test.

I REST MY CASE

There is a term that researchers use for evidence called strength of association. Strength of association is why, when penicillin was first used in the early 1940s, no physician withheld it from a patient with pneumonia because the anecdotal evidence demonstrating the effectiveness of the drug was so overwhelming.

In the case of gluten, strength of association is looking impressive. It's clear that when so many physicians report sustained positive results in patients on a gluten-controlled diet, their improvement is not likely to be due to the placebo effect.

I am not suggesting we don't conduct randomized studies. What I am suggesting is that we don't discount the anecdotal evidence and fail to help people in the meantime.

As I did with Harry, on occasion I have recommended a gluten-free diet to patients with diabetes or prediabetes (metabolic syndrome) who I suspect may have a gluten sensitivity. I do this hoping that they will feel so much better generally that they will continue to stay away from the refined carbohydrates and other junk foods that had fueled their elevated blood sugars. And my plan often works.

But . . . not everyone feels better off gluten.

Several spouses of gluten-sensitive patients have participated in our Gluten Solution Program to be supportive, even though they had no gluten-associated symptoms. Other than the weight loss they experienced on the program (which, of course, made them happy), they reported no other benefits.

To me, these are the exceptions that prove the rule. Not everyone is gluten sensitive, but those who are feel *genuinely* better.

CHAPTER 8

IT STARTS EARLY

"A PARENT IS ONLY AS HAPPY AS HIS UNHAPPIEST CHILD" IS AN OLD expression that I believe resonates with all parents. And children with gluten sensitivity are often very unhappy. Can you imagine how bad you'd feel if you found out that your child's chronic health issues could have been solved much earlier simply by modifying his or her diet? Alternatively, think how great you'd feel if you made a simple change in your child's diet and it alleviated his or her problems.

Both situations are true for parents of children with gluten sensitivity, a condition that is often undiagnosed, misunderstood, and mismanaged.

As frustrating as an unrecognized case of gluten sensitivity can be to any adult, it can be doubly hard on children and their parents. All too often, gluten-sensitive children are mislabeled as hyperactive, treated for mood disorders or depression, or subjected to a battery of uncomfortable medical tests. Parents feel helpless. No matter how many specialists they take their children to see, their kids never seem to get better. Their children may fall behind in school and lack the stamina to engage in afterschool activities or keep up with their friends. This, in turn, makes the children unhappy and their parents anxious.

In Chapter 6, I described President John Fitzgerald Kennedy's difficult childhood—which was fraught with pain, fatigue, and frequent absences from school. Back then, there were no simple tests for celiac disease, and no one would have known to treat him with a simple gluten-free diet in any case.

Gluten sensitivity as a source of chronic symptoms in childhood wouldn't be considered for many decades.

In contrast, today the diagnosis for celiac disease can be made with a fairly easy series of tests, and gluten sensitivity can be diagnosed by simply removing—or cutting way back on—gluten from your child's diet and observing the results. It is a shame to have a child experience so much misery for a problem that can be so easily controlled! That is why it's important for parents to learn to recognize the symptoms of gluten sensitivity in children, and why every family needs to be conscious of the telltale signs and symptoms.

MISUNDERSTOOD, MISDIAGNOSED, AND MISMANAGED

Let me tell you about Olivia, a patient of my colleague Dr. Natalie Geary. Before Olivia went to see Dr. Geary, her undiagnosed case of gluten sensitivity had put her and her family through years of unhappiness.

Olivia was a bright, slightly overweight 7-year-old who often complained of stomachaches, which led to frequent absences from school. She also tended to be moody and irritable. Worried sick about her daughter, Olivia's mother asked her pediatrician to test Olivia for likely medical problems that could be causing her symptoms. This even included a test for parasites.

When the pediatrician couldn't find a physical cause for Olivia's problems, he sent her for an evaluation with a child therapist who promptly diagnosed ADHD (attention-deficit hyperactivity disorder) and prescribed Adderall, a drug typically used to treat this problem. Olivia's symptoms did not improve, so her mother then consulted a gastroenterologist, who performed a few more studies and decided that Olivia had "functional abdominal pain," often a code for somatization of emotional stress. Remember, this means the symptoms are "all in Olivia's head." Sound familiar?

Despite the tests, medication, and visits to therapists, Olivia did not get better. Desperate to find a way to help her daughter, Olivia's mother decided to switch pediatricians and sought help from Dr. Geary, who detected some interesting patterns in the child's symptoms during the very first visit. First, she learned that Olivia rarely complained of stomachaches, was in a better mood, and simply felt much better over the summer when the family went on vacation in Maine. When Dr. Geary asked detailed questions about Olivia's diet, she learned that during the school year, Olivia ate pretty much the same food every day: a bagel for breakfast, pizza for lunch, and pasta for dinner. But in Maine, while she would still eat the bagel for breakfast, the rest of her meals consisted of fresh seafood and vegetables from a nearby farm stand. No pizza and almost no pasta.

Because of the improvement in Olivia's symptoms while she was in Maine, Dr. Geary suspected gluten sensitivity, which was likely being triggered by gluten overload due to excessive intake of wheat-based products at home and at school. She told Olivia's mother that she thought Olivia's school-year problems might be rooted in her high-wheat diet and suggested that the entire family make changes in their eating style, which could be beneficial for all of them.

The solution was as simple as switching from the bagel to wheat-free (gluten-free) waffles for breakfast and swapping the pasta at night for lean protein (like chicken, lean cuts of beef, fish, and tofu), fresh vegetables, and whole-grain brown rice. On this new regimen, Olivia could still occasionally eat pizza at lunch like the other kids at her school so that she didn't feel stigmatized by having to eat differently than her classmates.

When she and her mother returned for a follow-up visit with Dr. Geary a month later, Olivia was smiling, calm, and talking happily about school and friends. The best news was that she had not missed a day of classes since starting this new way of eating. And since her dietary changes were made during the school year, Olivia's marked improvement and happy mood could not be attributed to her being under less stress during the summer. Dr. Geary was pleased to see that Olivia's mother, who had been a bundle of nerves at their last meeting, looked well rested and was relieved by her daughter's progress.

SENSITIVE AT AN EARLY AGE

Olivia's story is typical of the many children with gluten sensitivity who go undiagnosed for years. Generally, the onset of symptoms is subtle: As children are weaned off breast milk or formula, they are usually transitioned to jar foods or freshly prepared puréed vegetables and rice cereal that contain little if any wheat. They start to develop symptoms around the age of 2 when they begin eating regular table food with their family, including bread, pasta, bagels, muffins, and pizza—all sources of gluten. At around the same age, children begin to exercise their will over what they eat, often fixating on a few foods and refusing the rest. They tend to favor foods like chicken nuggets (breaded), pasta, hot dogs (with a bun), and other wheat-based products. Parents of children with gluten sensitivity may not see a sudden change in their children's behavior or health, however, until the youngsters are a little older and in even more control of their diet. It's at this point that many children quite literally "overdose" on wheat or other gluten-containing grains.

Some symptoms of gluten sensitivity in children include:

- Gastrointestinal issues like nausea, abdominal pain, heartburn, constipation, or diarrhea
- Agitation and mood swings
- Asthma
- Runny nose and postnasal drip

- Ear infections
- Extreme changes in weight
- Fatigue
- Headaches
- Joint pain
- Skin rashes like eczema

Gluten sensitivity is not something that you outgrow. You *adapt*. This is an important distinction: Adults tend to adapt to unpleasant physical sensations unless those sensations are so extreme as to compromise the ability to function. So the bloating, abdominal discomfort, mild aches, pains, and headaches are written off to other causes: "I ate too much last night," "I need a vacation," "I'm stressed."

Because children do not have the same ability to adapt as adults, they complain that their stomach hurts, but when they are taken to the pediatrician, nothing abnormal is found on the exam. The kids are irritable, but it is blamed on a lack of sleep. They have a rash (eczema) that is attributed to "allergy." They have attention issues and are prescribed Adderall. The truth is that by the age of 5, many children—perhaps as many as 40 percent—have a gluten sensitivity, mild to moderate, that goes undiagnosed. And it often gets progressively worse as they get older and spend more time away from home making independent food choices, which often involve highly processed, wheat-based fast food.

Parents who do all the right things, like breast-feeding and serving only organic food, and who have no history of allergy in their families, cannot prevent their children from developing gluten sensitivity if the organic fare includes bread and wheat-based cereals. But gluten sensitivity does depend in good measure on the *quantity* of gluten ingested. That is why we are seeing such an epidemic of gluten-related problems now, in both children and adults.

GLUTEN AWARE IS GOOD FOR THE ENTIRE FAMILY

Becoming a gluten-aware family is easier than you think. And there is a good chance that if you have a gluten-sensitive child in your family, you will feel better cutting back on gluten yourself. It doesn't have to be a hassle. When you are all on the same program, and the house is stocked with tasty alternatives, including plenty of healthy gluten-free snacks (rapidly growing children need three nutritious meals *and* three snacks a day up to age 8 to thrive), no one will feel deprived or punished.

Studies show that the time to teach children healthy eating habits is before the age of 9. After that, it is difficult to impose dietary changes or restrictions because a child perceives it as a punitive measure. So the earlier you make the dietary changes in your household, the better. When children are young, they are malleable, and they imitate their parents—and, as I have learned, their teachers as well.

In 2004, the Agatston Research Foundation began our Healthy Options for Public Schoolchildren (HOPS) study in Osceola, Florida. We changed the food in selected elementary school cafeterias and initiated a nutrition education program. While our focus was not on gluten-free food, the emphasis on fruits, vegetables, lean sources of protein, and some whole grains definitely decreased gluten overload. The children in the schools with the program achieved a healthier weight and had higher test scores than the kids in schools without the program. Whether a decrease in gluten resulting from the decrease in processed carbohydrates played a role, we can only speculate. Our program certainly showed that children feel and perform better eating fewer processed carbohydrates and more fruits and vegetables. But perhaps our most important finding was that children from kindergarten to sixth grade will embrace healthy eating if they are involved in a program that includes food tastings and nutrition education. And the earlier it starts, the better.

So parents, don't be afraid. Kids really are adaptable. And if your child is gluten sensitive or has celiac disease, you can successfully help him make— and accept—the dietary changes he needs to be healthy.

We also know that healthy eating habits begun in childhood have a direct impact on a child's long-term health. The risk of diabetes and metabolic syndrome is markedly decreased in children who are of normal weight and physically fit. But gluten is often a metabolic deadweight. Many children and adults feel sluggish, tired, and slightly uncomfortable after a meal that includes gluten-laden foods. As a result, they are less likely to exercise on a regular basis. In addition, in Dr. Geary's experience, removing or reducing gluten in the diet of sensitive children clearly reduces the inflammatory response. This means that these kids have less mucus production (and therefore fewer ear infections), less stomach discomfort, a healthier appetite, and a better ability to focus and stay still. It also means fewer visits to the pediatrician.

GLUTEN AWARE, NOT GLUTEN PHOBIC

Dr. Geary's critical message for parents is this: Unless your child has true celiac disease, gluten is not a poison; it's just something to be mindful of, and you don't need to be the food police. As I've explained throughout this book, gluten-related disorders can range from severe (celiac disease) to mild. So if your child is somewhat gluten sensitive and is headed to a birthday party (i.e., pizza, cake, cookies), the best approach is not to tell her, "No, you can't participate in the fun." Just the opposite. It's to plan ahead and recognize that she will likely get a wheat overload that day, so for breakfast and dinner it's best to have zero wheat.

Certainly, you do not want your child to feel socially isolated or "sick" at the party, and parents who send a child with special foods to social events do not always realize the psychological impact that has on the child. Better to plan ahead and then let her enjoy herself.

BECOME AN INTENTIONAL GLUTEN EXPERT

Gluten sensitivity is at the root of so many health problems that it can be difficult to pinpoint the source. That's why, as I discussed earlier, gluten-related disorders are called the "great imitators," and that's why these problems often persist for decades, from childhood well into adulthood, before gluten is identified as the culprit.

The good news is, none of this has to happen. Not to your child, not to any child. And not to you.

The great news is that gluten sensitivity is a problem that you can fix.

But the real challenge is learning to recognize gluten sensitivity when you see it, and why I call upon all parents to become "intentional gluten experts." Make it a point to educate yourselves about the signs of gluten sensitivity and be on the alert if you feel that your children may be falling prey to gluten overload.

If you suspect that this may be a problem, it's easy enough to prove or disprove your suspicions. Just try removing—or cutting way back on—gluten from your child's diet and see if he or she feels better. A small minority of children should have no wheat at all, but for most kids, moderation will significantly resolve their discomfort. The proof will be a rapid improvement in your child's physical symptoms, mood, and behavior. And remember, unless your child has celiac disease, no food that contains gluten is completely off-limits.

The point is, every child should be given the best nutrition possible, as early as possible, to lay the foundation for a long and healthy life. That's why becoming a gluten-aware parent is critical.

CHAPTER 9

JUNK FOOD
BY ANOTHER NAME

I RECENTLY OPENED AN ISSUE OF A MAJOR DIETETICS JOURNAL TO see an article headlined "Gluten-Free Diet: Imprudent Dietary Advice for the General Population?" Clearly, the two authors were tackling a provocative question on many people's minds, including my own.

The article covered the recent popularity of eating gluten free, but its bottom line was that unless you have celiac disease, gluten sensitivity, or a wheat allergy, a gluten-free diet is unnecessary and may cause you to miss out on fiber and some important nutrients like niacin, thiamine, and riboflavin. If you have a gluten-related condition, it is important to include gluten-free whole grains in your diet to make up for some of these missing nutrients. The article also pointed out that many gluten-free products are long on calories and short on nutrition.

This critique is representative of numerous others suggesting that the gluten craze is moving ahead of the science. I agree with several of their points, particularly their analysis of the perils of many gluten-free foods.

But the growing gluten awareness does *not* have to be stopped. It simply needs to be nurtured with accurate information and education.

In my first South Beach Diet book, I described my one-time infatuation with a brand of cookies that were considered to be "heart healthy" solely because they were fat and cholesterol free. Back then, nobody was concerned about whether a product was made with whole grains or refined grains, as long as it was low in fat. And when food manufacturers added nutrient-poor starches and extra sugars to their products to compensate for removing the fat and cholesterol, it was not considered a problem.

In those dark days of "all fat is bad," the entire nation was fixated on squeezing every drop of fat and cholesterol out of our food supply. So, like millions of other Americans, I would blissfully gobble up these tasty, overly sweetened, fat-free miracles in the mistaken belief that I was eating a healthy snack. Not infrequently, in the late afternoon I would feel just terrible— light-headed, weak, and shaky. No problem. I headed for the doctors' lounge, which had a "healthy" supply of fat-free muffins. Blueberry was my favorite.

Eventually, I realized what was happening to me, my patients, and the American public. I was suffering from the classic symptoms of reactive hypogly- cemia, a condition caused by a surge in blood sugar, followed by a steep drop. Those fat-free so-called healthy cookies were low-fat, bad-carb junk food in disguise. This revelation and others led to the creation of the South Beach Diet.

The South Beach Diet has always emphasized the difference between high-fiber, nutrient-rich, slow-burning, low-sugar good carbs and highly pro- cessed, low-fiber, fast-burning, high-sugar, nutrient-poor bad carbs. As we now know, bad carbs produce the rapid spikes and subsequent drops in blood sugar that trigger the food cravings that can lead to obesity, insulin resistance, type 2 diabetes, and chronic disease—even cancer. In contrast, good carbs are digested slowly, provide a steady source of energy, and contain beneficial nutrients, including fiber, vitamins, and minerals, that are removed in the processing of refined products.

South Beach dieters have heard this story before. Choosing good carbs over bad is an integral part of the diet and is now in the mainstream of reliable dietary advice. Add in good unsaturated fats and lean sources of protein (not forgetting that vegetables and fruits are good carbohydrates) and you have the sound principles of healthy eating that will endure in current and future national diet guidelines.

But I now find myself in the position of playing Paul Revere once again. So heed my warning: *The bad carbs are coming back! The bad carbs are coming back!* Just as in the days of the no-fat craze, bad carbs are being marketed under the cover of good health. And if you are among the thousands of people tantalized by gluten-free products, you may be unknowingly contributing to their resurgence.

GLUTEN FREE CAN PACK ON THE POUNDS

There's a growing public perception that anything labeled "gluten free" is good for you, but many people, like my patient Carla, learn the hard way that gluten free can lead to trouble if you make bad gluten-free choices.

About a year ago, Carla came to me for a cardiac risk evaluation because she had high cholesterol levels. When I reviewed her medical history, I was struck by the long list of her other issues, including thyroid problems, rashes, anemia, chronic abdominal symptoms, arthritis, and some other conditions. Thirty years earlier, she had even been told she had lupus, though no serious complications had ever developed.

I am confident that by now you recognize this potpourri of seemingly unrelated diagnoses to be consistent with one unifying diagnosis—a gluten-related disorder.

Carla's tests for celiac disease were negative, but she did have a low vitamin B_{12} level along with a very low vitamin D level, which might have been a cause of her osteopenia. She also suffered from reflux esophagitis, with some resultant damage to the lower esophagus.

As I'm sure you've already guessed, I suggested that Carla go gluten free for a month, but she was in a hurry that day and did not have time to consult with our nutritionist, Marie Almon. Instead, she decided she would go off gluten on her own.

Carla proceeded to avoid gluten-containing foods and quickly felt better. But it wasn't quite the happy ending she had hoped for. When she came to see me for a follow-up visit, she was very upset because she had gained 10 pounds.

At that point, I *insisted* that Carla have a nutritional consultation with Marie, who quickly figured out why she had gained the weight. Carla had been indulging in many of the highly refined, gluten-free foods like cookies, crackers, and pretzels that are made with ingredients such as white rice flour or potato starch. These high-glycemic, gluten-free ingredients were causing swings in her blood sugar that kept her coming back for more. (Remember how low-fat cookies sent me running for blueberry muffins?) Little did she realize that many of these products, though gluten free, were very high in sugar and starch, which are often added to make gluten-free foods taste like those made from the traditional refined carbohydrates that we now know contributed to our epidemics of obesity and diabetes in the first place.

Armed with her new knowledge, Carla got on track with *healthy* gluten-free eating and experienced gradual but steady weight loss. She still had to avoid gluten—and most of those packaged gluten-free products—but she could enjoy high-fiber, gluten-free grains like quinoa and brown rice and plenty of vegetables, fruits, and legumes that are "naturally" gluten free. Carla turned things around and lost the 10 pounds and then some.

A few months later, Carla's husband, Dick, came in for his visit and commented that they had just returned from a cruise. My initial reaction was "Uh-oh!" Even the healthiest eaters can go "overboard" on a cruise. I was afraid to ask how much weight Carla had regained.

To my relief, I learned that Carla had lost even more weight. When I inquired about how she had managed to do this, Dick told me that Carla was much more active than she had ever been before. He told me that one night while on the cruise, rather than wait on a long elevator line to go up five flights to their stateroom, Carla suggested that they use the stairs instead. Dick was astonished to watch Carla take the lead and bound up the steps.

For him, there was no doubt. Her newfound energy and endurance were the result of her new gluten and South Beach Diet awareness, including getting rid of the gluten-free junk food that had previously tempted her. I was happy to agree.

SO WHERE DID THINGS GO WRONG?

Why would food manufacturers make gluten-free products that are almost nothing but refined flour and sugar?

Here it is helpful to understand why these products were created originally—for people with celiac disease who needed an alternative to the gluten-laden breads and baked goods being eaten by the rest of us. Remember, celiac sufferers must avoid even minuscule amounts of foods containing gluten, or their condition will worsen. Their first three dietary priorities must be: no gluten, no gluten, and no gluten.

Celiac patients are often quite thin or sometimes malnourished, due to the poor absorption of calories and nutrients across the inflamed walls of their small intestine. Unless they have type 1 diabetes, the sugar and starch in a gluten-free cookie is of little concern. At the time, the only things that mattered in evaluating a gluten-free product were that it had no gluten and tasted as good as it could.

Although it's clear that even the thinnest celiac patient shouldn't have been eating too many of these nonnutritive gluten-free products to begin with (there are far healthier ways to put on some weight if you need to), there weren't a whole lot of healthier packaged options out there years ago. Unfortunately, there still aren't many high-fiber, nutritious gluten-free choices, although some manufacturers are making an effort to improve their products from a nutritional standpoint.

Just as the high-glycemic, fat-free products of the 1980s and 1990s contributed so mightily to our diabetes and obesity epidemics, many of these gluten-free products have the potential to do the same thing today. They continue to flood the market because of popular demand and lack of consumer awareness.

This is why, whether you have celiac disease or gluten sensitivity, you must learn how to read package labels and become an educated food consumer. Junk food is junk food. And gluten-free junk food by any name is no exception.

PART II

THE
SOUTH BEACH DIET
GLUTEN SOLUTION
PROGRAM

CHAPTER 10

THE SOUTH BEACH DIET GLUTEN SOLUTION PROGRAM

THE SOUTH BEACH DIET IS NOT JUST A DIET, IT'S A LIFESTYLE.
Millions of successful South Beach dieters can tell you that ultimately it's about knowing how to make the right choices most of the time. Your healthy weight is maintained because you have learned what works for you.

The South Beach Diet Gluten Solution Program is simply an extension of our time-tested plan. The same principles of eating a varied diet consisting of nutrient- and fiber-rich vegetables, fruits, and whole grains, as well as lean protein and good fats, still hold true here. You'll just be giving up all gluten for a few weeks to determine if you have any gluten sensitivity.

If you are experiencing any of the symptoms described in the first part of this book, which may be gluten related, this program should help. If you're feeling pretty good but you're curious to see if you might feel even better, this program will give you the answer. Either way, you will be losing weight and getting healthier on the South Beach Diet for the next 4 weeks. Everyone will benefit from that—gluten sensitive or not.

If you're lucky enough to already be at your optimal weight but you suspect you may be gluten sensitive, this program can benefit you, too. When I designed my good carbs, good fats diet almost 20 years ago to help my cardiac and diabetes patients improve their blood profiles, lose weight, and avoid a heart attack or stroke, America was getting fatter and sicker following the low-fat, high-carb diet recommended at the time. Back then, fat was the enemy, and the idea that gluten might be connected to many of our health problems, including obesity, was not on the radar.

Today, wheat has been targeted as the enemy, and some people have gone a little overboard avoiding it. Just as people were wrongly fat phobic back in the 1990s, they're wrongly gluten phobic today. That's why I have created the South Beach Diet Gluten Solution Program: to clear up the confusion about gluten, to help you figure out whether you need to be concerned about gluten at all, and then to help you make the best food choices for better health if it turns out you do have a gluten sensitivity.

ALL THAT AND HEALTHY WEIGHT LOSS, TOO

You'd be surprised at how many people have put on weight eating too many of the sugary and starchy, highly processed, fiberless—yet gluten free—products so widely available today. Empty-calorie foods are a bad choice, gluten free or not. If you follow our Gluten Solution Program carefully, you should lose 8 to 10 pounds in the next 2 weeks for starters if you begin the program on Gluten Solution Phase 1 (GS Phase 1, for short). Then, if you continue to follow the program, you'll lose even more weight—1 to 2 pounds a week—on Gluten Solution (GS) Phase 2 until you reach a weight that's healthy for you. And the best part is that you'll keep that weight off because you'll have learned how to make the right food choices most of the time.

One more important thing. In 2003, I wrote, "The South Beach Diet is not low-carb." That was the first line of my first book, and it holds true today. The South Beach Diet is about good carbs—even for the gluten sensitive. Remember this: Gluten free is not grain free. Just as we recommend nutrient- and fiber-rich whole grains on the South Beach Diet (along with plenty of vegetables, fruits, beans, and other good carbohydrates), we aren't giving up on all of those good whole grains on the Gluten Solution Program. That's because there are plenty of healthy whole grains—amaranth and buckwheat and brown rice, to name a few—that don't contain gluten but do contain fiber and other important nutrients that are hard to get in other foods. In fact, it's extremely difficult to meet the recommended 25 to 30 grams of fiber a day without eating some whole grains. You'll find a full list of these grains and the flours made from them in our GS

Phase 2 Foods to Enjoy List on pages 126 to 128. And after 4 weeks, you'll be adding back some gluten-containing foods as your sensitivity allows.

As with my original diet, the beauty of the Gluten Solution Program is that it gives you flexibility. It teaches you where gluten can be found, then it gives you the freedom to experiment once you've determined the degree of your sensitivity. If you turn out to be only moderately gluten sensitive, as so many of my patients are, you may soon be enjoying that piece of whole-wheat bread or that side of whole-wheat pasta again (in moderation, of course) before you know it. You'll have come to understand what triggers your bloat or your brain fog or your joint pain, and you will have become gluten aware, though not necessarily gluten free.

Now that's a lifestyle, not a diet.

FIRST THINGS FIRST

If you were to walk into my office tomorrow with abdominal pain, fatigue, foggy mind, joint pain, tingling in the extremities, or any of the other symptoms commonly associated with both celiac disease and gluten sensitivity, I would test you for celiac disease before suggesting that you try the Gluten Solution Program. As I described in Chapter 3, this involves drawing blood to check for anti-tTG and other antibodies that are produced when intestinal cells are damaged and for the genes linked to celiac disease (HLA-DQ2 and/or HLA-DQ8). Depending on the results, a confirming biopsy may also be necessary. At the same time, I also test for nutritional deficiencies common in people with celiac disease, namely iron, folic acid, vitamin B_{12}, and vitamin D.

You may be wondering, "Why do I have to go through all this? Can't I just give up gluten and see what happens?" There are two important reasons why testing is necessary. First, in order for the blood tests and biopsy (if needed) to be accurate, you can't be gluten free at the time the tests are taken. Remember, the celiac disease blood tests look for antibodies that show your immune system's response to the gluten in your diet. If you're not eating foods containing gluten at the time of testing, your system won't be producing antibodies for the blood tests to identify. Intestinal biopsies go back to a normal or near-normal appearance if you have been gluten free.

In addition, patients who are gluten sensitive but who do not have celiac disease may experiment with foods containing gluten once they've been off gluten for a month or more and are feeling better. If you have celiac disease, you must be gluten free, *completely gluten free*, for life, or risk serious health complications. Since 97 percent of those with celiac disease don't even know they have it, ruling out this disease is extremely important.

If you have already begun to cut gluten from your diet, you will have to return to eating gluten again for a while or your body won't be making any antibodies against it. This is essential for a proper diagnosis. Particularly if you think you have celiac disease, it is critical to work with a knowledgeable doctor who can provide guidance about reintroducing gluten and monitor you before you do your baseline tests.

But let's be optimistic and assume that you don't have celiac disease, which is true for most of my patients. If that's the case, you can move on to the South Beach Diet Gluten Solution Program.

A QUICK GUIDE TO THE SOUTH BEACH DIET GLUTEN SOLUTION PROGRAM

As with the South Beach Diet, you can start our Gluten Solution Program on either GS Phase 1 or GS Phase 2.

WHO STARTS ON GLUTEN SOLUTION PHASE 1?

If you have more than 10 pounds to lose and cravings for sugary and starchy foods as well as symptoms of gluten sensitivity, you should begin the program on GS Phase 1. You will follow the GS Phase 1 plan for 2 weeks and see how you feel.

During the 2 weeks on GS Phase 1, you won't be eating any wheat, barley, or rye, and you will do your best to avoid any product that contains gluten. In fact, you won't be eating *any grains at all*, or fruits for that matter, because we want to get the blood sugar swings that cause your cravings under control. What you will be eating is three wholesome meals a day and at least two snacks as well as dessert, and that means you won't be hungry. (See our Meal Plans for GS Phase 1 on pages 107 to 120 for suggestions.)

This is exactly like Phase 1 of the South Beach Diet. The only difference is that we have eliminated those few items, like soy sauce and soy products, imitation crabmeat, and (surprisingly) blue cheese, because of their potential gluten content. Our GS Phase 1 Foods to Avoid List on pages 105 to 106 shows you these and other foods you need to stay away from.

By the end of the first 2 weeks, you should have lost 8 to 10 pounds, or maybe even more if you exercise regularly (which is critically important for your physical and mental health). Your cravings should have subsided, and hopefully your symptoms will have begun to diminish. If you still have cravings, you can stay on Phase 1 for 1 or 2 more weeks, if necessary. If not, you can move on to the first 2 gluten-free weeks of Phase 2.

I have found that symptoms such as bloating, diarrhea, reflux, and fatigue can disappear in a few days to a couple of weeks in some gluten-sensitive individuals. Other symptoms, such as arthritic complaints, may take longer.

But let's assume you feel great after just 2 weeks on GS Phase 1. At this point, you can enter GS Phase 2 to continue your weight loss at a slow and steady pace (you'll be losing 1 to 2 pounds a week) until you reach a weight that's healthy for you. Now you can begin to reintroduce *gluten-free* starches as well as fruits gradually over the next 14 days (working up to three *gluten-free* starches and three fruits a day). I show you how to do this on pages 122 to 123 and in our Meal Plans for GS Phase 2 on pages 131 to 144. You'll also be able to enjoy gluten-free alcohol, like red and white wine and certain spirits, in moderation.

You won't be reintroducing foods containing gluten yet, because research and my experience show that it takes at least 4 weeks off of gluten before reintroducing it to discover if a person is really gluten sensitive.

Okay. Now let's assume you've been on the Gluten Solution Program for 30 days. If you've been "good," you've probably lost 12 to 14 pounds, and most if not all of your symptoms will have likely subsided. What's next? If your weight loss is progressing well and your symptoms are relieved (but you still need to lose more weight), you can begin to reintroduce some gluten gradually, swapping gluten-containing starches for the gluten-free starches you've already been eating, as long as these foods are the high-fiber options that have always been allowed on Phase 2 of the South Beach Diet. (I give you some specific examples of how to do this reintroduction on pages 122 to 123.) Which gluten-containing foods you can reintroduce, if any, will depend on how you feel. Some highly gluten-sensitive people will experience an immediate intestinal reaction, typically bloating and abdominal pain, from eating just a little gluten. Irritability and fatigue may also recur quickly. Those who are less sensitive may be fine with some gluten but will still have to experiment to see which gluten-containing foods and how much of these foods trigger symptoms and/or cravings. Remember, like all starches, these foods still need to be limited if you want to continue your slow and steady weight loss. If you truly are gluten sensitive, you will know if a particular food affects you and will continue to avoid it.

It's important to note that if after 30 days off of gluten you are still suffering from the same symptoms you had before you started our program, then it's likely you aren't gluten sensitive and you will have to talk with your doctor about further testing. The good news is, you will have lost weight, and that alone will have a positive impact on your overall health. You will certainly have more energy from not lugging around those extra pounds.

Once you've lost the weight you've needed to, whether it is after 30 days or a more extended period on Phase 2, then you can enter GS Phase 3, the lifestyle phase of the diet, where you will continue to maintain your healthy weight. Again, how much gluten you can have, if any, will depend on just how gluten sensitive you are, which you will have determined on Phase 2. Because you are now at a healthy weight, on Phase 3 you will be able to enjoy all the healthy foods that your body can tolerate, and even the occasional empty-calorie indulgence, as long as you are able to sustain your weight loss and improved overall health.

WHO STARTS ON GLUTEN SOLUTION PHASE 2?

If you have fewer than 10 pounds to lose and no cravings but do have gluten-sensitivity symptoms, you will begin the Gluten Solution Program on Phase 2 and stay gluten free but not grain free for 4 weeks.

This means you can have any of the gluten-free foods listed on the GS Phase 1 Foods to Enjoy List (pages 99 to 104) plus any of the foods on the GS Phase 2 Gluten-Free Foods to Enjoy List (pages 126 to 128). Because you're not carrying that many extra pounds and you don't have cravings, you can start by having three fruits and three gluten-free starches the first week. However, if you find you're not losing about a pound or two a week, you should cut back and follow the gradual fruit and starch introduction described on pages 122 to 123 instead.

If after 30 days off gluten you are feeling great and your gluten-sensitivity symptoms have subsided, you can begin to reintroduce some gluten-containing starches, swapping them for the gluten-free starches you've already been enjoying, and see how you feel. If you are still suffering from the same symptoms you had before you started the gluten-free diet, then it's likely you aren't gluten sensitive and you will have to work with your physician to discover what might be causing your symptoms.

WHO STARTS ON MODIFIED GLUTEN SOLUTION PHASE 2?

If you have no weight to lose at all and no cravings, but believe you might be gluten sensitive because you have symptoms, you can do what I call Modified GS Phase 2—that is, a gluten-free version of Phase 3, our maintenance phase.

This means that you'll follow our GS Phase 2 plan and eliminate gluten for 4 weeks to see if your symptoms disappear. But because you are already at a healthy weight, you won't have the limitations on fruits and starches required for those who have weight to lose. And you'll also be able to enjoy the GS Phase 2 foods we suggest eating only rarely. At the end of 4 weeks, you can begin to experiment with adding some gluten-containing foods back into your diet and then see how you feel (turn to page 124 for suggestions on how to do this). You will know quickly whether a food triggers symptoms.

Modified GS Phase 2 is about learning to make healthy food choices for life. So if you've been living on sugar-free soda and a candy bar for lunch, your diet will change radically—and for the better—as you learn to enjoy the wide range of wholesome foods we recommend for better health. If, by chance, you start to lose weight following our program, you can simply increase the amount of the healthy foods you're eating. If you start to gain weight, cut back on the starches—not the vegetables and low-fat protein. Refer to the recommendations made for the unmodified GS Phase 2.

MORE ABOUT THE PHASES OF THE GLUTEN SOLUTION PROGRAM

On the following pages, I explain the three phases of the South Beach Diet Gluten Solution Program in more detail, provide 14 days of suggested gluten-free Meal Plans for GS Phase 1 and GS Phase 2, and give you complete lists of Foods to Enjoy and Foods to Avoid for both of these phases. While it is very difficult to avoid gluten in all of its hidden forms—and you may ultimately not need to—it's better to start out with more information than less. That's why our South Beach Diet registered dietitian, Marie Almon, spends a lot of time with my patients going over the lists of common gluten-containing foods and explaining how to read food labels (see page 160), which is a very important part of learning to be gluten aware.

Once you've become familiar with our suggested Meal Plans (which feature the recipes on pages 199 to 229 in Part III), you'll need to become a gluten-aware shopper and cook. We provide tips for both in Chapter 11, "The Gluten Aware Kitchen," in Part III. Remember, gluten free doesn't mean sugar or fat free. As I described in Chapter 9, many gluten-free products can be just as bad for your health and your waistline as junk food.

GLUTEN SOLUTION PHASE 1: LOSE WEIGHT AND FEEL BETTER FAST

I gave you the short version of who should be on which phase of our Gluten Solution Program above, but it bears repeating along with a few more details. If you have a substantial amount of weight to lose, experience significant cravings for sugary foods and refined starches, and also suffer from symptoms of gluten sensitivity, GS Phase 1 is where you need to start. During this phase, you'll jump-start your weight loss and stabilize your blood sugar levels to minimize cravings. You'll also begin to feel better fast by avoiding gluten and eating a diet consisting primarily of *naturally gluten-free* foods: unlimited vegetables, including plenty of salads; healthy lean protein (fish and shellfish, chicken and turkey, lean cuts of meat, plain soy products); loads of beans and other legumes; reduced-fat cheeses; eggs; low-fat dairy; and nuts and other good unsaturated fats, such as extra-virgin olive oil and canola oil.

YOU'LL NEVER BE HUNGRY

There's no way you'll be hungry when you look at our sample GS Phase 1 Gluten-Free Meal Plans on pages 107 to 120 and realize that you're eating six times a day! Three wholesome meals, two strategic snacks, and even dessert. If you've never eaten breakfast before, consider this. Studies show that those who skip breakfast tend to eat more poorly throughout the day than those who don't. And that's why breakfast skippers also have bigger waistlines! The best breakfast consists of some lean protein and fiber-rich carbohydrate to keep your blood sugar stable and your hunger under control until midmorning, when you should enjoy your first snack of the day.

If you haven't been snacking regularly, now is the time to start. Studies show that it takes relatively few calories to prevent cravings but many more to satisfy them once they occur. And that's why not just one but two snacks a day is important. As with breakfast, the best snacks contain some good carbs and lean protein.

What you won't be eating on GS Phase 1 are starches (bread, pasta, rice), *with or without gluten,* or sugars (including fruits and fruit juices). While giving up bread, pasta, pizza, and fruit may seem like a hardship at first, most people find that their cravings begin to diminish after just a few days. By the end of 2 weeks, they're begging me to stay on Phase 1 forever, not just because they've lost weight but because they don't have bloat or brain fog or indigestion anymore.

But staying on GS Phase 1 forever is a mistake. While you will certainly lose weight rapidly and hopefully feel much better on this phase, I don't want you to miss out on the numerous vitamins, minerals, and other nutrients (including additional fiber) that come from reintroducing whole fruits and gluten-free whole grains into your diet on GS Phase 2. If you were to continue indefinitely on Phase 1 and deny yourself these foods, you wouldn't be learning how to make good food choices in the real world and, more important, you'd be missing out on many of the health-giving phytonutrients these additional foods have to offer.

Furthermore, if you were to continue with the limited number of foods we allow on GS Phase 1, your diet would get dull over time. And once food boredom sets in, you're much more likely to revert to your old eating habits. For a diet to truly become a lifestyle—one that allows you to sustain weight loss and garner all the related health benefits—there has to be variety and satisfaction in your eating plan. That's another reason why we move most people on to GS Phase 2 after just 2 weeks. It's this lifestyle approach that has allowed so many people to be so successful on the South Beach Diet for so many years.

WHAT CAN I EAT ON GS PHASE 1?

On the following pages, you'll find a list of the GS Phase 1 Gluten-Free Foods to Enjoy and GS Phase 1 Foods to Avoid, along with 2 weeks of sample GS Phase 1 Gluten-Free Meal Plans. You'll be pleased to see nearly all the healthy foods we've always recommended on Phase 1, *just not those containing gluten.* Keep in mind that the Meal Plans are just guidelines. Feel free to mix and match similar Foods to Enjoy from the list as you desire.

It's important to note that when you are on the South Beach Diet, gluten aware or not, we never ask you to weigh, measure, or count what you eat in ounces, calories, or grams of fat or carbohydrate. Weighing, measuring, and counting are simply a nuisance when you're leading a busy life. But even though we don't encourage you to count calories, we do want to remind you that calories do count: It's the *quality* of those calories that naturally leads to appropriate hunger satisfaction. When you are making the right food choices, and eating all of your meals and snacks each day, counting isn't necessary and portion control will usually take care of itself.

PROTEIN

Start with a small portion (2 oz. for breakfast, 3 oz. for lunch/dinner), eat slowly, go back for seconds if still hungry. Be careful of any prepackaged meat, poultry, or fish products, such as burgers or canned seafood, which may contain fillers, including wheat flour, wheat starch, bread crumbs, or hydrolyzed wheat protein.

BEEF

Lean* cuts, such as:

> Bottom round
>
> Eye of round
>
> Flank steak
>
> Ground beef
>
> > Extra-lean
> >
> > Lean sirloin
>
> London broil
>
> Pastrami, lean
>
> Sirloin steak
>
> T-bone
>
> Tenderloin (filet mignon)
>
> Top loin
>
> Top round
>
> **Lean meat has 10 g or less total fat and 4.5 g or less saturated fat per 100 g portion.*

POULTRY

Choose cuts without the skin or remove it when cooking or before eating.

> Chicken breast, all cuts
>
> Cornish hen
>
> Duck breast
>
> Ground breast of chicken
>
> Ground breast of turkey
>
> Turkey bacon, gluten-free
>
> Turkey breast, all cuts
>
> Turkey pastrami, gluten-free
>
> Turkey pepperoni, gluten-free
>
> Turkey sausage, low-fat, gluten-free (3–6 g fat per 60 g serving)

SEAFOOD

Limit your intake of fish high in mercury and other contaminants. These include marlin, swordfish, shark, tilefish, orange roughy, king mackerel, bigeye and ahi tuna, and canned albacore tuna—use light tuna instead.

> Fish (all types)
>
> Salmon roe
>
> Sashimi
>
> Shellfish (all types)
>
> Tuna, water-packed light in cans or pouches, and salmon and other water-packed fish

PORK

> Boiled ham (check label for gluten)
>
> Canadian bacon (check label for gluten)
>
> Loin, chop or roast
>
> Smoked ham, natural uncured (check label for gluten)
>
> Tenderloin

VEAL

> Chop
>
> Leg, cutlet
>
> Leg, roast
>
> Top round

LAMB

Eat occasionally and remove all visible fat.

> Center cut
>
> Chop, loin, rib, or shoulder
>
> Roast, loin

GAME MEATS

Buffalo (bison)

Elk

Ostrich

Venison

DELI MEATS

Choose all-natural, lower-sodium, and nitrite- and nitrate-free meats; always check labels to confirm that a product is gluten free.

Chicken breast, regular, smoked, or peppered

Ham, boiled, and all-natural uncured smoked (avoid sugar-cured, maple-cured, and honey-baked)

Turkey breast, regular, smoked, or peppered

Roast beef, lean

VEGETARIAN MEAT ALTERNATIVES

Unless otherwise stated, look for products that have 6 g or less fat per 2–3-oz. serving. Most veggie burgers and many vegetarian meat substitutes contain gluten in the form of soy sauce made from wheat, texturized wheat protein, wheat gluten, bulgur wheat, or wheat flour. Read labels carefully.

Tempeh—¼ cup suggested serving size; check label carefully for gluten

Tofu (all varieties without gluten-containing seasonings)—½ cup suggested serving size

Yuba (bean curd in sticks or sheets)

CHEESE (Fat-free, low-fat, or reduced-fat)

All cheeses should have 6 g or less fat per ounce. Here's a sampling:

Cheddar

Cottage cheese, 1%, 2%, or fat-free

Farmer cheese (and light farmer cheese)

Feta

Goat cheese (chèvre)

Mozzarella

Parmesan

Provolone

Queso fresco

Ricotta, nonfat or part-skim

Sheep's milk cheese

Soy cheese (read label carefully)

Spreadable cheese, light (¾ oz. wedge, all flavors)

String cheese, part-skim

Swiss

EGGS

The use of whole eggs is not limited unless otherwise directed by your doctor. Egg whites and egg substitutes are okay if marked gluten free.

DAIRY AND DAIRYLIKE PRODUCTS

Except for evaporated milk and half-and-half, 2 cups allowed daily, including nonfat or low-fat plain yogurt.

Almond milk, unsweetened

Buttermilk, low-fat (1%) or light (1% or 1.5%)

Coconut milk beverage, unsweetened, plain (boxed, not canned, and approximately 45 calories per cup)

Evaporated milk, fat-free (2 Tbsp.)

Greek yogurt, nonfat (0%) plain

Half-and-half, fat-free (2 Tbsp.)

Kefir, nonfat and low-fat plain

Milk, fat-free or 1%

Nonfat dry milk powder, instant

Soy milk, unsweetened, or low-sugar plain or vanilla (4 g or less fat per 8-oz. serving). Avoid products that contain high-fructose corn syrup.

Yogurt, nonfat or low-fat plain

BEANS AND OTHER LEGUMES

Fresh, dried, frozen, or canned without added sugar. Start with a ⅓- to ½-cup serving size. Check labels carefully for gluten, since even some dried bean products may have been exposed to wheat. If you are highly sensitive to gluten, avoid legumes stored in bulk bins, since cross-contamination is possible.

Adzuki beans
Black beans
Black-eyed peas
Broad beans
Butter beans
Cannellini beans
Chickpeas (garbanzos)
Cranberry beans
Edamame
Fava beans
Great Northern beans
Hummus (2 oz. or ¼ cup)
Italian beans
Kidney beans
Lentils (any variety)
Lima beans
Mung beans
Navy beans
Pigeon beans
Pinto beans
Refried beans, fat-free, canned
Soybeans
Split peas
White beans

VEGETABLES

May use fresh, frozen, or canned without added sugar. Eat a minimum of 2 cups with lunch and dinner, and at least ½ cup with breakfast as often as possible. Check labels carefully on frozen or canned products, since some may be high in sodium and have gluten additives.

Artichoke hearts
Artichokes
Arugula
Asparagus
Bok choy
Broccoli
Broccolini
Broccoli rabe
Brussels sprouts
Cabbage (green, red, napa, Savoy)
Capers
Cauliflower
Celeriac (celery root)
Celery
Chayote
Collard greens
Cucumbers
Daikon radishes
Eggplant
Endive
Escarole
Fennel
Fiddlehead ferns
Garlic
Grape leaves
Green beans
Hearts of palm
Jícama
Kale
Kohlrabi
Leeks
Lettuce (all varieties)
Mushrooms (all varieties)
Mustard greens
Okra

VEGETABLES *(cont.)*

Onions

Parsley

Pepperoncini

Peppers (all varieties)

Pickles (dill or artificially sweetened)

Pimientos

Radicchio

Radishes

Rhubarb

Sauerkraut

Scallions

Sea vegetables (seaweed, nori)

Shallots

Snap peas

Snow peas

Spinach

Sprouts (alfalfa, bean, broccoli, lentil, radish, sunflower)

Squash, spaghetti

Squash, summer
  Yellow
  Zucchini

Swiss chard

Tomatillos

Tomatoes (fresh and all varieties of canned, jarred, and dried with 3 g sugar or less per serving)

Tomato juice, low-sodium

Turnip greens

Vegetable juice blends, low-sodium

Water chestnuts

Watercress

Wax beans

NUTS AND SEEDS

Limit to one serving per day as specified. Avoid seasoned or coated nuts, which may contain gluten or sugar.

Almonds—15

Brazil nuts—4

Cashews—15

Chestnuts—6

Chia seeds—3 Tbsp. (1 oz.)

Coconut, unsweetened—¼ cup

Edamame, dry roasted—¼ cup

Filberts—25

Flaxmeal (ground flaxseed)—3 Tbsp.

Flaxseed—3 Tbsp. (1 oz.)

Hazelnuts—25

Macadamias—8

Peanut butter, all-natural, and other nut butters (look for brands with 1 g sugar or less per 2 Tbsp.)—2 Tbsp.

Peanuts, dry roasted or boiled— 20 small

Pecans—15

Pine nuts (pignoli)—1 oz.

Pistachios—30

Pumpkin seeds—3 Tbsp. (1 oz.)

Sesame seeds—3 Tbsp. (1 oz.)

Soy nuts—¼ cup

Sunflower seeds—3 Tbsp. (1 oz.)

Tahini—2 Tbsp.

Walnuts—15

FATS/OILS

Up to 2 Tbsp. of the following fats/oils are allowed daily. Monounsaturated oils are particularly recommended.

MONOUNSATURATED OILS

Canola

Olive (particularly extra-virgin)

POLYUNSATURATED OILS OR A BLEND OF MONOUNSATURATED AND POLYUNSATURATED

Corn

Flaxseed

Grapeseed

Peanut

Safflower

Sesame

Soybean

Sunflower

OTHER FATS/OILS

Avocado—$\frac{1}{3}$ whole = 1 Tbsp. oil

Coconut oil, extra-virgin—1 Tbsp.

Cream cheese, light—2 Tbsp. (use occasionally)

Cream cheese alternative, dairy-free, made from soy—2 Tbsp. (use occasionally)

Guacamole—$\frac{1}{2}$ cup = 1 Tbsp. oil

Margarine (see vegetable oil spread)

Mayonnaise, low-fat or light—2 Tbsp. (avoid varieties made with high-fructose corn syrup)

Mayonnaise, regular—1 Tbsp.

Olives (small green)—15 = $\frac{1}{2}$ Tbsp. oil

Olives (small black)—8 = $\frac{1}{2}$ Tbsp. oil

Salad dressing, prepared—2 Tbsp. (use those that contain 3 g sugar or less per 2 Tbsp.; best choices contain canola or olive oil—check labels carefully for gluten)

Sour cream, light and reduced-fat—2 Tbsp. (use occasionally)

Vegetable oil spread (margarine)—2 Tbsp. (choose brands that do not contain trans fats; no stick margarine)

SEASONINGS AND CONDIMENTS

Check labels on all seasonings or condiments to confirm that a product is gluten free; spice blends often contain gluten additives.

All pure herbs and spices that contain no added sugar

Arrowroot

Barbecue sauce, sugar-free

Broth, gluten-free beef, chicken, vegetable (preferably fat-free, low-sodium, or less-sodium)

Chile peppers, fresh and dried

Chile paste

Chile sauce, sugar-free

Chipotles in adobo

Cocktail sauce, sugar-free

Cooking sprays (such as olive oil, canola oil)

Espresso powder

Extracts (pure almond, pure vanilla, or others)

Horseradish and horseradish sauce

Hot pepper sauce

Ketchup, sugar-free

Lemon juice

Lime juice

Liquid smoke

Mustard, all types, except honey mustard; check yellow mustard and mustard powder carefully

Pepper, ground and whole peppercorns (black, cayenne, pink, white, and pepper blends)

Salsa (check label for added sugar and gluten)

Vinegar, all except malt vinegar

Wasabi, powdered or paste

Use the following only occasionally for flavor; check all labels to confirm that the product is gluten free; also check the label for added sugar or monosodium glutamate (MSG).

Coconut milk, lite, unsweetened, for cooking—$\frac{1}{4}$ cup max.

Cream cheese, fat-free—1 Tbsp.

Shoyu—$\frac{1}{2}$ Tbsp. (check label carefully for gluten)

Sour cream, fat-free—1 Tbsp.

Sriracha sauce—1 tsp.

Steak sauce—$\frac{1}{2}$ Tbsp.

Taco sauce—1 Tbsp.

Tamari soy sauce—1 Tbsp. (check label carefully for gluten)

Whipped topping, light or fat-free dairy—2 Tbsp.

Worcestershire sauce—1 Tbsp. (check label carefully for gluten)

SWEET TREATS

Limit to 75–100 calories per day.

Candies, hard, sugar-free

Chocolate powder, no-sugar-added

Chocolate syrup, sugar-free

Cocoa powder, unsweetened baking type, labeled 100% cacao and gluten-free

Drink mix, sugar-free and nutrient-enhanced

Fruit-flavored pops, frozen, sugar-free

Fudge pops, frozen, no-sugar-added (check labels carefully for added gluten)

Gelatin, sugar-free

Gum, sugar-free

Jams and jellies, sugar-free

Syrups, sugar-free

Some sugar-free products may be made with sugar alcohols (isomalt, lactitol, mannitol, sorbitol, or xylitol), which are permitted but not encouraged on the South Beach Diet. They may have associated side effects of gastrointestinal distress if consumed in excessive amounts.

SUGAR SUBSTITUTES

All sweeteners except these sugar substitutes are off-limits on Phase 1.

Acesulfame K

Agave nectar (1 Tbsp. daily maximum)

Aspartame (NutraSweet, Equal)

Monk fruit natural no-calorie sweetener (Nectresse, Monk Fruit in the Raw)

Saccharin (Sweet'N Low)

Stevia

Stevia and erythritol (Truvía)

Sucralose (Splenda)

Some sugar substitutes may be made with sugar alcohols (isomalt, lactitol, mannitol, sorbitol, or xylitol) and are permitted but not encouraged on the South Beach Diet. They may have associated side effects of gastrointestinal distress if consume in large amounts.

BEVERAGES

Almond milk, unsweetened (limit to 2 cups daily as part of total dairy servings)

Buttermilk, low-fat (1%) or light (1% or 1.5%); limit to 2 cups daily as part of total dairy servings

Caffeinated and decaffeinated coffee and tea (drink caffeinated in moderation)

Club soda

Coconut milk beverage, unsweetened, plain, and boxed, not canned, with approximately 45 calories per cup (limit to 2 cups daily as part of total dairy servings)

Diet soda and drinks, caffeinated and decaffeinated sugar-free (drink in moderation)

Herbal teas, pure (peppermint, chamomile, etc.); watch out for herbal teas containing barley malt or other forms of gluten

Kefir, nonfat and low-fat plain

Milk, fat-free or 1% (limit to 2 cups daily as part of total dairy servings)

Seltzer

Soy milk, unsweetened, or low-sugar plain or vanilla (4 g or less fat per 8-oz. serving). Avoid products that contain high-fructose corn syrup. (Limit to 2 cups daily as part of total dairy servings.)

Sugar-free powdered drink mixes

Tomato juice, low-sodium

Vegetable juice blends, low-sodium

PROTEIN

BEEF

Brisket

Jerky, unless homemade without sugar

Liver

Prime rib

Rib steak

Skirt steak

FISH

Surimi (imitation crabmeat)

PORK

Bacon (except gluten-free Canadian)

Honey-baked, sugar-cured, and maple-cured ham

Pork rinds

POULTRY

Chicken, dark meat (wings, legs, and thighs)

Duck legs

Goose

Turkey, dark meat (wings, legs, and thighs)

VEAL

Breast

VEGETARIAN MEAT ALTERNATIVES

Most veggie burgers and many vegetarian meat substitutes contain gluten in the form of texturized wheat protein, wheat gluten, bulgur wheat, wheat flour, or soy sauce made from wheat. Unless a product is specifically labeled gluten free, avoid the following:

Seitan

Soy bacon

Soy burger

Soy chicken, unbreaded

Soy crumbles—¼ cup (2 oz.) suggested serving size (plain or seasoned)

Soy hot dogs

Soy sausage patties and links

Tofu with seasonings made with soy sauce or other gluten-based ingredients

CHEESE

American (processed cheese); may contain gluten

Blue, such as Roquefort, Stilton, Gorgonzola (sometimes made with mold cultured on gluten)

Full-fat cheeses

DAIRY AND DAIRYLIKE PRODUCTS

Ice cream (all types)

Milk, 2% or whole

Soy milk, with more than 4 g of fat per 8 oz. serving

Yogurt, artificially sweetened or low-fat flavored

Yogurt, frozen

FRUIT

Avoid all fruits and fruit juices on Phase 1.

VEGETABLES

Beets

Calabaza

Carrots

Cassava

Corn

Parsnips

Peas, green

VEGETABLES *(cont.)*

Potatoes, instant

Potatoes, sweet

Potatoes, white

Pumpkin

Squash, winter

Taro

Turnips (root)

Yams

STARCHES

Avoid all starchy foods on Phase 1, including gluten-free starches:

Bread, all types

Cereal, all types

Croutons, all types

Flour (all types, including pancake and waffle mixes)

Matzo

Oatmeal

Pasta, all types

Pastries and baked goods, all types

Rice, all types

FATS/OILS

Butter

Hydrogenated or partially hydrogenated oils

Solid vegetable shortening or lard

CONDIMENTS

Barbecue sauce, with sugar

Cocktail sauce, with sugar

Honey

Honey mustard

Jams and jellies, with sugar

Ketchup, with sugar

Malt vinegar

Maple syrup and other syrups, with sugar

Miso

Soy sauce

Teriyaki sauce

BEVERAGES

Alcohol of any kind, including wine and light beer

Carrot juice

Coffee, flavored, and coffee substitutes, like chicory blends that often contain gluten

Fruit juice, all types

Kefir, full-fat and flavored

Milk, full-fat and 2%

Powdered drink mixes containing sugar

Soda and other drinks containing sugar

Soy milk with more than 4 g fat per 8-oz. serving

Tea blends with barley malt added

DAY 1

BREAKFAST

6 ounces low-sodium vegetable juice blend

Ham and reduced-fat feta cheese omelet with chives

Coffee or tea (with 1% or fat-free milk and/or sugar substitute, optional)

MIDMORNING SNACK

Vegetable dippers with Indian-style yogurt dip (mix nonfat or low-fat plain yogurt with a little ground cumin, coriander, and turmeric)

LUNCH

Vegetarian chili

Large mixed green salad

2 tablespoons low-sugar, gluten-free ranch dressing or other low-sugar, gluten-free prepared dressing of your choice

MIDAFTERNOON SNACK

Chilled shrimp cocktail with spicy red pepper sauce (for the sauce, in a blender, combine 1 diced red bell pepper with 2 tablespoons reduced-fat sour cream, 1 clove garlic, and hot pepper sauce to taste)

DINNER

Grilled sirloin steak (grill extra for Day 2 lunch)

Sliced garden tomatoes with fresh basil

Grilled bell peppers and onions with minced garlic and balsamic vinegar (grill ahead and let marinate in the dressing for best flavor)

DESSERT

Mocha ricotta crème (combine ½ cup part-skim ricotta with ½ teaspoon unsweetened gluten-free cocoa powder, ¼ teaspoon pure vanilla extract, and sugar substitute of your choice to taste, if desired; serve chilled)

DAY 2

BREAKFAST

> 6 ounces low-sodium vegetable juice blend
>
> Quiche Lorraine Minis (page 206)
>
> Coffee or tea (with 1% or fat-free milk and/or sugar substitute, optional)

MIDMORNING SNACK

> 2 ounces hummus with red bell pepper strips

LUNCH

> Clear mushroom soup (gluten-free chicken broth and reconstituted dried mushrooms)
>
> Sliced steak on a bed of mixed greens (use leftover steak from Day 1 dinner)
>
> 2 tablespoons lemon vinaigrette or other low-sugar, gluten-free prepared dressing of your choice

MIDAFTERNOON SNACK

> 1 ounce reduced-fat Cheddar cheese cubes with grape tomatoes

DINNER

> Baked red snapper with lemon
>
> Sautéed green beans with a sprinkling of Parmesan
>
> Radicchio and endive salad
>
> 2 tablespoons Dijon vinaigrette or other low-sugar, gluten-free prepared dressing of your choice

DESSERT

> Peanut butter delight (in a blender, process ½ cup part-skim ricotta, 1 tablespoon all-natural peanut butter, ½ teaspoon pure vanilla extract, and sugar substitute of your choice to taste, if desired, until smooth; chill and serve)

DAY 3

BREAKFAST

6 ounces low-sodium tomato juice

Poached egg and salmon Florentine (1 poached egg with smoked salmon served on ½ cup spinach cooked in olive oil)

Coffee or tea (with 1% or fat-free milk and/or sugar substitute, optional)

MIDMORNING SNACK

Turkey and Swiss cheese roll-up

LUNCH

1 cup gluten-free tomato soup

Chopped salad with tuna and white beans (on a bed of chopped romaine lettuce, layer 6 ounces light tuna with chopped cucumber, celery, and radishes; ½ cup canned gluten-free white beans; and ⅓ cup diced avocado)

MIDAFTERNOON SNACK

Plum tomato halves topped with 1 ounce gluten-free reduced-fat turkey pepperoni slices (crisp the pepperoni in the microwave)

DINNER

Rotisserie chicken on a bed of mixed greens with up to ¼ cup toasted pistachios (buy supermarket rotisserie chicken breast and get extra for Day 4 lunch; remove all skin)

2 tablespoons balsamic vinaigrette or other low-sugar, gluten-free prepared dressing of your choice

Roasted artichoke hearts (toss thawed frozen artichoke hearts with a little olive oil, sea salt, and freshly ground black pepper and bake at 350°F until crisped)

DESSERT

½ cup nonfat (0%) plain Greek yogurt with a dash of pure almond extract

DAY 4

BREAKFAST

6 ounces low-sodium vegetable juice blend

2 eggs scrambled with sautéed chopped onion and gluten-free roasted red peppers (from a jar)

2 strips gluten-free turkey bacon

Coffee or tea (with 1% or fat-free milk and/or sugar substitute, optional)

MIDMORNING SNACK

Roast beef roll-up with horseradish

LUNCH

Gazpacho

Southwestern chicken salad (toss leftover chicken from Day 3 dinner with up to ½ cup canned black beans, ⅓ diced small avocado, chopped scallions, and prepared gluten-free salsa; serve on a bed of greens)

MIDAFTERNOON SNACK

Celery stalks stuffed with 1 wedge French onion and garlic light spreadable cheese

DINNER

Grilled salmon with lemon and capers (make extra for Day 5 lunch)

Sautéed zucchini and yellow squash

Jícama and red onion salad

2 tablespoons low-sugar, gluten-free green goddess dressing or other low-sugar, gluten-free prepared dressing of your choice

DESSERT

Iced vanilla coffee milk (combine strong decaf coffee, 1% or fat-free milk, pure vanilla extract, and sugar substitute of your choice, to taste, if desired; top with a dollop of fat-free or light dairy whipped topping)

DAY 5

BREAKFAST

6 ounces low-sodium vegetable juice blend

Mushroom and onion omelet (cook chopped mushrooms and diced onion in extra-virgin olive oil before filling)

Coffee or tea (with 1% or fat-free milk and/or sugar substitute, optional)

MIDMORNING SNACK

Caprese bites (cut 1 part-skim mozzarella cheese stick into 4 pieces; place each piece in a hollowed-out cherry tomato and microwave to melt cheese, if desired)

LUNCH

1 cup gluten-free bean soup of your choice

Easy salmon salad (toss leftover salmon from Day 4 dinner with diced cucumber, watercress, 1 tablespoon mayonnaise, and chopped dill)

MIDAFTERNOON SNACK

Vegetable sticks with avocado-cilantro guacamole ($\frac{1}{3}$ avocado mashed with $\frac{1}{3}$ cup reduced-fat cottage cheese, chopped onion, minced garlic, minced cilantro, and red pepper flakes)

DINNER

"Spaghetti" and Meatballs (page 216)

Mixed baby lettuces with shaved Parmesan cheese

2 tablespoons Dijon vinaigrette or other low-sugar, gluten-free prepared dressing of your choice

DESSERT

Dessert smoothie (blend $\frac{1}{2}$ cup unsweetened vanilla soy milk, $\frac{1}{2}$ cup nonfat plain Greek yogurt, a few almonds, and sugar substitute of your choice to taste, if desired)

DAY 6

BREAKFAST

6 ounces low-sodium vegetable juice blend

Portobello breakfast stack (top a portobello mushroom with a slice of tomato and broil 3 minutes; top the mushroom with scrambled eggs and minced chives)

Coffee or tea (with 1% or fat-free milk and/or sugar substitute, optional)

MIDMORNING SNACK

1 wedge light spreadable cheese with cucumber sticks

LUNCH

Cobb salad (top chopped romaine lettuce with diced gluten-free deli chicken, ⅓ diced small avocado, 2 strips crumbled cooked gluten-free turkey bacon, and chopped tomatoes and red onion)

2 tablespoons lime vinaigrette or other low-sugar, gluten-free prepared dressing of your choice

MIDAFTERNOON SNACK

½ cup roasted, lightly salted chickpeas and ½ cup 1% or 2% cottage cheese

DINNER

Pan-grilled cod with lemon wedges

Oven-roasted asparagus with minced garlic and freshly ground black pepper

Julienned vegetable salad with crumbled reduced-fat feta cheese

2 tablespoons red wine vinaigrette or other gluten-free low-sugar prepared dressing of your choice

DESSERT

1 ounce reduced-fat Gouda cheese with 15 pecan halves

DAY 7

BREAKFAST

6 ounces low-sodium tomato juice

1 or 2 eggs over easy topped with gluten-free tomato salsa

Coffee or tea (with 1% or fat-free milk and/or sugar substitute, optional)

MIDMORNING SNACK

1 ounce reduced-fat cheese cubes of your choice with crudités

LUNCH

Lump crabmeat salad (do not use surimi!) in a tomato bowl (mix 4 ounces lump crabmeat, ¼ cup finely diced bell pepper, and 1 minced scallion with 1 tablespoon mayonnaise and 1 tablespoon nonfat plain yogurt; serve in a hollowed-out tomato)

Sugar-free frozen fruit-flavored pop

MIDAFTERNOON SNACK

Latte with fat-free milk (sweetened with sugar substitute, if desired)

DINNER

Oven-roasted pork tenderloin (make extra for Day 8 lunch)

Mashed cauliflower with minced chives

Assorted grilled vegetables, such as asparagus, zucchini, and bell peppers

DESSERT

½ cup nonfat (0%) plain Greek yogurt with 1 tablespoon chopped pumpkin seeds

DAY 8

BREAKFAST

> 6 ounces low-sodium vegetable juice blend
>
> 1 or 2 eggs, any style
>
> Red and yellow grape tomatoes
>
> Coffee or tea (with 1% or fat-free milk and/or sugar substitute, optional)

MIDMORNING SNACK

> ½ cup nonfat (0%) plain Greek yogurt with a dash of pure almond extract

LUNCH

> Gluten-free tomato soup
>
> Sliced pork tenderloin (use leftovers from Day 7 dinner) on a bed of baby greens
>
> 2 tablespoons spicy vinaigrette dressing or other low-sugar, gluten-free prepared dressing of your choice

MIDAFTERNOON SNACK

> 2 tablespoons cashew butter with celery sticks

DINNER

> Baked catfish with lemon and paprika
>
> Spinach sautéed with garlic and olive oil
>
> Gluten-free red beans with hot sauce

DESSERT

> Part-skim ricotta sweetened with 1 tablespoon agave nectar

DAY 9

BREAKFAST

6 ounces low-sodium vegetable juice blend

2 scrambled eggs with 2 slices gluten-free Canadian bacon

Broiled asparagus spears

Coffee or tea (with 1% or fat-free milk and/or sugar substitute, optional)

MIDMORNING SNACK

Smoked salmon with a wedge of light spreadable cheese and capers
on endive leaves

LUNCH

Sirloin burger with 2 ounces melted reduced-fat Monterey Jack cheese,
Dijon mustard, and tomato on a bed of lettuce

Three-bean salad (combine equal amounts of gluten-free black beans,
kidney beans, and chickpeas with chopped red onion; toss with a low-sugar,
gluten-free prepared dressing of your choice; enjoy a ½-cup serving)

MIDAFTERNOON SNACK

4 ounces reduced-fat cottage cheese with bell pepper strips

DINNER

Grilled shrimp skewers (add veggies of your choice)

Radish, cucumber, and scallion salad

2 tablespoons low-sugar, gluten-free ranch dressing or other low-sugar, gluten-
free prepared dressing of your choice

DESSERT

1 ounce reduced-fat sharp Cheddar cheese and 30 pistachios

DAY 10

BREAKFAST

Wake-up energy shake (blend ½ cup unsweetened vanilla soy milk, ½ cup nonfat plain yogurt, 3 ounces firm silken tofu, and ¼ cup dry-roasted almonds until frothy; add sugar substitute of your choice to taste, if desired)

Coffee or tea (with 1% or fat-free milk and/or sugar substitute, optional)

MIDMORNING SNACK

Ham and provolone cheese roll-up

LUNCH

1 cup gluten-free lentil soup

Grilled tuna steak (marinate 1 hour in olive oil flavored with minced ginger and garlic; use for basting)

Steamed green and yellow beans with grated lemon zest

MIDAFTERNOON SNACK

1 part-skim mozzarella cheese stick (any flavor) with veggie sticks

DINNER

Chicken, bell pepper, and snow pea stir-fry

Fennel and red onion salad with chopped kalamata olives

2 tablespoons balsamic vinaigrette or other low-sugar, gluten-free prepared dressing of your choice

DESSERT

Lemon zest ricotta crème (combine ½ cup part-skim ricotta with ¼ teaspoon grated lemon zest and ¼ teaspoon pure vanilla extract, and add sugar substitute of your choice to taste, if desired; serve chilled)

DAY 11

BREAKFAST

6 ounces low-sodium vegetable juice blend

Scrambled eggs topped with chopped scallions and tomatoes and a dollop of nonfat (0%) plain Greek yogurt

Coffee or tea (with 1% or fat-free milk and/or sugar substitute, optional)

MIDMORNING SNACK

Celery, jicama, and/or cucumber sticks with 2 ounces hummus

LUNCH

Grilled turkey burger with tomato and onion on a bed of watercress

2 tablespoons gluten-free Thousand Island dressing or other low-sugar, gluten-free prepared dressing of your choice

MIDAFTERNOON SNACK

½ cup shelled edamame with a sprinkling of sea salt

DINNER

Grilled London broil

Spaghetti squash tossed with fresh lemon juice and freshly ground black pepper

Mixed green salad

2 tablespoons champagne vinaigrette or other low-sugar, gluten-free dressing of your choice

DESSERT

15 cashews and a wedge of light spreadable cheese

DAY 12

BREAKFAST

> 6 ounces low-sodium vegetable juice blend
>
> Cheddar cheese and spinach omelet
>
> Coffee or tea (with 1% or fat-free milk and/or sugar substitute, optional)

MIDMORNING SNACK

> Smoked salmon on cucumber rounds

LUNCH

> 1 cup gluten-free white bean soup
>
> Endive salad with toasted walnuts and reduced-fat goat cheese
>
> 2 tablespoons Dijon vinaigrette or other low-sugar, gluten-free prepared dressing of your choice

MIDAFTERNOON SNACK

> Baba ghannouj with veggie dippers

DINNER

> Spice-Rubbed Grilled Pork Chops (page 218) with sautéed Swiss chard
>
> Mixed green salad with cucumbers and bell peppers
>
> 2 tablespoons lemon vinaigrette or other low-sugar, gluten-free prepared dressing of your choice

DESSERT

> Yogurt and walnut parfait (½ cup nonfat plain Greek yogurt layered with chopped walnuts)

DAY 13

BREAKFAST

6 ounces low-sodium vegetable juice blend

Veggie scrambled eggs (sauté chopped mushrooms, zucchini, and onions in a little extra-virgin olive oil before scrambling with 2 eggs)

Coffee or tea (with 1% or fat-free milk and/or sugar substitute, optional)

MIDMORNING SNACK

2 ounces hummus with red bell pepper, celery, and cucumber sticks

LUNCH

Water-packed light tuna with tomato and onion slices on a bed of greens

2 tablespoons red wine vinaigrette or other low-sugar, gluten-free prepared dressing of your choice

MIDAFTERNOON SNACK

¼ cup dry-roasted soy nuts and 1 cup unsweetened coconut milk beverage

DINNER

Grilled lean lamb chop

Sautéed kale with garlic and red pepper flakes

Baked eggplant rounds with Parmesan cheese

DESSERT

Vanilla chill (blend 1 cup nonfat or low-fat plain yogurt, ⅔ cup plain unsweetened soy milk, 1 teaspoon pure vanilla extract, ice cubes, and a sprinkling of ground cinnamon until frothy; add sugar substitute of your choice to taste, if desired)

DAY 14

BREAKFAST

Morning mocha smoothie (blend ½ cup fat-free milk, 1 cup nonfat plain yogurt, instant coffee powder to taste, 2 tablespoons sugar-free chocolate syrup, and 6 ice cubes until frothy)

Coffee or tea (with 1% or fat-free milk and/or sugar substitute, optional)

MIDMORNING SNACK

4 ounces reduced-fat herbed cottage cheese with chopped green bell pepper in a red bell pepper cup

LUNCH

1 cup gluten-free soup of your choice

Chef salad (with 1 ounce each ham, turkey, and low-fat cheese on mixed greens)

2 tablespoons low-sugar, gluten-free French dressing or other low-sugar, gluten-free prepared dressing of your choice

MIDAFTERNOON SNACK

2 sliced hard-boiled eggs with chilled steamed asparagus spears and sea salt

DINNER

Grilled chicken, bell pepper, and red onion kebabs

Greek salad (diced cucumbers and tomatoes, kalamata olives, and 1 ounce reduced-fat feta cheese on a bed of romaine lettuce)

2 tablespoons balsamic vinaigrette or other low-sugar, gluten-free prepared dressing of your choice

DESSERT

Part-skim ricotta whisked with a dash of pure coconut extract and sugar substitute of your choice to taste, if desired

GLUTEN SOLUTION PHASE 2: ACHIEVING YOUR HEALTH AND WEIGHT-LOSS GOALS

As described earlier, you can move to GS Phase 2 from GS Phase 1, start the program on GS Phase 2, or do a Modified GS Phase 2 if you have no weight to lose and just want to feel better. On Phase 2, you will be delighted with the wide variety of foods you can reintroduce, including fruits, higher-fiber gluten-free breads and pasta, as well as many nutritious gluten-free grains. But you need to be careful. Just because you can have these foods doesn't mean you can go overboard. Whatever product you buy, it's important to read the label and monitor your reaction. As I noted earlier, many gluten-free packaged products can be just as high in saturated fat, sugar, and sodium as other junk food, and these products often contain high-glycemic refined ingredients like white rice flour or fillers like potato starch that can affect your blood sugar and trigger cravings. If you can't eat just a few gluten-free crackers, for example, without going back for half the box, this product spells trouble.

THE GIFT BASKET FROM HELL

This is exactly what happened to my patient, Margaret. Her family was so excited to see how much better she felt once she started eating gluten free that they sent her a "care package" of gluten-free cookies, pretzels, and crackers when she entered GS Phase 2 of our program. Margaret gradually ate them all without bothering to look at a single label and couldn't understand why she had stopped losing weight and why she was suddenly hungry all the time. Our nutritionist set her straight by giving her a crash course in label reading.

I am embarrassed to admit that I made this mistake when I first became interested in gluten. I had a field day ordering all kinds of what turned out to be high-glycemic, zero-fiber, gluten-free products online. My wife warned me about these snacks (she knows how my cravings always return when I eat foods made with refined flour). It took only a couple of weeks of mindlessly eating those little gluten-free cookies and pretzels (I broke my own rule about label reading and didn't look carefully at the ingredients list) before I had to loosen my belt a notch and realized that just because a label says "gluten free" doesn't mean it's good for you.

TAKE IT SLOWLY

In addition to overdoing it on gluten-free products, another big mistake that people often make, particularly when going from GS Phase 1 to GS Phase 2, is adding too many gluten-free whole grains, starchy vegetables, and fruits back into their diet too quickly. Even though these are "good carbs," they are still much higher in sugar than the lean protein and nonstarchy "good carb" vegetables that form the mainstay of the GS Phase 1 eating plan. And if, after spending 2 weeks eating a very low-sugar, low-starch diet on GS Phase 1, you suddenly flood your system with much more sugar, even in the form of good

THE GRADUAL REINTRODUCTION OF GOOD GLUTEN-FREE STARCHES AND FRUITS

Here's a quick guide to the gradual reintroduction of healthy gluten-free starches and fruits over 14 days on GS Phase 2. You can get a more specific idea of how to do this by looking over our sample GS Phase 2: Gluten-Free Meal Plans on pages 131 to 144. Remember, these plans are designed to inspire ideas for healthy meals and snacks. You don't have to follow them literally as long as you stick to the program guidelines.

Keep in mind as well that we've compressed the reintroduction of starches and fruits into 2 weeks, as these GS Phase 2 Meal Plans show. Some people can handle adding starches and fruits quickly without igniting cravings and consequently over-doing it; for others, it's too much too soon. Also, for some people, a rapid increase in fiber intake from the grains and fruits can cause gas, bloating, and diarrhea, and these issues can be mistaken for the symptoms of the gluten sensitivity they're trying to get rid of in the first place. So start here, and if you find the reintroduction plan is not working for you, go at your own pace and reintroduce grains and fruits more slowly to keep any digestive problems—and cravings—under control.

If you are doing a modified version of GS Phase 2 because you don't have crav-ings or weight to lose, you don't have to follow this gradual reintroduction and can begin GS Phase 2 with three fruits and three starches daily.

GS PHASE 2, WEEK 1

Days 1 to 7: 1 good gluten-free starch, 1 piece of fruit each day. Have one starchy good carb, like some quinoa cereal (see page 199) or a corn tortilla wrap, and one gluten-free carbs, it can sometimes trigger the same cravings that got you into trouble in the first place. That's why I recommend *gradually* reintroducing these good carbs into your diet.

Some people can work up to three good starches and three fruits a day (in addition to eating all the healthy food you've already been enjoying on GS Phase 1) in just 2 weeks. Others—especially those who find that they're still getting those occasional cravings—need to add these foods more slowly, perhaps sticking with two good starches and two fruits indefinitely, or three fruits and fewer starches if starchy carbs really stimulate cravings. In addition,

piece of fruit daily the first week. These good carbs can be added at any meal or as a snack. If you find that you're hungry an hour after eating a particular good carb, the next day try eating a different one—preferably one with more fiber—and add a little protein to the mix. For example, have a piece of reduced-fat cheese with an apple for your snack. Eating some protein along with fruit or gluten-free crackers helps prevent the sugar-induced insulin spike that can trigger food cravings.

GS PHASE 2, WEEK 2

Day 8: 2 good gluten-free starches, 1 piece of fruit. If you've done well on Phase 2, Week 1—in other words, you are continuing your slow and steady weight loss and you have no problems with cravings or digestive issues—you can start the second week by adding one more good starch to your diet. Continue to stick with one piece of whole fruit.

Day 9: 2 good gluten-free starches, 2 pieces of fruit. If you are feeling well on Day 8 and have no increased cravings or other issues, add a second piece of fruit today, so you are now up to two pieces of fruit and two servings of good starches daily.

Days 10 and 11: 3 good gluten-free starches, 2 pieces of fruit each day. If you're continuing to do fine with the added carbs, you can now add an additional good starch. At this point, you will be eating three servings of good starches daily and two pieces of fruit.

Days 12 to 14: 3 good gluten-free starches, 3 pieces of fruit each day. By now, your body should have adjusted to the additional good carbs. You will have learned how to make the right choices and monitor yourself. Most people will continue to lose 1 to 2 pounds a week by sticking with three starches and three fruits daily.

if you ever find that your weight loss isn't proceeding slowly and steadily or that you're regaining weight on GS Phase 2, you can go back to one good gluten-free starch and one fruit a day for a while.

Keep in mind that each of us has a different metabolism. One size does not fit all. That's why it is so important for you to learn how to monitor your own responses to new foods, and adjust accordingly. Your optimal diet is just that—yours. And it will always differ from that of friends and family.

It's also important to be aware that there are some foods that are still

REINTRODUCING GLUTEN

After 4 weeks, you will be able to reintroduce gluten to see if you are gluten sensitive. This reintroduction is really the only test available for gluten sensitivity to date. You will quickly find out just how sensitive you are and how much, if any, gluten you can have.

The best way to do this is to start by reintroducing *one* gluten-containing starchy carbohydrate in place of a gluten-free grain into your diet each day during the first week. Monitor your reaction to it carefully, not only for the return of symptoms but also for any return of hunger or cravings. For example, if you look at the Phase 2 Gluten-Free Meal Plans for the first week, you could substitute ¾ cup of low-sugar, high-protein whole-wheat cold cereal for the Irish oatmeal on Day 1, a small whole-wheat tortilla for the corn tortilla on Day 2, a slice of whole-wheat bread for the gluten-free muffin on Day 3, and so on. You should know quickly what foods, if any, trigger your symptoms, and if they do, just stop eating them. Then follow the rest of the food suggestions in the Meal Plans, if desired.

If you are fine with one serving of gluten each day for the first week, you can add a second daily serving of a gluten-containing carbohydrate the second week, working up to a maximum of three a day as the week progresses. Remember, you are swapping the gluten-containing starches for the gluten-free starches, not adding them on. For example, you could replace the gluten-free pita half on Day 7 lunch with half of a whole-wheat pita and swap the corn tortilla for a whole-wheat tortilla on Day 8 breakfast. On any day, you could have ½ cup of farro or barley or whole-wheat pasta instead of one of the gluten-free starch suggestions. And again, you must monitor yourself carefully for renewal of symptoms or cravings and for weight gain.

nearly always off-limits until GS Phase 3; even then, we recommend that you have them only occasionally. If you look at the GS Phase 2 Foods to Eat Rarely list on page 130, you'll see that it includes fruits that are high in natural sugar (such as watermelon, pineapple, dates, and figs) as well as certain vegetables, such as white potatoes and beets. These foods are likely to trigger cravings in susceptible people.

One thing that might surprise you if you're already familiar with the South Beach Diet is that we are now allowing corn and cornmeal on GS Phase 2 as part of our Gluten Solution Program because we want you to have as many options as possible when you're cooking at home or dining out. With wheat, rye, and barley off-limits, corn (which is actually a grain) becomes an important staple, and if you enjoy it in moderation (that's half an ear of corn, not a whole one), it won't significantly raise your blood sugar. You'll see that we use corn tortillas instead of whole-wheat tortillas in our Mushroom and Black Bean Bake recipe on page 208, and we use cornmeal to make the delicious Lemon Polenta Cake on page 225.

Some of my patients complain that losing just a pound or two a week on GS Phase 2 isn't fast enough for them. These are the people I need to constantly remind that slow and steady weight loss is the healthiest and most effective way to keep the weight off permanently. Furthermore, if they were to continue to lose weight rapidly on GS Phase 2, they would likely lose lean muscle mass, which could slow down their metabolism. Short-term success is not what the South Beach Diet is about. It's about learning to eat well, feel better, and keep the weight off for life.

WHAT CAN I EAT ON GS PHASE 2?

On the following pages, you'll find a list of the GS Phase 2: Gluten-Free Foods to Enjoy, GS Phase 2 Foods to Avoid, and GS Phase 2 Foods to Eat Rarely, along with 2 weeks of sample Gluten-Free Meal Plans that feature the GS Phase 2 recipes in this book. The Meal Plans show you how to gradually reintroduce fruits and additional gluten-free good carbohydrates into your diet over a 2-week period. You can experiment to see what works best for your continued weight loss.

GS PHASE 2: GLUTEN-FREE FOODS TO ENJOY

You can have all the Foods to Enjoy on GS Phase 1 and reintroduce these additional foods once you begin GS Phase 2.

PROTEIN

BEEF, PORK, POULTRY

Hot dogs (beef, pork, poultry) can be enjoyed occasionally (once a week) if they are at least 97% fat-free (3–6 g fat per serving). Check labels carefully for gluten.

CHEESE

Rice cheese (look for varieties that have 6 g or less fat per ounce)

FRUIT

Start with one serving daily, gradually increasing to up to three servings daily. Choose fresh, frozen, or canned without added sugar. Look at labels on dried fruits; some may have been dusted with wheat flour or wheat starch to prevent clumping.

Apple—1 small or 5 dried rings or 2 oz. applesauce

Apricots—4 fresh or 7 dried

Banana—1 medium (4 oz.)

Blackberries—¾ cup

Blueberries—¾ cup or 2 Tbsp. dried

Boysenberries—¾ cup

Cactus pear fruit (prickly pear)—1

Cantaloupe—¼ melon or 1 cup diced

Cherries—12 or 2 Tbsp. dried

Clementines—2

Elderberries—1

Gooseberries—¾ cup

Grapefruit—½

Grapes—15

Honeydew melon—⅛ melon or 1 cup diced

Kiwi—1

Loganberries—¾ cup

Mandarin oranges—2

Mango—½ medium (4 oz.)

Mulberries—¾ cup

Nectarine—1 small

Orange—1 medium

Papaya, yellow or green—1 small (4 oz.)

Peach—1 medium

Pear—1 medium

Plums—2

Pomegranate seeds—from 1 medium pomegranate

Pomelo—½

Prunes—4

Raspberries—¾ cup

Strawberries—¾ cup

Tangelo—1 small

Tangerines—2

DAIRY AND DAIRYLIKE PRODUCTS

See Phase 1 and enjoy 2 to 3 cups daily as indicated.

Limit artificially sweetened low-fat or nonfat flavored yogurt to 6 oz. per day; avoid varieties that contain high-fructose corn syrup or any other added sugars; check labels carefully for gluten

Rice beverage, all-natural, limit to ½ cup daily (check label carefully for gluten)

WHOLE GRAINS AND STARCHY VEGETABLES

Start with one serving daily, gradually increasing to up to three servings daily.

WHOLE GRAINS

Amaranth—½ cup cooked

Bagel, small, gluten-free—½ (1 oz.)

Bread—1 slice (1 oz.), gluten-free (choose brands with a minimum of 2 g fiber per serving)

Buckwheat—½ cup cooked

Cellophane noodles (mung bean threads)—¾ cup cooked

Cereal, cold, gluten-free—Choose low-sugar with a minimum of 2 g fiber per serving; serving sizes vary, so be sure to check the label to determine recommended amount.

Cereal, hot, gluten-free, not instant— Serving sizes vary, so be sure to check the label to determine recommended amount.

Corn—½ ear occasionally

Crackers, gluten-free, whole-grain— Follow serving size on packaging for 1 serving.

English muffin—½ muffin (1 oz.), gluten-free

Flour (including legume, nut, and seed flours)
  Almond flour
  Amaranth flour
  Black bean flour
  Brown rice flour
  Buckwheat flour (100% buckwheat)
  Coconut flour
  Corn flour, cornmeal
  Flaxseed meal
  Garbanzo bean (chickpea) flour
  Garbanzo-fava bean flour
  Hazelnut flour
  Millet flour
  Oat flour (gluten-free certified)
  Quinoa flour
  Sorghum flour

  Soy flour
  Teff flour
  White bean flour

Matzo, gluten-free—½ sheet

Millet—½ cup cooked

Muffins, gluten-free—1 small

Oats and oat products (gluten-free certified)

Pasta (gluten-free)
  Brown rice—½ cup cooked (3 g or more fiber per ½ cup)
  Couscous, brown rice—½ cup cooked (3 g or more fiber per ½ cup)
  Multigrain—½ cup cooked (2 g or more fiber per ½ cup)
  Quinoa—½ cup cooked (2 g or more fiber per ½ cup)
  Soy—½ cup cooked (2 g or more fiber per ½ cup)

Pita, gluten-free, whole-grain (1 oz.)— ½ pita

Popcorn—3 cups popped
  Air-popped, plain
  Stove-top, cooked with canola oil

Quinoa—½ cup cooked

Rice—½ cup cooked
  Basmati
  Black
  Brown
  Wild

Rice noodles—½ cup cooked

Shirataki noodles—¾ cup cooked

Soba noodles (100% buckwheat)— ¾ cup cooked

Tortilla, 100% corn—1 small

STARCHY VEGETABLES

Count as a starch/grain serving.
  Calabaza—¾ cup
  Cassava—¼ cup
  Potato, sweet—1 small
  Pumpkin—¾ cup
  Taro—⅓ cup
  Turnip (root)—1 small

STARCHY VEGETABLES (*cont.*)

Winter squash—¾ cup

Yam—1 small

OTHER VEGETABLES

Carrots—½ cup

Parsnips—½ cup

Peas, green—½ cup

FATS/OILS

Coconut oil spread, made with extra-virgin coconut oil (1 Tbsp.)

BEVERAGES

Most distilled alcoholic beverages made from gluten grains (bourbon, scotch and other whiskeys, gin, and vodka) are fine unless you are highly gluten sensitive. Watch out for distilled beverages with flavorings added after distillation. As for sake, which is made from fermented rice, look for the words *House of Gekkeikan* (traditional) or *Junmai* (pure) on the bottle. Other types of sake may have barley or wheat by-products added for flavor. Limit distilled beverages and sake to a 1½-oz. serving. The following beverages are fine:

Cava, extra-brut—1 glass, 4 oz.

Champagne, extra-brut—1 glass, 4 oz.

Ouzo—1 glass, 4 oz.

Prosecco, extra-brut—1 glass, 4 oz.

Rum—1 serving, 1½ oz.

Tequila—1 serving, 1½ oz.

Wine, red or white—1 or 2 glasses, 4 oz. each, permitted daily with or after meals

SPECIAL TREATS

Chocolate, dark—1 oz.; choose gluten-free brands that contain at least 70% cacao and the least amount of sugar

Pudding—4 oz.; fat-free, no-sugar-added, gluten-free

GS PHASE 2: FOODS TO AVOID

All of these gluten-containing foods must be avoided for 4 weeks on the Gluten Solution Program. At that point, you gradually introduce gluten. See page 124 for an introduction plan. Keep in mind that whether you are eating gluten grains or not, limit yourself to three servings maximum per day on this phase.

All baked goods and pastries containing gluten, including cakes, cookies, muffins (while baked goods may be labeled gluten free, they are not permitted on the South Beach Diet until Phase 3, and then only on occasion)

All breads with gluten, including bagels, English muffins, matzo, croutons

All bread crumbs containing gluten, including panko

All cereals containing gluten, including farina, cream of wheat

All pasta containing gluten, including couscous

All stuffings and dressings containing gluten

GLUTEN-CONTAINING GRAINS AND DERIVATIVES

Barley
- Barley enzymes
- Barley extract
- Barley grass
- Barley malt
- Barley pearls
- Hordeum vulgare (a type of barley)
- Miso (may contain barley)

Bran
- Rye bran
- Oat bran
- Wheat bran

Bulgur

Flour: all flour containing wheat, barley, rye, or any of their derivatives
- Bleached flour
- Graham flour
- Kamut (a fine whole-meal flour made from low-gluten, soft-textured wheat; also known as chapatti flour)
- Rye
- Semolina
- Spelt
- Dinkel (also known as spelt)
- Farro or faro (also known as spelt)
- Macha (spelt wheat)
- Wheat
- Durum
- Einkorn
- Emmer
- Hydrolyzed wheat protein
- Mir
- Sprouted wheat
- Triticale (a wheat/rye cross)
- Wheat berries
- Wheat germ
- Wheat oil
- Wheat protein
- Wheat starch

BEVERAGES

Beer, including gluten free; if light gluten-free beer is available (it was not as of this writing), it may be enjoyed on occasion on Phase 2

MISCELLANEOUS

Beef/chicken/fish/vegetable stock, broth, or bouillon (may contain wheat)

Cooking spray for baking (may contain wheat flour)

Communion wafers (may contain wheat)

Dextrin

Fu (dried wheat gluten sold as sheets or cakes used in Asian dishes)

Imitation bacon/seafood (may contain wheat)

Malt
- Malt flavoring
- Malt syrup
- Malt vinegar

Marinades/dressings (may contain malt/fillers)

Meat, poultry, seafood, or vegetables that are breaded, floured, served with a sauce made from wheat, or marinated in a wheat-based sauce such as soy or teriyaki; also self-basting poultry

Rice malt

Rice syrup, brown (it may contain barley)

Sauces and gravies, with gluten fillers

Seitan (a meatlike food derived from wheat gluten used in many vegetarian dishes)

Udon (wheat noodles)

Yogurt, flavored (most contain gluten fillers)

Some of the items listed below may be gluten free but should be eaten only rarely on Phase 2 of South Beach Diet or avoided entirely, if you'd prefer, due to their high glycemic index.

STARCHES AND GRAINS

Cornflakes

Oatmeal, instant (may be cross-contaminated; check labels carefully)

Potatoes
  Instant, plain (skip flavored entirely)
  White

Rice
  Jasmine
  Sticky
  White

Rice cakes

Rice crackers, plain

VEGETABLES

Beets

Potatoes, white

FRUIT

Look at labels on dried fruits; some may have been dusted with flour or starch to prevent clumping.

  Canned fruit, in heavy syrup

  Dates

  Figs

  Fruit juice

  Lychees

  Pineapple

  Raisins

  Watermelon

BEVERAGES

Brandy

Carrot juice

Liqueurs

Port

Sherry

MISCELLANEOUS

Honey—1 tsp.

Cane juice syrup—1 tsp.

Ice cream—100-calorie frozen bars and treats, on occasion; check labels carefully for gluten

Sucrose (table sugar, including raw sugar)—1 tsp.

GS PHASE 2: SAMPLE GLUTEN-FREE MEAL PLANS

DAY 1

BREAKFAST

6 ounces low-sodium tomato juice

4 ounces nonfat (0%) plain Greek yogurt

Gluten-free Irish oatmeal with ground cinnamon and chopped walnuts

Coffee or tea (with 1% or fat-free milk and/or sugar substitute, optional)

MIDMORNING SNACK

¾ cup sliced strawberries and a latte with fat-free milk (sweeten with sugar substitute, if desired)

LUNCH

Grilled shrimp on a bed of salad greens with chopped cucumber and cherry tomatoes

2 tablespoons lemony dill dressing or other low-sugar, gluten-free prepared dressing of your choice

MIDAFTERNOON SNACK

1 hard-boiled egg with carrot sticks

DINNER

Broiled sirloin steak with fresh mushroom "gravy" (cook mushrooms in gluten-free beef broth with herbs of your choice)

Roasted asparagus with minced shallots

Cannellini bean purée with chopped fresh sage and rosemary (choose gluten-free canned beans)

DESSERT

Chocolate mousse (4 ounces no-sugar-added, gluten-free chocolate pudding mixed with 2 tablespoons light or fat-free dairy whipped topping)

DAY 2

BREAKFAST

> 6 ounces low-sodium vegetable juice blend
>
> Open-face turkey breakfast stack (top a 100% corn tortilla with 1 slice tomato, 1 strip gluten-free turkey bacon, and 1 poached egg)
>
> Coffee or tea (with 1% or fat-free milk and/or sugar substitute, optional)

MIDMORNING SNACK

> 1 small Granny Smith apple with 1 ounce reduced-fat Cheddar cheese cubes

LUNCH

> 1 cup gluten-free black bean soup
>
> Spinach salad with diced tofu, chickpeas, sliced button mushrooms, and onions
>
> 2 tablespoons sherry vinaigrette or other low-sugar, gluten-free prepared dressing of your choice

MIDAFTERNOON SNACK

> 2 ounces hummus and red bell pepper slices rolled in Bibb lettuce

DINNER

> Baked lemon chicken on a bed of lentils
>
> Frisée salad with chopped black olives and a sprinkling of Parmesan cheese
>
> 2 tablespoons champagne vinaigrette or other low-sugar, gluten-free prepared dressing of your choice

DESSERT

> No-sugar-added, gluten-free strawberry pudding cup

DAY 3

BREAKFAST

6 ounces low-sodium tomato juice

2 hard-boiled eggs

Orange-Blueberry Breakfast Muffin (page 204)

Coffee or tea (with 1% or fat-free milk and/or sugar substitute, optional)

MIDMORNING SNACK

4 ounces nonfat (0%) plain Greek yogurt topped with slivered almonds

LUNCH

1 cup gluten-free split pea soup

Tomato stuffed with tuna salad (3 ounces canned light tuna, chopped celery and onion, and 1 tablespoon mayonnaise)

MIDAFTERNOON SNACK

1 slice lower-sodium boiled ham wrapped around 1 part-skim mozzarella cheese stick

5 green or black olives of your choice

DINNER

Roasted turkey breast topped with sautéed mushrooms (roast extra turkey for Day 4 lunch)

Steamed green beans with lemon and a sprinkling of sea salt

Bibb lettuce salad with diced cucumber and cherry tomatoes

2 tablespoons Thousand Island dressing or other low-sugar, gluten-free prepared dressing of your choice

DESSERT

No-sugar-added, gluten-free vanilla pudding cup

DAY 4

BREAKFAST

> 6 ounces low-sodium vegetable juice blend
>
> 1 slice gluten-free multigrain toast topped with 1 tablespoon light cream cheese, smoked salmon, cucumber and tomato slices, chopped red onion, and capers
>
> Coffee or tea (with 1% or fat-free milk and/or sugar substitute, optional)

MIDMORNING SNACK

> 15 grapes with 1 ounce reduced-fat Cheddar cheese

LUNCH

> 1 cup gluten-free lentil soup
>
> Sliced roast turkey on a bed of greens with ⅓ small avocado sliced on top (use leftover turkey from Day 3 dinner)
>
> 2 tablespoons low-sugar, gluten-free green goddess dressing or other low-sugar, gluten-free dressing of your choice

MIDAFTERNOON SNACK

> 4 ounces nonfat (0%) plain Greek yogurt with chopped cucumbers and peppers

DINNER

> Herbed pork tenderloin (spray pork with olive oil cooking spray and coat with ¼ cup mixed fresh herbs, such as rosemary, thyme, sage, and/or parsley; roast an extra pork loin for Day 5 lunch)
>
> Sautéed kale with garlic and a sprinkling of sea salt
>
> Spaghetti squash (microwave spaghetti squash and toss strands with a little extra-virgin olive oil and lemon zest)

DESSERT

> Sugar-free, gluten-free strawberry gelatin with chopped pecans and 2 tablespoons light or fat-free dairy whipped topping and an 8-ounce glass of 1% or fat-free milk

DAY 5

BREAKFAST

6 ounces low-sodium tomato juice

1 slice Toasted Walnut Bread (page 222)

½ cup 1% or 2% cottage cheese

Coffee or tea (with 1% or fat-free milk and/or sugar substitute, optional)

MIDMORNING SNACK

¾ cup blueberries with 4 ounces nonfat (0%) plain Greek yogurt

LUNCH

1 cup gluten-free vegetable soup (without pasta or potatoes)

Thinly sliced pork tenderloin over mixed greens (use leftovers from
Day 4 dinner)

2 tablespoons balsamic vinaigrette or other low-sugar, gluten-free prepared
dressing of your choice

MIDAFTERNOON SNACK

2 deviled egg halves

Jícama and cucumber slices

DINNER

Baked chicken breasts stuffed with reduced-fat feta cheese and sun-dried
tomatoes

Vegetable napoleon (stack slices of steamed eggplant with slices of tomato and
thin slices of part-skim mozzarella cheese; bake at 350°F until the cheese is melted)

Mesclun salad

2 tablespoons balsamic vinaigrette or other low-sugar, gluten-free prepared
dressing of your choice

DESSERT

No-sugar-added, gluten-free chocolate pudding cup

DAY 6

BREAKFAST

6 ounces low-sodium vegetable juice blend

Almond-Pear Quinoa Breakfast Cereal (page 199)

Coffee or tea (with 1% or fat-free milk and/or sugar substitute, optional)

MIDMORNING SNACK

4 ounces nonfat (0%) plain Greek yogurt with pure extract of your choice

LUNCH

1 cup gluten-free black bean soup

3-ounce can light tuna mixed with 1 tablespoon mayonnaise, chopped onion,
celery, and cucumber on a bed of shredded romaine lettuce with 2 tablespoons
herb vinaigrette or other low-sugar, gluten-free prepared dressing of your choice

MIDAFTERNOON SNACK

4 ounces reduced-fat herbed cottage cheese with veggie dippers

DINNER

Steak kebab with mushrooms, peppers, and onions

Caesar salad (no croutons)

2 tablespoons low-sugar, gluten-free Caesar dressing or other low-sugar,
gluten-free prepared dressing of your choice

DESSERT

Sugar-free, gluten-free lime gelatin topped with a sprinkling of toasted
almonds

DAY 7

BREAKFAST

6 ounces low-sodium tomato juice

2 eggs, any style

2 strips gluten-free turkey bacon

Coffee or tea (with 1% or fat-free milk and/or sugar substitute, optional)

MIDMORNING SNACK

1 wedge light spreadable cheese with veggie sticks

LUNCH

Grilled turkey burger in a whole-grain gluten-free pita half with Dijon mustard, sliced tomato, and red onion

Mixed greens sprinkled with reduced-fat feta cheese

2 tablespoons olive oil and vinegar or other low-sugar, gluten-free prepared dressing of your choice

MIDAFTERNOON SNACK

2 ounces hummus with grape tomatoes

DINNER

Homemade chili con carne

Cucumber and radish salad

2 tablespoons low-sugar, gluten-free ranch dressing or other low-sugar, gluten-free prepared dressing of your choice

DESSERT

2 grilled peach halves sprinkled with cinnamon and chopped toasted cashews

DAY 8

BREAKFAST

6 ounces low-sodium vegetable juice blend

Scrambled eggs in a 100% corn tortilla with salsa

Coffee or tea (with 1% or fat-free milk and/or sugar substitute, optional)

MIDMORNING SNACK

4 ounces reduced-fat cottage cheese with ¾ cup blueberries

LUNCH

Southwestern Cobb salad (chopped romaine lettuce with ½ cup gluten-free black beans, 1 chopped hard-boiled egg, 1 ounce shredded reduced-fat Monterey Jack cheese, 2 strips crumbled gluten-free turkey bacon, and diced radishes and yellow bell pepper)

2 tablespoons lime vinaigrette or other low-sugar, gluten-free prepared dressing of your choice

MIDAFTERNOON SNACK

Chilled shrimp with horseradish sauce

DINNER

Stir-fried beef with bell peppers, onions, and snow peas (make extra for Day 9 lunch)

¾ cup shirataki noodles

DESSERT

Gluten-free snack bar and an 8-ounce glass of 1% or fat-free milk

DAY 9

BREAKFAST

6 ounces low-sodium vegetable juice blend

Sausage and Scrambled Egg Breakfast Tostada (page 200)

Coffee or tea (with 1% or fat-free milk and/or sugar substitute, optional)

MIDMORNING SNACK

1 wedge light garlic-flavored spreadable cheese with celery sticks

LUNCH

Asian beef salad cups (fill lettuce "cups" with leftover beef and vegetables from Day 8 dinner, add extra shredded veggies, and drizzle with fresh lime juice)

4 ounces nonfat (0%) plain Greek yogurt mixed with a little agave nectar and a dash of powdered ginger

MIDAFTERNOON SNACK

1 Banana-Nut Snack Bar (page 227)

DINNER

Halibut baked with lemon slices

Steamed Brussels sprouts tossed with a sprinkling of sea salt and freshly ground black pepper

Watercress and red onion salad

2 tablespoons lime vinaigrette or other low-sugar, gluten-free prepared dressing of your choice

DESSERT

Baked apple with pistachios (stuff the cored apple with crushed pistachios)

DAY 10

BREAKFAST

6 ounces low-sodium tomato juice

Gluten-free Irish oatmeal with ground cinnamon and ¾ cup fresh blueberries

Coffee or tea (with 1% or fat-free milk and/or sugar substitute, optional)

MIDMORNING SNACK

2 ounces hummus with carrot sticks

LUNCH

1 cup gluten-free split pea soup

Grilled shrimp skewers

Tomato-Feta Quinoa Tabbouleh with Pumpkin Seeds (page 219)

MIDAFTERNOON SNACK

Baba ghannouj with veggie dippers

DINNER

Crispy Fish Fillets with Spicy Mayo (page 207)

Steamed Swiss chard tossed with extra-virgin olive oil and fresh lemon juice

Small baked sweet potato

DESSERT

Broiled "caramel rum" banana (cut a banana in half lengthwise and top with 1 tablespoon sugar-free, gluten-free caramel topping and a dash of pure rum extract; broil until heated through)

DAY 11

BREAKFAST

6 ounces low-sodium vegetable juice blend

Quiche Lorraine Mini (page 206)

Coffee or tea (with 1% or fat-free milk and/or sugar substitute, optional)

MIDMORNING SNACK

1 small Granny Smith apple with 2 tablespoons all-natural almond butter

LUNCH

Romaine hearts with 6 ounces pouched or canned salmon and grape tomatoes

2 tablespoons red wine vinaigrette or other low-sugar, gluten-free prepared dressing of your choice

MIDAFTERNOON SNACK

½ cup nonfat (0%) plain Greek yogurt with 1 medium sliced pear

DINNER

Broiled flank steak with grilled onions (make extra for Day 12 lunch)

Individual Eggplant Parmesan Stacks (page 210)

Arugula salad with fresh lemon juice

DESSERT

1 wedge Lemon Polenta Cake (page 225)

DAY 12

BREAKFAST

6 ounces low-sodium tomato juice

Breakfast "banana split" (cut 1 medium banana in half, top with 4 ounces artificially sweetened nonfat or low-fat vanilla yogurt, and sprinkle with crushed gluten-free granola)

Coffee or tea (with 1% or fat-free milk and/or sugar substitute, optional)

MIDMORNING SNACK

10 high-fiber gluten-free crackers with 2 tablespoons all-natural peanut butter

LUNCH

1 cup gluten-free bean soup of your choice

Sliced steak (use leftover steak from Day 11 dinner) with cucumber rounds and bell pepper strips on a bed of romaine lettuce with half of a gluten-free whole-grain pita

2 tablespoons lemon vinaigrette or other low-sugar, gluten-free prepared dressing of your choice

MIDAFTERNOON SNACK

1 cup diced cantaloupe sprinkled with 1 ounce crumbled reduced-fat feta cheese

DINNER

Turkey and Noodles in Broth (page 220)

Asian cabbage slaw (shredded bok choy and napa cabbage with mung bean sprouts)

2 tablespoons mustard vinaigrette or other low-sugar, gluten-free prepared dressing of your choice

DESSERT

Poached plum with black walnut whipped topping (combine 2 tablespoons light or fat-free dairy whipped topping with 1 teaspoon pure black walnut extract)

DAY 13

BREAKFAST

½ pink or red grapefruit

2 poached eggs on a bed of sautéed vegetables

Coffee or tea (with 1% or fat-free milk and/or sugar substitute, optional)

MIDMORNING SNACK

2 nectarine halves, each topped with a dollop of nonfat (0%) plain Greek yogurt flavored with pure vanilla extract

LUNCH

Chicken with Lemon-Scallion Sauce (page 212) with ½ cup brown basmati rice

Mediterranean salad (mixed greens with reduced-fat feta cheese cubes, diced cucumber and tomatoes, and kalamata olives)

2 tablespoons red wine vinaigrette or other low-sugar, gluten-free prepared dressing of your choice

MIDAFTERNOON SNACK

1 Pistachio Biscotti (page 226) with an 8-ounce glass of 1% or fat-free milk

DINNER

Mushroom and Black Bean Bake (page 208)

Sautéed broccoli rabe with garlic and red pepper flakes

DESSERT

3 large or 5 small strawberries dipped in melted dark chocolate (save extra strawberries for Day 14 midmorning snack)

DAY 14

BREAKFAST

6 ounces low-sodium tomato juice

Hearty Buttermilk Pancakes with Sautéed Apples (page 202)

Coffee or tea (with 1% or fat-free milk and/or sugar substitute, optional)

MIDMORNING SNACK

Strawberry smoothie (blend ¾ cup chopped strawberries, ½ cup low-fat plain yogurt, 1 teaspoon agave nectar, and 6 ice cubes until frothy)

LUNCH

Black Bean "Pizza" with Tomatoes and Artichokes (page 214)

Cucumber salad with radish sprouts

2 tablespoons balsamic vinaigrette or other low-sugar, gluten-free prepared dressing of your choice

MIDAFTERNOON SNACK

7 dried apricot halves chopped and mixed with 4 ounces reduced-fat cottage cheese with a sprinkling of ground cinnamon

DINNER

Pan-seared beef tenderloin strips with spicy gluten-free tomato salsa

Quinoa pilaf

Endive and radicchio salad

2 tablespoons homemade yogurt-horseradish dressing or other low-sugar, gluten-free prepared dressing of your choice

DESSERT

1 wedge Spiced Carrot Cake (page 228) or a Double-Chocolate Cupcake (page 224)

GLUTEN SOLUTION PHASE 3:
BETTER HEALTH AND A HEALTHY WEIGHT FOR LIFE

GS Phase 3 is the maintenance phase of the Gluten Solution Program. It's a flexible lifestyle with *you* in control. The symptoms of gluten sensitivity you were experiencing should have abated on GS Phase 2, and you are now at a weight that's healthy for you. If you had no weight to lose and were following Modified GS Phase 2 to see if you'd feel better off gluten, you now know if you do.

At this point, the eating principles you learned on GS Phase 1 and/or GS Phase 2 should be second nature. You should be familiar with the wide variety of wholesome foods that are naturally gluten free, and you will have learned the true meaning of being gluten aware because you know how your body reacts to these foods.

Remember, on GS Phase 3, nothing is absolutely off-limits. You have learned to monitor your body's response to particular foods, you know what triggers your cravings and/or your gluten-sensitivity symptoms, and you have learned to make the right choices for you.

If, given this new freedom, you find that you can't just eat a scoop of ice cream without devouring the entire pint or a piece of 100% whole-wheat bread without feeling bloated or getting cramps, it's a pretty good sign that you might want to avoid these foods altogether. You can always try to reintroduce small quantities later. Since no food is off-limits on GS Phase 3 unless you say it is, you can enjoy a decadent dessert on occasion, and when you do, you will probably find that you've satisfied your sweet tooth after just a few bites. At this point, you'll know just how gluten sensitive you are—if at all— and adjust your choices accordingly.

I like to tell my patients that GS Phase 3 isn't about abandoning a healthy diet and suddenly resuming your old unhealthy eating habits. If, by chance, you do find the number on the scale creeping up, it's probably because you're not paying as much attention to our healthy eating principles as you used to, or you're not getting enough exercise—or both. If you have put on 10 or more pounds or have started to have food cravings again (which I suspect may be responsible for your weight gain), you may need to return to GS Phase 1 for several days until your cravings subside. If your weight gain is minimal and you don't have cravings, just return to the GS Phase 2 eating plan that worked for you before.

If weight gain is not the issue and you simply "felt better" on GS Phase 2, it may mean that too much gluten has somehow found its way back into your diet. In this case, eliminate *all* gluten again—usually for just a couple of weeks—and see how you feel. After that, you can once again self-monitor, this time paying stricter attention to how much gluten you can tolerate and still feel well. It's important to remember that gluten is hidden in many packaged foods. Take a good look at the ingredient list on all products when shopping, and refer to the Food Lists and Meal Plans in this book for a refresher whenever you need it.

A REMINDER ABOUT THE IMPORTANCE OF EXERCISE

Regular exercise has always been an essential component of the South Beach Diet lifestyle, and it is equally important if you're following the South Beach Diet Gluten Solution Program. Because so many people with gluten sensitivities lack energy, have issues with joint pain, or suffer from a host of other ailments, keeping up with a regular exercise program may be difficult.

But avoiding exercise is a mistake. In fact, getting regular exercise on all phases of the Gluten Solution Program can make a big difference in how you feel and in how quickly you'll lose weight. Not only will exercise help with weight loss, shrink your belly fat, and increase your muscle tone, it will strengthen your bones, helping to prevent osteoporosis; slow the degenerative effects of aging, including arthritis and brain drain; reduce the risk of high blood pressure, diabetes, and metabolic syndrome (and thus the risk for heart attack and stroke); and strengthen your immune system. And if that's not enough, it will also boost your mood and give you more energy in general. I am not suggesting that you become an Olympian. Regular long walks are easy to accomplish, and they work.

THE GLUTEN-AWARE ATHLETE

Gluten sensitivity and athletic performance made headlines in 2011 when Novak Djokovic became the number-one tennis player in the world and announced that his improved stamina on the court was due to the fact that he had adopted a gluten-free diet.

In a *60 Minutes* interview in June 2012, he admitted having consumed bread, pasta, and pizza—particularly pizza—almost every day of his life before starting his new diet. He recommended that everyone give gluten free a chance.

Perhaps inspired by Djokovic's success, many other athletes, both male and female, involved in a wide range of sports—from golf and track to swimming and hockey—have started paying more attention to gluten. And that includes Andy Murray.

In August 2011, Murray—the 2012 winner of Olympic Gold and the US Open in tennis—converted to the gluten-free lifestyle, saying it gave him more energy and a faster recovery time. When you think about it, the 2012 US Open may have been the first major sporting event where both finalists were gluten free!

It certainly stands to reason that if you are gluten sensitive, fatigue, heartburn, joint pains, and brain fog will not help your athletic performance. And for those of you who just feel you need a burst of energy and sharper focus to perform better at the gym or to simply get through the day, it is worth giving the South Beach Diet Gluten Solution Program a try.

Oh, and once you do, please let me know if you win a "gold medal" or even a first victory over your brother, sister, or best friend.

MAKE THE MOST OF 20 MINUTES

I always recommend doing both cardiovascular conditioning (aerobics) and core strengthening (resistance exercise) on a regular basis, usually on alternate days, along with some stretching before and after. And you don't have to spend hours doing it. Studies show that you can improve your health by exercising for just 20 minutes a day. Keeping your workout short all but eliminates the "I don't have time to exercise" excuse. But you do have to maximize what you do in that time. Of course you should talk with your doctor before you

GLUTEN AND YOUR WEIGHT

The effect of a gluten-free diet on weight loss is perhaps one of the most discussed and confusing issues in the diet world today. One week you'll read an article saying that cutting out gluten helps you lose weight quickly; the next week, the story is that a gluten-free diet leads to weight gain. But the truth is, no one really knows. No researcher to date has conducted a study to examine the effect of a gluten-free diet on weight loss in the general population.

We do know that people with untreated celiac disease or serious gluten sensitivity are often underweight or even malnourished because they often suffer abdominal pain, heartburn, and/or bloating after meals, which can cause them to limit their caloric intake. In addition, inflammation or damage to the lining of the small intestine may result in decreased absorption of calories from foods. After starting a gluten-free or gluten-aware diet, sensitive individuals may actually gain weight when their intestinal symptoms improve and they are better able to absorb nutrients.

For the rest of us, whether we are gluten sensitive or not, removing gluten from our diet often does lead to weight loss, but that has little to do with gluten per se. If your standard diet is high in refined, processed grains or in empty-calorie junk foods, you'll drop pounds because you eliminated those foods, not simply because you cut out gluten. Keep in mind that processed, low-fiber wheat products are associated with weight gain, obesity, and poorly controlled diabetes, because they stimulate wide swings in blood sugar that result in increased hunger and caloric intake. In fact, the major cause of the epidemics of obesity and diabetes in America and around the world is the rampant overconsumption of processed carbohydrates from fast food and junk food. Lack of exercise is

make any sudden change in your level of activity, especially if you are age 50 or older, have been inactive, have difficulty keeping your balance, have periods of dizziness, or have known heart problems.

When it comes to aerobics, I've found that interval training—which means alternating short bursts of intense activity with easier recovery periods—lets you burn more fat and calories in just 20 minutes than you would doing 40 minutes of steady-state exercise. And you'll keep your metabolism revved up for a while even after you stop exercising. Doing interval another big contributor, as is the destruction of our gut flora due to the overuse of antibiotics, among other factors.

You won't lose weight by saying good-bye to gluten, though, if you simply replace gluten-containing processed foods with gluten-free processed foods. In fact, you might gain. Many packaged gluten-free products are made with white rice or potato flours, lots of sugar, and plenty of additives and preservatives (read more about gluten-containing junk foods in Chapter 9) to enhance taste and texture. They're just as likely to cause the swings in blood sugar that contribute to weight problems as highly refined wheat-based products.

One of our most important South Beach Diet principles is to substitute high-fiber, nutrient-rich good carbohydrates, including vegetables, whole fruits, and whole grains, for nutrient-poor, highly processed, high starch- and sugar-based carbs. This is important for any healthy diet, whether the carbohydrates contain gluten or not.

If you turn out to be gluten sensitive after following the South Beach Diet Gluten Solution Program for 4 weeks and you also need to lose more weight, continuing with this program is your healthiest route to weight loss success. Furthermore, if your reaction is like that of so many of my gluten-sensitive patients, long-term compliance won't be an issue. The renewed energy you'll feel, along with relief from nagging symptoms such as headaches or joint pain, will keep you on track and inspire you to work in more exercise.

If you aren't gluten sensitive, but still have weight to lose, or if you simply want to maintain a healthy weight by eating well, then following the original South Beach Diet guidelines, which include the full complement of whole grains, with and without gluten, is your prescription for success.

walking outdoors, or on a treadmill, elliptical machine, or stationary bike indoors, is a great way to get started. You can also do intervals while swimming or riding a regular bike.

But let's stick with walking, which almost everyone can do. First, you'll warm up for 5 minutes by walking at a slow to moderate pace. Then you'll alternate short bursts of walking fast (for 15 to 30 seconds, say) with short recovery periods of slower walking (enough to catch your breath). Depending on your conditioning, you can do any number of intervals within 20 minutes.

As your endurance improves, you can spend more time doing the fast walking and less time in the slower recovery periods, gradually adding more repetitions at higher intensity. And, of course, you can always do longer workouts if you like. End your exercise session with a 2-minute cooldown at a slow pace.

On the days when you're not doing intervals, I recommend doing some core-strengthening exercises to target the vital muscles in your back, abdomen, pelvis, and hips. These are the muscles that are critical for improved posture, flexibility, balance, and stability. Since core exercises involve using several muscle groups in one fluid movement and also use your own body weight as resistance, they are good for strengthening and toning the peripheral muscles in your arms and legs. When you have a strong core, you'll find that day-to-day tasks like lifting grocery bags and luggage become much easier and that you are less likely to succumb to the many injuries related to poor muscle tone.

Let's not forget that an important cause of our obesity and diabetes epidemics is the "sitting disease," not just lack of exercise. There's no question that spending most of the day and evening in front of a computer or TV screen is dangerous to our health and our waistlines. So get up from your desk and couch and move. Just walking down the hall to chat with co-workers rather than calling or e-mailing, or doing jumping jacks or arm raises during TV commercials, can make a big difference to your health and well-being over time.

STICK WITH IT

Some people believe that once they have achieved their goal weight and start to feel better, they can stop exercising. Nothing could be further from the truth. Exercise is essential to maintaining your weight loss and good health over the long term. But if you really want to stick with it, you need to integrate an exercise program seamlessly into your lifestyle. Make exercise a habit by working out at the same time and in the same place every day, or at least on most days of the week. And don't forget to keep up the good work on those business trips and vacations, too. If you do have to miss a day, don't beat yourself up about it. Just pick up where you left off.

For a complete interval walking and core-strengthening program, see my book *The South Beach Diet Supercharged*.

PART III

REAL-LIFE GLUTEN SOLUTIONS

Now that you've read parts I and II of this book, you should have a good understanding of how gluten could be affecting your health and how you can lose weight and feel great once you start the South Beach Diet Gluten Solution Program.

Many of you will turn out to be moderately gluten sensitive; some of you will need to give up gluten entirely or almost entirely; still others of you will not need to give it up at all. The key to being gluten aware is understanding where you fit on that gluten spectrum.

In this section of the book, I show you how to shop for gluten-free foods and how to cook gluten-free meals during the first 4 weeks of the program and beyond, if need be. To help make it easy, I've supplied 20 healthy and delicious gluten-free recipes that fit the South Beach Diet principles. Of course, you're not limited to these. Many South Beach Diet–friendly recipes—such as turkey chili and brown rice pilaf—are gluten free and are dishes you probably make already!

I also give you tips for gluten-aware dining in all kinds of restaurants and for traveling gluten aware by train, plane, ship, and automobile so you can navigate your way through the real world as seamlessly as possible as you follow our program.

Keep in mind that these chapters provide strategies, not rules. Every person who adopts the Gluten Solution Program will have a different experience, but the goals are the same for all—to determine if and how gluten is affecting your health and to lose weight, if necessary, for a healthier and happier life. Please remember, if you have been diagnosed with celiac disease, you must be *completely* gluten free, not just gluten aware. And you must follow the advice of your celiac physician.

CHAPTER 11

THE GLUTEN-AWARE KITCHEN

THOSE WHO KNOW ME WELL KNOW THAT I AM A DOCTOR, NOT A cook, but I love a good meal. And I believe that dining at home as often as possible—sitting down at the table and not standing up—is the healthiest way for you and your entire family to eat. Maria Rodale, the CEO of Rodale Inc., once interviewed me for "A Visit to My Kitchen," her blog on the Huffington Post. Among the questions she asked me was "What's the one thing in your kitchen you just couldn't live without?" My immediate answer: "The refrigerator." I told her that it's because I've never gotten out of my habit of coming home after work or after a golf or tennis match and opening the fridge to see what's in there.

Fortunately, my wife makes sure our refrigerator is always stocked with berries and other fruits, cut-up veggies, hummus, all-natural peanut butter, and plenty of other healthy snack options. That certainly hasn't changed since our whole family has become gluten aware. Because we follow the South Beach Diet philosophy at home, it means that we have never had a lot of gluten-containing bread, cakes, cookies, or muffins around anyway. So we were already inadvertently gluten aware, and creating a gluten-aware kitchen didn't take too much effort on our part. That said, we now read labels on all products more carefully to make sure we don't get too much hidden gluten in our diet.

The first step to creating a healthy South Beach Diet kitchen is always the same, whether you are gluten aware or not—evaluate what you have and get rid of the bad stuff.

ASSESS YOUR CUPBOARDS, FRIDGE, AND FREEZER

You should permanently purge your cupboards, fridge, and freezer of all the unhealthy, highly processed sugary and starchy foods we advise you to avoid—the full-fat ice cream, the candy bars, the chips, the pretzels—you know (or you can probably guess) the drill.

You will also be removing or putting away *all foods that contain gluten*, at least until you've been gluten free for 4 weeks on GS Phase 1 and/or GS Phase 2. See our Gluten-Free Foods to Avoid lists for GS Phase 1 (pages 105 to 106) and GS Phase 2 (pages 128 to 129) and also check labels (see "Finding Gluten on a Food Label," page 160).

If you are beginning our program on GS Phase 1, you will also need to *temporarily* remove all *gluten-free* grains and products made with them (cereals, pastas, and so on) from your diet until you enter GS Phase 2. Phase 1 of the South Beach Diet has always been more or less gluten free because it is grain free. It's just that now, in order to truly test for gluten sensitivity, you will need to be aware of gluten hiding in less obvious places like seitan and soy sauce—and remove those products as well. The same is true for wine and other gluten-free types of alcohol, which are not allowed on GS Phase 1.

Here's a quick checklist of the foods that should ideally be *removed from your kitchen*, at least for Phase 1. When you've determined your level of gluten sensitivity and reached your weight-loss goals, some of these items may find their way back (in moderation, of course).

BAKED GOODS All baked goods must disappear on GS Phase 1. This includes breads, bagels, rolls, cakes, cookies, crackers, cupcakes, muffins, and waffles, gluten free or not, even if they're made with healthy flours.

BEVERAGES All fruit juices, sugary sodas, wine, beer, spirits, and any other sugary drink particularly with high-fructose corn syrup. Red and white wine and certain spirits can be introduced on GS Phase 2.

CANDY All candy, except sugar free. Gluten-free dark chocolate can be reintroduced on GS Phase 2.

CEREALS All cereals are off-limits on GS Phase 1. Low-sugar, high-fiber, gluten-free cereals can be enjoyed on GS Phase 2, with additional cereals added after 4 weeks of being gluten free.

CONDIMENTS, DRESSINGS, AND SEASONINGS All condiments that are not gluten free, particularly soy sauce (check labels). Also barbecue sauce, honey mustard, ketchup, and any other condiment or sauce made with corn syrup, molasses, or sugar.

DAIRY AND CHEESE Whole and 2% milk, full-fat soy milk, full-fat yogurt, and ice cream; cheeses made with anything but 1%, part-skim, or fat-free milk; full-fat cheeses.

FATS/OILS All solid vegetable shortening or lard, butter, and hydrogenated or partially hydrogenated oils.

FLOUR All flours and packaged products made with flour (such as pancake and waffle mixes) must be removed from your kitchen for GS Phase 1. Gluten-free flours and cornmeal must go on GS Phase 1, too, but can be reintroduced on GS Phase 2.

FRUIT No fruit on GS Phase 1, period. No fresh fruits, dried fruits, canned fruits in syrup, or sugared jellies or jams are permitted during GS Phase 1. Fresh and dried fruits are reintroduced on GS Phase 2 along with sugar-free jams and jellies. As explained, you give up these foods for only 2 weeks in order to get control of swings in blood sugar and cravings. Even nutritious fruit has sugar.

MEAT AND POULTRY Anything processed using sugars (honey-baked or maple-cured ham, for instance); fatty fowl such as goose and duck legs; pâté; dark-meat chicken and turkey (legs and wings); processed fowl such as packaged chicken nuggets or patties; beef brisket, liver, rib steaks, skirt steak, bacon (except Canadian and turkey), bologna, pepperoni (except turkey), salami, and other fatty meats.

PASTA All pasta is banished on GS Phase 1. Gluten-free pasta can be reintroduced on GS Phase 2.

POTATOES AND OTHER STARCHY VEGETABLES White and instant potatoes and beets are gone, to be enjoyed only occasionally once you've lost the weight you need to. You can reintroduce carrots, corn, sweet potatoes, winter squash, and other starchy vegetables on GS Phase 2.

RICE All rice, including white rice, jasmine rice, and sticky rice, is off-limits on Phase 1. You can introduce white basmati rice, converted rice, parboiled rice, brown rice, and wild rice on GS Phase 2.

SNACK FOODS All unhealthy packaged snacks are off-limits (such as cheese puffs, chips, pretzels, and cookies, even if they're gluten free). You can enjoy high-fiber, high-protein, low-sugar, gluten-free snack bars on GS Phase 2.

SOUP All powdered soup mixes (many are full of trans fat and sodium) and any soups containing cream, hydrogenated oils, or gluten starches.

SWEETENERS Remove white sugar, brown sugar, honey, molasses, and corn syrup as stand-alone products permanently. You can use agave nectar in moderation on GS Phase 1 and stevia, monk fruit natural no-calorie sweetener, and other sugar substitutes, if you so choose.

VEGETARIAN MEAT SUBSTITUTES Get rid of seitan, soy bacon, soy burgers, soy chicken, soy crumbles, soy hot dogs, soy sausage, and tofu with seasonings that might contain gluten.

BE AWARE: GLUTEN IS EVERYWHERE

Once you've cleaned out the bad stuff from your kitchen, you'll need to shop for the good stuff. But being a gluten-aware grocery shopper isn't always easy. As you can see from the GS Phase 1 Foods to Avoid list on pages 105 to 106 and the GS Phase 2 Foods to Avoid and Foods to Eat Rarely lists on pages 128 to 130, gluten is found everywhere under a variety of names. Unless you know how to read a food label (see page 160), you could end up spending hours in the grocery store searching for the gluten-free products.

To make matters even more complicated, as of this writing the FDA has yet to establish a standard for putting the words "gluten free" on packaging, although at the time this book went to press, the agency was slated to do so. Right now the only "rule" is that labels have to be "truthful with no misleading information." Because of this lack of uniform regulation, today you can find "gluten free" on everything from bottled water to bags of apples, which only makes people wonder about the similar products that *don't* say that. Part of the proposed new regulations will prevent putting these words on products that are *naturally* gluten free.

Another aspect of the FDA ruling, if passed as currently proposed, is to define gluten free as an end product that contains less than 20 parts per million of gluten (or less than 0.007 of an ounce of gluten for every 2.2, pounds of food). While this level was chosen because it's the generally accepted safe threshold for gluten for people with celiac disease, it is more than some people with celiac disease or a serious gluten sensitivity can tolerate. That's why a number of watchdog gluten-free certification organizations have their own standards. For example, the Gluten-Free Certification Organization will certify products as gluten free only if they are under 10 ppm, the same standard the nonprofit National Foundation for Celiac Awareness uses. The Celiac Sprue Association Recognition Seal appears only on products that are under 5 ppm and that are "completely free of wheat, barley, rye, oats, their crosses and derivatives in product, processing and packaging (WBRO-free)."

Confusing? You bet. In fact, it's a little bit like the Wild West out there right now when it comes to the inconsistency in gluten-free labeling and certification, especially since the labeling is and will continue to be voluntary even when the regulations are passed. In other words, a product could be gluten free and a manufacturer can decide not to label it as such. So even with a government ruling, it's still going to be up to you to be an educated consumer.

And consumers we are. According to various market research estimates, in 2012 alone Americans will spend some $4 billion to $7 billion on foods labeled gluten free, with sales currently growing at a double-digit pace annually. Walmart and Target, as well as regional and national supermarket chains like Publix and Kroger, to name some of the popular shopping destinations, now carry a wide selection of gluten-free products, and most supermarkets provide shopping lists of gluten-free items on their Web sites (including that bottled water and those apples!). But take care: Just because there are thousands of gluten-free products available doesn't mean every one of them is good for you. I've said it before and I'll say it again: Many of these products are simply nonnutritious, empty-calorie, blood-sugar-raising, gluten-free refined starches that can be just as unhealthy as junk food. And there's more. Just as sugar was added to so many "fat-free" products during the "fat-free" craze of the 1980s and 1990s, many manufacturers now add sugar, along with fat and salt, to gluten-free products to help with flavor and texture. That's why reading the ingredient list and the Nutrition Facts panel on packages is so important.

SHOP SMART

Another downside to many gluten-free products: They can be rather expensive. Who wouldn't get sticker shock picking up a small loaf of gluten-free

FINDING GLUTEN ON A FOOD LABEL

Checking product labels is essential if you really don't want gluten to creep into your diet. On the South Beach Diet, we strongly recommend looking at both the Nutrition Facts panel and the ingredient list to ensure you're buying nutritious foods that aren't highly refined and that don't have high levels of saturated fats, trans fats, sugars, or sodium. Once you've found a product that meets these requirements, you'll also have to search the label for gluten in its obvious and hidden forms.

Even though government-regulated gluten-free labeling hasn't become a reality as I write this, by law, food manufacturers under FDA jurisdiction do have to identify *in plain English* any ingredient from a list of eight major food allergens. This means that if a food contains milk, eggs, fish, crustacean shellfish, tree nuts, peanuts, *wheat*, or soybeans, the label is required to say so. This identification can be done in one of two ways: 1) by listing the allergen in the ingredient list in parentheses after a food, or 2) by adding a "Contains" statement at the end of the ingredient list. In the first instance, enriched flour in the ingredient list would have parentheses next to it that clearly states (*wheat*); lecithin would have (*soy*); whey would have (*milk*); and so on. With the second option, you'd simply see Contains: Wheat, Soy, and Milk. Some manufacturers choose to do both. But because gluten is not only found in wheat—and barley, rye, and oats are not covered by the labeling law—you will still have to read the ingredient list carefully if the "Contains" option is all that's used. Most careful gluten-aware buyers use the "Contains" statement only as a quick way to eliminate a product, not as a quick way to determine if it is safe.

Luckily, rye is not used in that many foods, and the label usually lists it simply bread and discovering that it costs $6—or being asked to pay $3.84 for a 12-ounce box of gluten-free pasta? (Manufacturers say the prices reflect the increased costs of the processing required to remove the gluten.)

But my advice to them is always the same: Don't skimp on your food budget. While some healthy foods can be pricey, the reality is that when you stop buying junk foods and replace them with high-quality nutritious foods, your grocery dollars will go further. The healthiest diet, including one that cuts back on or eliminates gluten, should always be based on eating a wide variety of whole foods. And many of these, like beans, eggs, and brown rice, fit into

as "rye" when it is there. Barley may be listed as barley malt or as malt, malt syrup, malt extract, malt flavoring, or simply as "flavoring." As for oats, you can assume that if they are listed without the words "gluten free" next to them, they may be contaminated with wheat.

Some manufacturers also voluntarily add a line to the food label that reads something like this: "Manufactured in a facility that also produces products made with wheat" or "Manufactured on equipment that also produces products that contain wheat." Depending on your level of gluten sensitivity, this type of cross-contamination warning may or may not affect your decision to buy the product.

So these are the basics. But gluten can still hide in the ingredient list under various other guises. Some of the words to watch out for include *binder* or *binding*, *thickening* or *thickener, emulsifier, edible starch, gum base, filler, modified food starch* (this is usually made from corn, but if it contains wheat, it must say so) or *modified starch, special edible starch, triticale, rusk, wheat alternative,* and *maltodextrin* (even though this word begins with *malt*, it is gluten free and is usually made from corn, potato, or rice; if wheat is used, the label would have to say *wheat maltodextrin* or *maltodextrin* [*wheat*]). Another potential gluten-containing ingredient, hydrolyzed vegetable protein (HVP), must specify the vegetable or grain it's made from, such as hydrolyzed wheat protein, which is not gluten free, or hydrolyzed soy protein, which is.

Phew. It almost makes me want to skip the grocery store altogether—and I don't even shop that often. The bottom line here is: If in doubt, call the manufacturer. Many products list the phone number right on the package, and most producers are used to fielding questions about gluten.

even the leanest food budget. In contrast, once you begin to rely heavily on overly processed, highly refined convenience foods, gluten free or not, you'll start to lose out on key nutrients, including B vitamins, vitamin C, calcium, and fiber, which are all essential for good health. Think of it this way: Spending money on nutrient-rich groceries today can mean less spent on doctor visits later.

That said, there are some budget-conscious shopping tips that can save you money when you're shopping gluten aware:

Plan meals a week at a time. Creating a shopping list based on the ingredients needed for your gluten-aware meals will save you both time and money. What's more, when you follow a shopping list, you're less likely to toss unnecessary items or impulse buys into your cart, which you may or may not ever use or will regret later. Be flexible enough to take advantage of any sale items that you know you'll use immediately or that can be stored or frozen. And remember, if you're cooking for your family and you're the only one with a gluten sensitivity, it's not worth buying expensive specialty products just for you. Better to buy foods that are naturally gluten free and cook meals that the whole family can enjoy.

Eat before you shop. Never go food shopping hungry. You will be more vulnerable to the sights and smells of food and end up with a shopping cart full of items you wouldn't succumb to if your hunger were in check. As I just said, gluten-free crackers aren't necessarily healthy crackers. Eat a healthy meal or snack before setting foot in the store.

Use coupons. Many large companies—Betty Crocker, Boar's Head, General Mills, Zatarain's, and Heinz, to name a few—offer coupons on products that don't contain gluten. Check out their Web sites and Facebook pages to download the coupons. Or visit aggregating sites such as BeFreeForMe.com and Glutenfreemall.com. Some have daily alert newsletters to let you know about good offers. But again, check out the products carefully before ordering.

Buy in bulk. Many supermarkets will special order a case of your favorite healthy gluten-free product and give you 10 percent off. Buying in bulk at a health-food store (watch out for product cross-contamination) or online is another good way to save, but only if you'll actually use all of what you buy. Some of the best buys are for gluten-free grain, nut, and bean flours in bulk, but you need a place to store them, and nut flours go rancid quickly if not placed in the freezer. To find the best prices, including estimated shipping costs (which can be considerable), use the Shopping button under the More tab on Google.com. Pick a product like Bob's Red Mill Organic Amaranth Flour, for example. You'll be amazed at the range of prices for this one product.

Shop beyond the conventional supermarket. When it comes to naturally gluten-free produce, in particular, some of the best buys may not be found in your regular market. If you haven't done so already, consider joining a food co-op or a community-supported agriculture group for discounts, and be sure to shop your local farmers' markets and farm stands, where seasonal fruits and vegetables, dairy products, eggs, meat, and poultry can be cheaper than at the grocery store. Also, don't forget to check out ethnic markets for good buys on 100% soba noodles, 100% corn tortillas, and so on.

BUY THIS, NOT THAT

Here's a short list of what's generally safe—and what's not—in your supermarket when it comes to gluten-aware shopping. Many supermarkets have gluten-free aisles, but you should still check labels, including the ingredients list. If you're still unsure, look online for the nutritional analysis or call the manufacturer before buying. Remember: The fresher the food, the more likely it's gluten free. The more processed or convenient the food, the riskier it is. Also watch out for deli meats and cheeses that may have been cross-contaminated by being sliced on the same equipment as gluten-containing meats or cheeses. Check out our Gluten Solution Phase 1 and Phase 2 Gluten-Free Foods to Enjoy and Foods to Avoid and Eat Rarely lists on pages 99 to 106 and 126 to 130 for more specifics.

PRODUCE

Enjoy: All fresh fruits and vegetables and frozen and canned fruits and vegetables with no additives.

Watch out for: Prepackaged fruits and vegetables (including frozen and canned) that contain additives, sauces, or fillers with gluten. Certain dried fruits (like dates) may have a flour dusting to prevent clumping (look for packages that say 100% pure fruit). Even though 100% fruit juices are gluten free, we don't recommend drinking fruit juices on any phase of the South Beach Diet. We prefer that you eat the whole fruit.

MEATS, SEAFOOD, AND POULTRY

Enjoy: Fresh meats, poultry, and fish that have been kept away from gluten cross-contamination at the store. (Grain-fed beef, poultry, and fish have not been shown to create gluten problems in most gluten-sensitive people.) Frozen meat, fish, and poultry with no additives or fillers. Gluten-free lean deli meats from manufacturers such as Boar's Head, Applegate, Hillshire Farm, or Wellshire Farms (avoid sugar-cured, maple-cured, and honey-baked ham altogether). Canned and pouched light tuna as well as salmon and sardines (check labels for broth additives in some brands, however).

Watch out for: Fresh or packaged meats, poultry, or seafood that is breaded or marinated with a gluten mixture. Self-basting poultry. Any deli meats, reduced-fat hot dogs, sausages, or other smoked, cured, or processed meats that have modified starches, which are used to bind water.

DAIRY PRODUCTS

Enjoy: Reduced-fat and fat-free milk, light (1% or 1.5%) buttermilk, and plain nonfat or low-fat yogurt. "Real" 100% pure cheeses, including nonfat and part-skim ricotta and some brands of reduced-fat cottage cheese. Fresh eggs, egg whites, and most egg substitutes.

Watch out for: Canned and tub cheese spreads. Beer-washed cheeses and blue cheese unless otherwise marked. Cheeses that have been presliced in the deli department rather than by the manufacturer may be cross-contaminated. Some brands of light sour cream, reduced-fat flavored yogurt, yogurt with "mix ins," reduced-fat flavored cottage cheese, and other flavored dairy products.

GRAINS, FLOURS, BREADS, CRACKERS, CEREALS, PASTA, AND OTHER STARCHES (GS PHASE 2 AND GS PHASE 3)

Enjoy: Grains and flours that are naturally gluten free such as almond, amaranth, bean, brown rice, buckwheat, coconut, cornmeal, flaxmeal, grits, lentil, millet, quinoa, soybean, teff, and wild rice, for example. Breads and crackers made with these grains. Oats, if clearly marked gluten free (Bob's Red Mill, Cream Hill Estates, and GF Harvest all offer certified gluten-free oat products). Pasta made from corn, brown rice, quinoa, amaranth, bean, and chickpea flours. One hundred percent buckwheat (soba) noodles. Corn tortillas (read the label, since some brands may contain wheat).

Watch out for: All flours and products made with wheat, barley, or rye. Flavoring agents or fillers in baked goods (which you shouldn't be buying anyway). Baking powder, which may contain wheat starch. Most cereals, including granolas, which often have malt flavoring made from barley. Wild rice blends that may contain barley. Flavored popcorn.

BEANS AND OTHER LEGUMES

Enjoy: Most gluten-free canned and dried legumes (read labels carefully).
Watch out for: Flavored canned legumes and canned baked beans. Dried beans that have been processed in factories that also process wheat, rye, and barley (this will be marked on the label). Rinsing and soaking dried beans (even canned varieties) may help minimize any gluten contamination.

SOY PRODUCTS

Enjoy: Traditional soy foods such as plain tofu, edamame, and some types of miso and tempeh (read labels carefully). Many brands of unsweetened soy milk.
Watch out for: Soy milks containing barley malt. Soy sauce (look for wheat-free tamari). Seitan and soy-based veggie burgers, which contain "vital wheat gluten," the ingredient that gives these foods the texture and taste of meat. (See page 105 for more problem soy foods.)

SOUPS

Enjoy: Look for low-sodium chicken, beef, and vegetable broth labeled gluten free (choose organic or free-range, if available).

Watch out for: Canned soups and chicken, beef, and vegetable broths containing flour or hydrolyzed wheat protein.

OILS, VINEGARS, AND SALAD DRESSINGS

Enjoy: Olive, canola, peanut, corn, grapeseed, safflower, sesame, sunflower, walnut, and other unsaturated oils. Extra-virgin coconut oil (a healthy saturated fat). Balsamic, rice, rice wine, wine, and apple cider vinegars. Most trans-fat free vegetable oil spreads are gluten free, but do check labels. Many Kraft, Newman's Own, and Walden Farms salad dressings do not contain gluten fillers or barley malt. Look for prepared dressings with 3 grams of sugar or less per 2 tablespoons.

Watch out for: Malt vinegars and other vinegars made with barley. Distilled white vinegar can be made from grapes, corn, wheat, or other sources. Salad dressings made with fillers or barley malt. Some nonstick cooking sprays may contain wheat flour.

NUTS AND SEEDS

Enjoy: All plain nuts and natural nut butters. Most seeds, including sunflower and flaxseed, but not rye and barley seeds.

Watch out for: Seasoned nuts and seeds that have been coated with a flavoring agent or processed on equipment that has also processed wheat. Check labels on dry-roasted nuts. Also avoid nuts with sugary coatings.

CONDIMENTS, SEASONINGS, AND EXTRACTS:

Enjoy: Fresh and dried herbs, whole or ground spices, garlic powder, and onion powder. Heinz ketchup, French's mustard, Hellmann's and Best Foods mayonnaise, and Lea & Perrins Worcestershire sauce are just some of the condiments now sold gluten free. Extracts made without barley malt: Look for *pure* vanilla, lemon, peppermint, and so on.

Watch out for: Soy sauce, unless marked gluten free. Seasoning mixes, including chili and taco seasoning packets.

ALCOHOLIC BEVERAGES (GS PHASE 2 AND GS PHASE 3)

Enjoy: Many people with gluten sensitivity can safely drink distilled alcoholic beverages, even those that are made from gluten-containing grains, such as scotch, whiskey, and gin. Distilling generally removes the gluten protein gliadin from spirits made from wheat, rye, and barley. If you are highly gluten sensitive, however, you may be able to consume only potato-based vodka (avoid the flavored varieties), rum (made from sugar cane), and tequila (made from agave). You can also have red and white wine, certain types of sake, ouzo, brut or extra-brut champagne, prosecco, or cava.

Watch out for: Because beer (made from barley malt) is brewed, not distilled, it's off-limits (and that includes the light beer we generally allow on Phase 2 of the South Beach Diet). Gluten-free beer, which is just as caloric as regular beer, is also not recommended on the South Beach Diet (as of this writing, light gluten-free beer isn't available). Sweet wines: While they don't contain gluten, they are very high in sugar and should not be consumed on the South Beach Diet.

NONALCOHOLIC BEVERAGES

Enjoy: Unflavored coffee and plain black, green, oolong, white, and red tea. Most pure herbal teas (chamomile, peppermint, and so on) are fine, but some blends may have malt or barley malt or natural or artificial flavors added. Club soda, seltzer, and mineral water. See also "Dairy Products," above.

Watch out for: Some varieties of flavored instant coffee and some brands of flavored regular coffee; the flavoring may have a base derived from gluten grains. Certain brands of flavored teas may also have natural or artificial flavorings that contain gluten; check labels on all tea, since cross-contamination is possible. Some brands of carbonated water may contain barley malt.

SWEETENERS

Enjoy: Granular sugar substitute, stevia, agave nectar, monk fruit natural no-calorie sweetener.

Watch out for: Sugar, honey, molasses as stand-alone products. They do not contain gluten but are not recommended as sweeteners on GS Phase 1 and GS Phase 2, the weight-loss phases of the program.

COOKING GLUTEN AWARE

If you've already been cooking the South Beach Diet way, you know that many of the healthy recipes available in our cookbooks and on SouthBeachDiet.com are gluten free. You can be certain that all of the Phase 1 recipes we've ever published in our books and on our Web site are grain free, as are many of our Phase 2 recipes. If you're truly gluten free, however, you will have to take care to use gluten-free versions of soy sauce and other ingredients that may appear in these previously published recipes.

Furthermore, the same healthy cooking techniques we've always recommended—steaming, roasting, baking, grilling, sautéing (in olive oil, not butter!)—apply to gluten-aware cooking. The key to delicious and healthy gluten-free meals is to keep them simple, using a variety of fresh ingredients.

It really isn't hard to transform recipes made with foods containing gluten into those without. Instead of tabbouleh made with barley, for example, you can use quinoa. Instead of tacos made with wheat tortillas, you can use 100% corn tortillas. Instead of making baked goods with whole-wheat flour, you can choose from a wide range of gluten-free flours made from grains like amaranth and buckwheat and from beans and nuts as well. There's no question that baking can be the biggest challenge for a gluten-free cook who's also South Beach Diet savvy. In addition to avoiding the gluten, you'll have to avoid the butter and white sugar, as always. And if you are serious about losing weight, you don't want too many baked goods around anyway until you reach Phase 3, when they can be enjoyed on occasion.

The other good news is that unless you are extremely gluten sensitive, you won't have to overhaul your kitchen by buying a dedicated toaster, colander, sifter, baking pans, cutting boards, and other utensils to prevent cross-contamination. You probably will want to mark containers for your gluten-free grains and designate a pantry shelf or area of the refrigerator to gluten-free items, but overall, your kitchen really doesn't need two sets of everything.

Those with celiac disease, however, do have to worry about even the slightest crumb getting into the peanut butter jar, so creating a "shared" kitchen is a must. Celiac.org has excellent information for doing so.

To get started cooking in your gluten-aware kitchen, we've included 20 gluten-free recipes that are all recommended in either our GS Phase 1 or GS Phase 2 Meal Plans. See pages 199 to 229 and enjoy. Also, feel free to use your favorite healthy gluten-free recipes, if you prefer.

CHAPTER 12

DINING OUT GLUTEN AWARE

I'D LIKE TO TELL YOU ABOUT MY FRIEND CHARLIE, A 58-YEAR-OLD man who truly loves restaurant dining (he often dines out twice a day). Charlie had been experiencing recurring heartburn and acid reflux since he was in his twenties, and he basically ignored the problem until it got so bad that it began to affect his enjoyment of food. His doctor told him he might have "yeast overgrowth" and to take a probiotic along with a proton-pump inhibitor (Prilosec, Prevacid, Nexium) to reduce his stomach acid and his reflux. While the heartburn did go away, he began to feel what he described as "weird and bloated." He took himself off the proton-pump inhibitor and stayed on the probiotic and felt better but not perfect.

Wandering around a health-food store one day, Charlie noticed a probiotic green drink supplement that advertised itself as a "the ultimate gluten-free superfood." Even though the probiotic he was already taking was gluten free, he switched to this one. The term *gluten free* intrigued him.

This was a year or so ago, when the gluten-free craze was just taking America by storm. After doing some reading, Charlie decided going gluten free was worth a try, even if it meant changing his typical restaurant diet (he wasn't about to give up dining out, but he could make a valiant attempt to give up three of his all-time favorites: pizza, pasta, and whole-wheat bread).

Within a month of avoiding the obvious sources of gluten, Charlie felt so much better that he even stopped taking the green supplement. He still felt great. No heartburn and no reflux—without the probiotic. Today, 1 year later, he continues to be gluten aware, enjoying the occasional backslide for a few bites of his partner's homemade desserts (he's even gotten his partner to bake gluten free for the most part). In restaurants, however, Charlie prefers not to "experiment" with foods he's unfamiliar with for fear of the return of the heartburn that he now calls the "Gluten Revenge." These days, he pretty much plays it safe and sticks with grilled meats, poultry, and seafood with plenty of veggies (no sauces). After 30 years of stomach problems, he says he plans to be gluten aware forever. And his pants fit better, too.

GOURMET GLUTEN FREE

As it happens, Charlie lives in Asheville, North Carolina, a thriving small city that has one of the best completely gluten-free restaurants in the country, Posana Café. Charlie doesn't have to worry about anything he orders when he eats there, which is often. When you look at Posana's menu, though, the fact that the dishes are gluten free isn't the first thing you notice. They just look delicious (the chef, Peter Pollay, was classically trained at the Culinary Institute of America).

I'd like to think of Posana as a model for more restaurant menus and chefs of the future, especially since so many of us have some degree of gluten sensitivity, but as Chef Pollay points out, running a 100 percent gluten-free restaurant means sourcing all the ingredients from providers who will absolutely guarantee that their product is gluten free. And because it's so time consuming, this is next to impossible for most restaurateurs. Even so, Pollay's menu at Posana, which changes regularly to feature the freshest seasonal ingredients, shows that eating gluten free doesn't mean giving up all the foods you love. Check it out at Posanacafe.com.

GOOD-BYE, BREAD BASKET

Today, you can go into almost any restaurant from a pizza joint to a classic French bistro and find (or at least ask for) gluten-free options—provided you're an educated eater. In fact, the more you know about where gluten lurks beyond the bread basket, the easier it will be to order around it. While you may decide, like Charlie did, that experimenting isn't worth the potential health repercussions, once you've figured out where you are on the gluten spectrum and how much gluten triggers your symptoms, you may be able to have that occasional serving of semolina pasta primavera or help yourself to a whole-wheat roll. I leave that to your own discretion. If you have celiac disease, however, you already know how ultracareful you must be when dining out, since cross-contamination is common when gluten-free foods are prepared on the same grill, in the same pasta water, or in the same tortilla warmer, for example, as those with gluten. If you're not a celiac sufferer or highly gluten sensitive, you don't have to obsess about cross-contamination. Just use your best judgment and order appropriately.

But before we get into some specific strategies for eating out gluten aware, I want to remind you of some basic dining principles that have helped our South Beach dieters navigate restaurants for years as they stay healthy and keep the weight off. These are strategies that will stand you in good stead in any restaurant—whether you are trying to avoid gluten or not. Not surprisingly, it's estimated that people consume about 500 more calories eating in a restaurant than they would if they ate a similar meal at home. And if you dine out three times a week, which many individuals and families do, that can quickly add up to 78,000 extra calories a year!

If you think banishing the gluten-filled bread basket will cut those stats, you are right, but there are other things you can do as well to keep the pounds from piling on:

Snack before you go. Going to a restaurant hungry is asking for trouble. The menu arrives, your eyes widen, and everything on it suddenly looks delicious. On the South Beach Diet, there's a reason why we recommend eating a protein- and fiber-rich midmorning and midafternoon snack. It prevents the drop in blood sugar that causes you to suddenly become ravenous and crave every sugary and starchy carb that comes your way. So before going out to Luigi's Italiano, enjoy some veggie sticks with a little hummus, or an apple and a little cheese, or some all-natural peanut butter. You'll avoid entering the restaurant ravenous.

Say, "More broccoli, please." Never feel shy about asking for double green vegetables or a tossed salad rather than the white rice or mashed potatoes that often accompany entrées. Yes, rice and potatoes are gluten free, but . . . they can raise your blood sugar. Your best bet is to skip the starchy sides altogether and request broccoli *and* green beans. If you must have a starch, make sure it's a sweet potato or a gluten-free grain like quinoa or brown rice or wild rice.

Forget fried. I have a friend who sees the words "fried calamari" on a menu and all diet rules are off. Needless to say, she hasn't lost the weight she's wanted to, and even though she's gluten aware, she manages to tell herself that there's "almost no gluten" in the crispy calamari batter. The point is this: Get the word *fried* out of your vocabulary, period; fried foods are not South Beach Diet–friendly. Simply ask for grilled, roasted, baked, steamed, or sautéed instead. This goes for the gluten sensitive and nonsensitive alike.

Have a nonalcoholic drink first. Having a cocktail before or wine with a meal can certainly enhance the dining experience, but too much alcohol can disrupt even the healthiest of dining intentions ("I'll have the chocolate mousse cake, please"). Rather than ordering a cocktail as soon as you sit down, I recommend asking for still or sparkling water with a slice of lemon or lime for flavor. Then slowly drink the entire glass. This helps fill you up and makes you less likely to overeat during the meal. On the South Beach Diet, we recommend no more than one alcoholic drink a day for women and two for men beginning on GS Phase 2 to preserve not just your waistline but your health as well. Enjoy a glass of red or white wine with your food (not on an empty stomach); both are gluten free, and the resveratrol in red wine has plenty of healthy benefits. For more gluten-free beverages, see the GS Phase 2 Gluten-Free Foods to Enjoy list on pages 126 to 128.

Follow the Three-Bite Rule: The South Beach Diet Three-Bite Rule for decadent desserts has worked for years for many successful Phase 2 dieters who must have their cake and eat it, too. For you gluten-free dessert fans, this rule can help as well, since gluten-free pastries are by no means low in fat or sugar. The rule is this: When you just can't resist a tempting dessert at a restaurant, or on a special occasion, try to limit yourself to three bites. Savor each one, then pass your dessert plate to a fellow diner or the busboy. You'll find that having just a few bites is extremely satisfying, and you won't feel deprived or crave more. If you are like me and know you have a problem with just three bites, order some berries (without the whipped cream or with just a dollop) for dessert.

STRATEGIES FOR DINING OUT

Now that you've reviewed the South Beach Diet Gluten Solution Program in Part II, you have a good idea about which foods contain gluten. You also understand that to determine whether you are gluten sensitive (and to potentially feel better while getting your weight loss jump-started), you'll need to eliminate gluten from your diet for 4 weeks. You don't have to skip dining out altogether for this time, but you will have to be more careful in your ordering.

Once you are on GS Phase 2, you'll still be watching your gluten for at least 2 more weeks, but you will have more foods available to you. Here are some simple strategies you can employ to make avoiding gluten easier during the first 4 weeks of the program. After that, you'll begin to introduce some gluten-containing foods and you'll understand how to navigate the menu in any restaurant—not just those with gluten-free offerings.

Plan ahead. It's easier to dine gluten aware if you have done your homework—and technology can help. Today many restaurants post their menus online (but don't always trust what you read, and be sure to check the date when the Web site was last updated). You can also type "gluten-free restaurant" and the city you're in (or traveling to) to come up with some options. Still, look at the restaurant's menu carefully, because some restaurants list themselves as "gluten-free friendly," meaning that not everything they serve is gluten free. The Gluten Intolerance Group of North America (gluten.net) is just one of many sites that have a restaurant database. This organization currently provides the only Gluten-Free Food Service accreditation in the world. If a restaurant displays the GFFS logo, it means the eatery has met strict gluten-free standards. The group also runs a Gluten-Free Restaurant Awareness Program (GFRAP) to help restaurants tailor their menus for gluten-free options.

To search for restaurants when you're out and about, you can download one of the many restaurant-finder apps, such as the Gluten Free Ultimate Solution from G-Free Foodie, which provides locations of gluten-free restaurants via GPS. Glutenfreetravelsite.com also has a mobile version of its Web site that works on any handheld device, including the BlackBerry. For more information on restaurant finders and other resources, see pages 231 to 236.

You should also keep in mind that just because your Web search or app shows that Domino's is now offering gluten-free pizza and that Wendy's and Burger King have gluten-free fries prepared in wheat-free oil, it doesn't mean you have a license to head immediately to the drive-thru or and forgo our South Beach Diet principles. It's great to know these options are available, especially when traveling, but remember that a french fry touted as gluten free is still a french fry.

Join a gluten-free dining club. If you're looking for company on your gluten-aware dining journey, consider joining a gluten-free dining club. You'll make friends who have similar dietary interests; discover new restaurants; share recipes, products, connections to doctors; and more. New York City's Celiac Disease Meetup Group (meetup.com/Celiac), for example, has more than 1,500 members, including not just those with celiac disease but also people with gluten sensitivities, wheat allergies, and more. Atlanta (meetup.com/atlantagfdinnerclub) and Washington, DC (meetup.com/celiacdisease-112), also have active meet-up groups. If you can't find a support group near you, register on the Meetup.com Web site to be notified when a group does start up. Depending on where you end up on the gluten spectrum, this may seem a bit much, but you will have expanded your gluten education and likely improved your social life as well.

Reserve an early table. As you've no doubt already experienced, restaurants' peak dining hours can be wildly busy, with orders coming in frantically and chaos in the kitchen. When you dine early, you minimize the risk that your order will get mixed up and you're more likely to get special attention from the servers and the chef. Let the reservationist know when you call that you have a gluten sensitivity and that you may have special questions about the menu that could take some time (ask that she note your special diet on your reservation).

Keep it simple for your server. Even though you've chosen a restaurant because you've determined it has gluten-free options, your server (who may have been hired yesterday) may not have a clue what you're talking about when you say you can't eat gluten. If you get a blank stare, tell the person you have a medical condition that does not allow you to eat certain grains, specifically wheat, barley, and rye, and any foods made with these grains, like soy sauce.

Depending on the ethnicity of the restaurant you've chosen, using a gluten-free restaurant card that tells the server in the appropriate language what you can't eat could help, especially if you're dining abroad. Consider downloading the free Gluten Free Restaurant Cards app produced by Celiac Travel from the iTunes store. It explains what eating gluten free means in close to 40 languages, including Cantonese and Mandarin. You can also download the restaurant cards for free in a PDF format at celiactravel.com. The cards are created for people with celiac disease, so they may be a little over the top for the gluten sensitive. But if you are really trying to avoid gluten in a restaurant, semantics don't matter.

Go to the top. If your server can't answer your questions to your satisfaction, don't be shy about asking to speak to someone in charge, or better yet, the chef. Inquire as to whether there are thickeners in the sauces, ask what's in the marinades and salad dressings and what flours are used in the desserts, and so on.

Watch out for substitutions. Just because a meal is guaranteed to be gluten free doesn't mean it will taste good. This is often the case when you're swapping something that normally contains gluten, like pasta or a pizza crust, for a gluten-free version. My friend Priscilla discovered this when she dined not long ago at an upscale Italian restaurant in Miami.

Priscilla had been gluten free for almost a month after I had advised her to go on our Gluten Solution Program to see if it would help resolve her bloating and migraines. Upon scanning the restaurant menu, she was delighted to see a notation that the "chef will substitute gluten-free pasta for regular pasta in any dish." As it happened, her server was a co-owner of the restaurant, and when she happily ordered the gluten-free linguine with a simple olive-oil-based clam sauce, he immediately recommended that she not do so, warning, "The gluten-free pasta isn't nearly as good as the regular."

Determined to stay gluten free for the last week of our program, Priscilla ordered the gluten-free linguine anyway. As the owner had suggested, she was very disappointed. Later she asked him why the chef even bothered to put gluten-free pasta on the menu if it didn't taste good. The owner's reply: "Because everybody's doing it."

Priscilla did the right thing by sticking with the program. But she won't order that pasta again. If you dine out a lot, you'll likely encounter the same problem when it comes to the issue of gluten-free food quality. You may always want to play it safe and order a dish that is naturally gluten free, like grilled or broiled fish or poultry.

MENU SAVVY

The good news about gluten-aware dining is that you can enjoy almost any cuisine, if you take care. But wherever you go, there are some general ordering guidelines to keep in mind, particularly during the gluten-free phases of our program. Once you've determined how gluten-sensitive you are (if at all), you'll know how careful you need to be.

◆ Skip most soups, since so many use flour as a thickener; instead, ask for clear broth or consommé with no flour additives.

◆ Watch out for the sauces and marinades, which are typically made with gluten-containing thickeners or may have gluten-containing soy sauce or teriyaki sauce added.

◆ Question how the salad dressing is made (does it have barley, binding agents, soy sauce, preservatives?).

◆ Beware of gravies, imitation seafood, casseroles, stews, potpies, and anything breaded, flour coated, or fried.

◆ Avoid white rice. While it is gluten free and ubiquitous across most cuisines, we don't recommend it on the South Beach Diet because it can raise blood sugar and cause cravings. Choose basmati (it's white, but lower on the glycemic index) or brown rice, black rice, or wild rice instead.

◆ Watch out for all baked desserts, which likely contain wheat flour but may also contain malt and rye. We don't recommend them on the South Beach Diet anyway.

◆ Think plain. No matter what cuisine you choose, you can usually find grilled or roasted meat, seafood, poultry, and some kind of steamed or grilled vegetable (ask for it without sauce and with lemon or lime on the side). Ordering this way works on all phases of our program.

The guidelines below highlight the dishes to enjoy and avoid in various types of restaurants while being gluten aware and following our basic South Beach Diet principles for healthy eating. If you're not sure if a food is allowed on GS Phase 1 or GS Phase 2, see our GS Gluten-Free Foods to Enjoy and GS Foods to Avoid lists on pages 99 to 106 and 126 to 130.

STEAK HOUSE

Enjoy: Clear soup or consommé; vegetable, bean, or meat-based soups without pasta, white potatoes, or thickeners. Tossed or Caesar salad with oil and vinegar (no croutons) or shrimp cocktail. Lean cuts of grilled steak (top sirloin, filet mignon, tenderloin), grilled chicken, fish, shrimp, or pork chops with a side of steamed veggies. A baked sweet potato is a great option instead of a white baked potato on GS Phase 2.

Avoid: The bread basket. All fried appetizers. All pasta unless gluten free. No bun with your burger. No steak fries or breaded onion rings; they're off-limits on the South Beach Diet.

If you're into chain steak houses, Outback Steakhouse has a menu marked with a "GF" next to many of its dishes. Check it out online.

JAPANESE

In Japanese restaurants, soy sauce is used in all types of dishes from teriyaki and sukiyaki to tofu dishes, so always ask before ordering.

Enjoy: Clear soup, edamame, tossed salad (avoid the miso dressing!), and seaweed salad. Sushi (with brown rice on Phase 2) or sashimi. Yakitori (grilled chicken kebabs). Shabu-shabu, in which you dip meats or vegetables into simmering water or broth (but watch out for the special sauces that come with it). Soba noodles, which are made from buckwheat, in moderation. On GS Phase 2 and beyond, any sake from the House of Gekkeikan or any labeled "Junmai" (which means pure) are safe. Other forms of sake may be flavored with barley and are therefore off-limits.

Avoid: Anything made with miso, since it could be made from barley, not soy. Anything breaded and fried, including all tempura. Unagi, an eel dish usually made with soy. Imitation crabmeat (surimi). Fried dumplings (pot stickers). All teriyaki dishes.

ITALIAN

Enjoy: Antipasto with grilled vegetables and beans. Minestrone without pasta or potatoes. Escarole and bean soup. Steamed artichokes with balsamic vinaigrette. Mozzarella and tomatoes. Steamed mussels and clams (watch the sauces). Grilled and baked chicken, meat, and seafood (watch the toppings). Chicken cacciatore (made without wheat flour). Shrimp scampi (made with olive oil). On GS Phase 2, you can begin to enjoy thin-crust gluten-free pizza with a veggie topping, as well as gluten-free pasta dishes, if available (just make sure the water it's cooked in is not the same water the wheat pasta was cooked in); stick with plain tomato or marinara with a vegetable or meat sauce. Risotto (only on occasion and on Phase 3, since we don't recommend white rice on the South Beach Diet). Polenta (cornmeal) dishes.

Avoid: Soups that contain potato or pasta. Skip the white and whole-wheat bread, pizza, and pasta and enjoy only whole-grain gluten-free versions on Phase 2 in moderation. Avoid all cream-based pasta sauces, which might be thickened with wheat flour. Avoid scaloppine dishes and mozzarella in carrozza, which are breaded.

FRENCH

Enjoy: Simply prepared poached or grilled meat, seafood, and poultry without sauces. Fish or chicken *en papillote* (cooked in its own juices in parchment). Poulet aux fines herbes. Plain veggies or veggies steamed or sautéed in olive oil. Ratatouille and salad Niçoise (ask for the salad without the white potatoes unless you're well into Phase 2 or beyond). Provençal fish stew, if it's not thickened with flour. On GS Phase 2 and beyond, enjoy a glass of wine with your meal.

Avoid: Skip the baguettes and breakfast croissants. Watch out for anything served au gratin, meunière, velouté, demi-glace, béchamel, beurre manié, croquette, cordon bleu, or *en croute*, which all mean gluten (or cream or butter!) in disguise. Ask for any sauce on the side when unsure. No frites (french fries).

CHINESE

Ordering gluten free in a Chinese restaurant can be very tricky, since so many dishes are made with soy sauce. That said, there are items you can order with special care. If you're highly gluten sensitive, avoid sharing, which is typical in Chinese venues.

Enjoy: Egg drop soup (if it's not thickened with flour), clear soup, and hot and sour soup (if not thickened). Steamed, stir-fried, roasted, or broiled meat, seafood, or poultry. Fresh vegetables prepared with a small amount of meat, fish, or poultry. Chow fun (wide rice noodles) and mei fun (thin rice noodles) in moderation on Phase 2 with steamed vegetables or chicken, meat, or seafood added, but no soy sauce. Tofu dishes (the plainer the better, and watch the soy). Dishes that are seasoned with rice wine, rice vinegar, dried mushrooms, sesame oil, and chili paste.

Avoid: Miso soup, which could be made with barley miso. Anything deep-fried like noodles or General Tso's chicken (which has a flour-based batter and wouldn't be recommended on the South Beach Diet, period). Imitation ("vegetarian") meat and seafood ingredients (including imitation crab, or surimi). Moo shu pancakes, wontons, dumplings, and lo mein noodles, which are typically made with wheat flour. Any dishes with brown sauce or black bean sauce. Watch all condiments, including plum sauce, hoisin sauce, sweet and sour sauce, and especially soy sauce.

THAI AND VIETNAMESE

Enjoy: Dishes that are stir-fried, sautéed, or steamed with herbs such as Thai basil or lemon grass. Most curries.

Avoid: All battered and fried dishes. Anything made with nam pla (Thai soy sauce), brown sauce, oyster sauce, or garlic sauce. Imitation crab.

INDIAN

Enjoy: Tandoori chicken, fish, and shrimp. Vegetable side dishes. Papadum, an Indian flat bread made from lentils. Dal (a dish made with lentils and/or various other kinds of beans), raita (yogurt dip), vegetable salads, curries, and some masala-style dishes.

Avoid: All fried dishes, including samosas and pakoras. All wheat-based breads, including naan, roti, paratha, poori, and chapati. Dishes made with maida (refined wheat flour) and with rava or suji, types of semolina wheat flour. Dishes flavored with asafetida powder, a pungent spice redolent of onion and garlic, which may contain wheat gluten.

GREEK AND MIDDLE EASTERN

Enjoy: Greek salad with feta, olives, or anchovies and an olive oil and vinegar dressing. Hummus (chickpea dip), tzatziki (a dip traditionally made with cucumber, garlic, and yogurt), and baba ghanoush (eggplant dip). Grilled or broiled seafood (all kinds including squid, octopus, shrimp, and sardines) prepared simply with lemon juice, herbs, and olive oil. Lean lamb chops and leg of lamb (occasionally). Chicken, beef, or seafood skewers (souvlaki). On GS Phase 2, ouzo, a wine made from pressed grapes, herbs, and berries.

Avoid: Pita bread. Bulgur (tabbouleh) and couscous. Pastitsio (a Greek version of lasagna) and orzo. Moussaka (usually topped with béchamel sauce, which is made with butter, flour, whole milk, and sometimes bread crumbs). Spanokopita (cheese and spinach pie made with phyllo dough). Gyro meat (which may contain hidden wheat) and the pita it comes in. Falafal (breaded ground chickpea mixtures). Desserts made with phyllo.

MEXICAN

Enjoy: Tortilla soup with corn tortilla strips. Jícama salad or green salad with oil and vinegar dressing. Freshly made guacamole. Fresh (not from a jar) salsa. Beans, beans, beans; just not refried. Grilled chicken, seafood, or veggie dishes like carna asada (watch the sauce) and fish Veracruz-style (with tomatoes, onions, and peppers). Tomatillo sauce and mole sauces may be fine (but ask about thickeners). Chicken, beef, seafood or veggie enchiladas, fajitas, or tacos made with corn tortillas (make sure they don't have wheat flour added). Ask if the fajita marinade is made with soy sauce. A shot of tequila is fine on GS Phase 2.

Avoid: All fried items, including the fried tortilla chips (ask for a fresh corn tortilla to dip in the guacamole and salsa instead). No whole-wheat tortillas. Skip the beer (even the gluten-free beer) and avoid all the sweet drinks like mojitos and margaritas (gluten free but high in sugar).

FAST-FOOD AND CHAIN RESTAURANTS

We don't recommend most fast food on the South Beach Diet, whether you are gluten aware or not. But there may be times when it's the only choice (like on a long road trip). Today, a number of fast-food chains describe their gluten-free options on their Web sites. Here's how Chipotle Mexican Grill, for example, described its offerings for their gluten intolerant/celiac disease clientele on its Web site as of this writing:

> *Most people wanting to avoid gluten can eat anything we serve except for our large and small flour tortillas, and possibly our red tomatillo salsa (there is a small amount of distilled vinegar in it which some gluten-oriented Web sites still say might be problematic, although most don't). Everything else is fine to eat for most people wanting to avoid gluten, including our crispy corn tacos and our corn chips [two SBD no-nos!]. However, you should know that it's possible our corn may have a small amount of gluten from potentially co-mingling with gluten-containing grains in the field. If you are highly sensitive and would like us to change our gloves, we would be happy to do that at your request. Additionally, because our folks work with wheat tortillas all day long, there may be the possibility of cross-contact in our restaurants. We encourage you to carefully consider your dining choices.*

It's clear that they're trying hard and most people will do just fine in one of their venues. However, if you have celiac disease or are highly gluten sensitive, you must exercise the same caution you would wherever you're dining out.

You also need to be careful in chain restaurants, which generally develop specific guidelines for every recipe so they can maintain consistency among franchises. As a result, recipes may be made using premixed seasoning blends and prepared foods that can't be adapted for a special diet. Many may contain wheat, barley, or rye.

BON APPÉTIT!

While gluten-aware dining may seem daunting at first, you'll soon learn to negotiate all manner of menus with confidence. And if you follow our South Beach Diet eating principles, you'll stay trim, too.

Just a final reminder: When you do have a wonderful meal and you get the service you need from the waitstaff and kitchen, write a nice review on their Web site so others can benefit from your gluten-aware dining experience.

CHAPTER 13

THE GLUTEN-AWARE TRAVELER

MY FRIEND LINDA HAS BEEN TO ITALY MANY TIMES BEFORE, AND HER motto always was: When in Rome, do as the Romans do. In other words, eat pasta and bread and lots of it. But her most recent trip was different. Over the past year, Linda had been suffering from fatigue and lack of mental focus—what she called "brain drain." At first she thought she was working too hard as a software engineer, but the problem continued even after she cut back on her hours and made an effort to get more sleep. She was tested for anemia and low vitamin D and was fine on both counts. It was only when a friend suggested she try eliminating gluten from her diet for a while that she began to feel normal again. In fact, she started feeling better after just a few weeks, and her newfound energy and clarity were what prompted her to book her trip. And there was no way she was going to let her new gluten-free diet slide and take the chance of feeling lousy again.

Her best-laid plans began to disintegrate on the plane, however. Linda had requested a gluten-free dinner when she booked her ticket online with a major carrier. When the flight attendant brought her meal, she was dismayed to see pasta with tomato sauce, a salad with a glutinous salad dressing, a white roll, and a cookie for dessert. She immediately protested, only to learn that all the gluten-free meals (which consisted of chicken breast with no seasonings, boiled vegetables and white rice, a green salad with vinaigrette dressing, a plain rice cake, and fresh fruit) had been distributed to others and that there were no more to be had.

Linda's complaints landed on deaf ears, and she had to resort to a few gluten-free snacks she'd smartly brought from home. By the time the plane landed in Rome, she was starving. So she did what she had promised herself she wouldn't do and grabbed a panini on the way out of the airport. A few hours later, she felt the old brain fog return, and she knew it wasn't just jet lag. For the rest of the trip, she negotiated her gluten-aware way through various Italian eateries (surprisingly not hard to do these days, since so many Italians have been diagnosed with celiac disease, perhaps due to their heavy intake of pasta and other gluten-containing foods), but that little glitch at the start of the trip had literally left a bad taste in her mouth. Before heading back on the same carrier, she called the airline numerous times to make sure the problem didn't happen again. And it didn't.

I can sympathize with Linda. I travel frequently for medical meetings. Like most people who spend time in airports (or train stations), I often find it a challenge to eat healthy when I'm on the road. I get bored during flight delays and sometimes nibble a few too many sugary and starchy snacks to kill time or for "instant gratification." When I arrive at my destination, I'm often jet lagged and immediately head to the hotel and order room service. But before the meal is delivered, there's the minibar calling, "Open me, Dr. Agatston." I know that it knows that I know there's chocolate in there. Yes, I am the doctor who created the South Beach Diet, but traveling is often stressful and exhausting, and I am human and I do love chocolate. But I have a strict rule: No minibar! At least most of the time.

Now that I have cut back on gluten-containing foods in my diet (I do have to confess I don't read the chocolate bar labels that carefully), I find it more challenging to eat healthfully while traveling. Where are those gluten-free snacks when I need them? I've always recommended carrying healthy snacks when traveling, but now I'm even more careful. When I have a long layover and I am forced to have a meal in an airport, I check my iPhone for where to dine. Unfortunately, most of the recommendations are for fast-food or family-dining chains, which have smartly taken advantage of the gluten-free craze. But as I said in the last chapter, fast food is a last resort on the South Beach Diet if you want to stay lean and healthy. Think of it this way: Do you really want to eat french fries or a sat-fat-laden cheeseburger without the bun just because it's labled GF on a fast-food menu? I don't. And hopefully you don't either. I provide some solutions below.

TRAVELING "ON THE BEACH"

Even the most ardent South Beach dieters know it: Most people gain weight on trips, simply because they feel it's escape time and they deserve to indulge, gluten aware or not. Whether you are traveling for business or vacationing alone or with your family, it's important to keep some basic South Beach Diet principles in mind if you want to stay healthy and keep the pounds off:

Carry our Gluten-Free Foods to Enjoy and Foods to Avoid lists for either GS Phase 1 (pages 99 to 106) or GS Phase 2 (pages 126 to 130), depending which phase you're on. This handy reference, which you can copy from this book or download from southbeachdiet.com/glutensolution, is a quick reminder of what you can and can't eat on each phase of our South Beach Diet Gluten Solution Program. If you are on GS Phase 1 of the diet, you may prefer to wait until you enter GS Phase 2 before traveling if you can. You'll simply have more food options to choose from, including gluten-free grains like brown rice, buckwheat, and quinoa as well as fruits and additional starches introduced after Phase 1. Once you've been gluten free for 4 weeks and are testing the reintroduction of some gluten-containing foods, continue to read labels carefully to avoid products high in fat, sugar, and sodium.

Don't leave home hungry. If you fuel up with a good meal at home before you start your trip, you'll be less likely to purchase one of those tempting cinnamon buns at the airport or train station or overindulge on the free drinks and salty, high-fat snacks so common in the airline passengers' clubs.

Snack between meals. It's easy to get off schedule when you're traveling, but if you skip your midmorning or midafternoon snack, you are much more likely to find yourself ravenous when you finally can sit down to a meal. While you are gluten free during the first 4 weeks of the program—and after, if you've determined you need to be—bring convenient protein- and fiber-rich gluten-free snack foods in containers or 1-quart resealable plastic bags. Try cut-up vegetables (carrots, celery, broccoli), individual reduced-fat mozzarella sticks, lean ham or turkey slices, individual 2-ounce containers of hummus, some nuts, or a filling high-fiber, protein-rich gluten-free snack bar. For additional phase-friendly snack ideas, see pages 190 to 191. Most airports will allow food (not liquids) through the TSA screening if it's packed right (see page 189 for more on the Transportation Security Administration rules).

Hydrate on water, not cocktails. Thirst often mimics hunger. But hydrating doesn't mean drinking four gluten-free vodka and tonics on the 15-hour direct flight from JFK to Johannesburg or indulging in a few too many sugary mojitos on the foredeck of your cruise liner to Barbados. Buy some bottled water as soon as you get through screening at the airport, or bring an empty reusable bottle and fill it up. And always carry plenty of water with you in a cooler in the car or in your travel bag on the train. If you're following a healthy eating plan, what you drink is just as important as what you eat. And on the South Beach Diet, certain beverages (like sugary sodas, fruit juices, and most mixed drinks) are not recommended. Starting on Phase 2 of the South Beach Diet, you can enjoy alcohol in moderation—one alcoholic beverage a day for women, and one or two a day for men. More than that not only adds additional empty calories but can also sabotage your willpower. For alcohol options that are both gluten free and South Beach Diet friendly, see page 128.

Allow yourself the occasional indulgence. Vacations in particular are a time to relax and have the occasional treat, not a time to stress about being absolutely perfect on a diet. If you have been gluten aware for a while, you will already know how much of which foods trigger your symptoms. While a bit of indulgence is well deserved, you don't want to return home 5 pounds heavier or sick from gluten overload. If you get carried away, be sure to return to your healthy eating habits at the next meal.

Find time for exercise. Any vacation or business trip can easily disrupt a regular exercise schedule, but that doesn't mean you should skip exercise altogether. In fact, it is the perfect antidote to those occasional indulgences and it makes you feel good. If you belong to a national-chain gym, ask about getting access to their various club locations. Many hotels will also offer passes to a local gym or fitness center. Another alternative is to avail yourself of the hotel gym or workout room. Most major hotels have at least a bike, a treadmill, or an elliptical machine along with free weights, and many have a pool. If possible, get out and walk if there are sidewalks or climb the hotel stairs if need be. And if all else fails, exercise in your room (packing portable exercise bands and/or an exercise DVD is easy; these items take up little room in your suitcase).

MORE TRAVEL BASICS

No matter where you travel or by what conveyance, planning ahead is important, especially when it comes to avoiding or cutting back on gluten. There's no worse time to get a stomachache, diarrhea, bloating, or a skin rash than when you're on a romantic vacation or important business trip.

Whatever your destination, a good first step is to review travel Web sites, forums, and chat boards to read comments from others who have been where you're going (see pages 234 to 235 for a list of some of the best). You can then make the healthiest choice of an airline or cruise line, for example, and also make a list of restaurants that have gluten-free options in the places you plan to visit. If you're traveling to a country where another language will be spoken, you can learn the words for "wheat, barley, and rye" and just make your own determination of what you can and can't have. If you have celiac disease, of course, you may want to download the appropriate gluten-free dining card or travel dining app (see page 233). You'll also need to consider the nutritional guidelines for the phase of the South Beach Diet Gluten Solution you're on and plan accordingly. Tip: Don't start GS Phase 1 while you're traveling. Why make it more difficult?

If you know where you're staying and plan to be there for a while, you may want to ship nonperishable gluten-free foods such as gluten-free crackers and cereal, gluten-free dried fruit, and unseasoned nuts to your destination directly from home or from an online source, so that you don't have to pack them or shop for these foods when you get there. If that doesn't work, request a mini fridge for your hotel room and shop for some items as soon as you arrive.

IF YOU'RE TRAVELING BY AIR

Getting meals on planes these days is hard enough for people who don't have special dietary needs. With so many airlines cutting costs, you can barely get a standard meal much less a GFML (that's the airline code for gluten-free meal) or snack without paying a premium. This is particularly true if your flight is less than 4 hours in duration, which eliminates most domestic flights (some transcontinental flights do offer gluten-free meals to premium-, first-, and business-class passengers only). The TSA also has strict regulations about what you can and can't bring on a plane in the way of food (see page 190), so it's important to be regulation aware as well as gluten aware. Here are some pointers:

Reserve your special meal(s) well ahead. Nearly all airlines require at least 24 hours' notice for special meals, and many change their policies frequently. If you are traveling while on the first 4 weeks of the program, or you are highly gluten sensitive, it's best to request your gluten-free meal(s) when you book your flight, then follow up, ideally with a reservationist, closer to departure to make sure your request has actually been noted. Check glutenfreetravelsite .com/glutenfreeairlines or glutenfreepassport.com/allergy-gluten-free-travel/ airline-meal-codes for carriers that offer gluten-free meals.

Don't always trust what's on your plate, though. Use your instincts: If you think that a roll that comes with your meal is questionable, don't eat it. Also keep in mind that if anything changes with your itinerary, the odds that your special meal will follow you to your new flight are slim to none. If you are gluten aware, just use your head about what to eat whenever you fly. You should know what foods trigger a gluten reaction.

Bring your own food. If you don't want to take the chance that you'll go hungry on a long flight like poor Linda, have a backup plan. Most travelers who want to avoid gluten bring their own food on board in a carry-on, even if they have reserved a special meal. That way, if there's a flight change or delay, you'll at least have your healthy snacks on hand to prevent hunger and cravings. And you won't have to take chances with questionable airport food.

The TSA regulates all food items brought through security and will literally toss anything that doesn't comply with their guidelines. Here's what those guidelines are in a nutshell: Whole unprocessed foods (like whole fruits and vegetables) don't have to be wrapped. All other prepared or processed foods like cold cuts, cheese, hard-boiled eggs, fruit salad, or sandwiches must be placed in hard-sided clear containers or be wrapped in plastic wrap (not foil), since all food must go through the x-ray machines, and the TSA doesn't want messes.

What many people don't realize, however, is that the TSA's 3-1-1 liquids rule applies to liquid and semiliquid foods in carry-on baggage. Liquids and

GLUTEN-FREE AIRLINE SNACKS

Here are some ideas for South Beach Diet–friendly gluten-free airline snacks by phase that shouldn't be a problem to carry on if they're wrapped properly. Remember: Bringing snacks and meals on a flight *is not a license to eat everything in your bag.* Follow the healthy eating guidelines outlined in the Gluten Solution Program.

PHASE 1

Lean, reduced-sodium deli meats (turkey and chicken breast, roast beef, boiled ham) or your own sliced leftovers

Raw veggies, such as celery sticks, green or red bell pepper strips, cauliflower and broccoli florets, edamame

Hard-boiled eggs

Part-skim mozzarella cheese sticks, light spreadable cheese wedges, and other reduced-fat cheeses

Nuts in a jar or bag, not cans (limit to a ¼-cup serving)

Sunflower seeds (limit to a ¼-cup serving)

Hummus (only if in 3-oz. containers or less and packed with liquids; keep cool once scanned)

Pouched light tuna (3-oz. pouch, must be packed with liquids)

Olives (15 small green or 8 small black as a serving)

gels may be carried on if they're at or under the required 3.4-ounce volume, provided that all such containers fit into a single transparent 1-quart resealable plastic bag. According to the TSA, soft or pourable foods that count as liquids include peanut butter, jelly, pudding, hummus, applesauce, cottage cheese, cream cheese, mayonnaise, ketchup, yogurt, dips, salad dressings, soups, and more. If you include your peanut butter and jelly or cream cheese or mayo in a sandwich, however, they are no longer liquids! Some of these foods, like hummus, are now being sold in 2-ounce containers; others, like mayonnaise, salad

Travel-size squeeze packets of low-sugar, gluten-free salad dressings, nut butters, mayonnaise, and so on

Sugar-free, gluten-free candies and gum

PHASE 2

Everything on Phase 1 plus the following:

Carrot sticks

Fresh fruit

Gluten-free dried fruit

Gluten-free, whole-grain, high-fiber crackers

Gluten-free, protein- and fiber-rich low-sugar meal bars and snack bars

Gluten-free whole-grain bread and wraps

Corn tortillas with gluten-free black bean spread (wrapped well)

Gluten-free instant oatmeal (ask for hot water on board)

High-fiber, gluten-free cereal with 3 g sugar or less per serving

Air-popped plain popcorn

Gluten-free dark chocolate (limit to 1 oz. per day)

dressings, and all-natural peanut butter, are available in travel-size packets online at minimus.biz/Gluten-Free.aspx. Overall, it's probably not worth siphoning your yogurt into a 3-ounce bottle, especially since you may still want to bring a few toiletries on board in that single 1-quart plastic bag.

Also keep in mind that depending on the airline, the liquid prohibition can extend to partially melted frozen foods and to ice packs, whether they are gel or liquid. If you need to keep any of your food cold, you may have to toss the ice pack before you go through screening, then fill extra resealable plastic bags with real ice before you board. A friendly flight attendant might give you some ice for your cooler bag, but you can't count on it. Your best bet may simply be to pack foods that can stay at room temperature for some period of time without spoiling.

Needless to say, what foods you'll be allowed to bring on a flight can vary widely among airports and TSA agents. It will also depend on customs, which regulates the transportation of food across international and state borders, regardless of whether such food is carried on or is packed in checked baggage. For example, travelers are not allowed to bring citrus fruits into the United States. In some cases, you may be able to consume such foods in flight, but for countries like Canada that have a US prescreening process, prohibited foods will likely be confiscated before you get on.

Many terminals are improving their healthy food offerings, and you may be able to buy a number of gluten-free foods after passing through screening. But don't count on every airport having good options.

IF YOU'RE TAKING A CRUISE

Food and drink—a lot of it—is available morning, noon, and night on cruise ships. I've had plenty of embarrassed patients on the South Beach Diet tell me that they gained 10 pounds in 7 days on a cruise because they conveniently "forgot" our healthy eating and exercise principles while on board. Being both gluten aware and weight conscious (aka health conscious) while cruising takes even more commitment than usual, but you'll feel better during the cruise and certainly better at the end of your vacation if you don't go too crazy.

Just because you've prepaid for all of your meals doesn't mean you need to devour all five courses at dinner or pay a regular visit to the midnight dessert buffet. Think three moderate, gluten-aware meals a day and a healthy mid-morning and midafternoon snack. Skip the sugary cocktails with pink umbrellas, don't drink the gluten-free beer (too many calories), and never reach for those fatty, salty "drink more" snacks!

And do not skip exercise. On bigger ships, visit the fitness center, ice-skating rink, rock-climbing wall, and the swim-against-the-current pool. If you're on a smaller vessel, take interval walks around the promenade deck to enjoy the sea air. Then dance the night away (many cruise ships have multiple lounges with bands playing everything from salsa to ballroom). Finally, on days in port, try to book an active excursion, like hiking or scuba diving or horseback riding. Some ports may be perfect for renting bikes, and you can always walk around the town or city if it's safe. With a little effort, you can turn your cruise into an opportunity to come back fitter and health-ier than ever.

Okay, now let's get to some gluten-aware cruise tips, which start with choosing the right ship:

Call a travel agent. All the major cruise lines, including Celebrity, Carni-val, Cunard, Disney, Holland America, Norwegian, Princess, and Royal Caribbean, as well as boutique lines like Silversea, Seabourn, P&O, and Azamara Club, cater to passengers with gluten sensitivities. But your experi-ence can vary widely. You can get cruise gossip and tips from other gluten-sensitive cruisers by reviewing the message boards on cruisecritic.com or look at the cruise reviews on glutenfreetravelsite.com. Once you've done a little advance research, use a travel agent. This may seem like going back to the dark ages, but the agent will likely have personal connections with var-ious lines and will make sure that your special dietary request is properly recorded. Every line is different, but some will actually order your favorite brands of certain gluten-free products if they are informed early enough, which can mean up to 90 days in advance for some trips. A travel agent can help with that and also book any pre- or post-hotel stays in places that accom-modate special diets.

If you do make your own reservation online, most cruise lines have a place to add your dietary request in the personal information section. This should help ensure that the chef and maitre d' have advance knowledge that you are gluten sensitive.

Bring some food on board. If you are on Phase 2, take a bag of gluten-free crackers, protein- and fiber-rich snack bars, cereal, and bread, or naturally gluten-free foods like nuts or fruit. You can also pick up gluten-free food from grocery stores at the ports where you dock. Remember, bringing liquor on board is not allowed.

Meet the dining room staff. Make a point to meet with the maitre d' or dining room host your first day on board to discuss your diet and to learn more about all of the dining options. Most large ships have specialty restaurants—steak house, Asian fusion, Italian—where you can dine for a surcharge, and some of these venues may be a better bet for eating gluten aware than the general dining room.

Many ships will allow you to see the next day's menus ahead of time. If that's the case, you can go over the menu with the maitre d' to special order the meal that's right for you. One cruise line promotes its gluten-free dining capabilities this way: "We are able to make quite a lot of menu items gluten free, such as roasts, fish and seafood, sauces, salads, appetizers, and desserts. Our executive chef can daily recommend a wide variety of gluten-free dishes from our featured menu. Furthermore, we are also able to make gluten-free bread and muffins as we use gluten-free flour onboard if specially requested." That's the kind of ship you want to be on.

Beware of the buffet. Most gluten-aware cruisers know better than to help themselves to anything except fresh fruit, veggie sticks, and cheese (preferably reduced-fat varieties) from the buffet. The poached salmon and roasted meats are also good bets. If you're highly gluten sensitive, you can assume there will be cross-contamination in any of the more complicated dishes. While the breakfast buffet may seem tempting, with some liners offering gluten-free pancakes, waffles, and cereal, your stomach and waistline are much better off with some fruit and a veggie omelet or eggs over easy cooked to order in the dining room.

Plan your shore trips. Research the various destinations on your cruise so that when you go ashore for your day visits, you are able to sample the local food. If you have celiac disease or are highly gluten sensitive, bring a gluten-free dining card along (see page 176) in the language of the country you're visiting so your server will understand what gluten free means.

IF YOU'RE TRAVELING BY TRAIN

As with cruising, traveling by train requires planning ahead. On most train lines, including Amtrak, you will have to bring your gluten-free food with you. Train travel does provide far more flexibility than planes for carry-on luggage, since the TSA restrictions on liquids and foods don't pertain. Just make sure you pack perishables in a cooler or insulated bag.

If you're traveling abroad, check out raileurope.com. Certain high-speed train lines, including Eurostar, have online booking for gluten-free meals if you do it 48 hours in advance. Many people prefer to take food along, since eating (and drinking) is allowed on European trains.

Again, if you've determined that you aren't highly gluten sensitive, you can monitor your intake of gluten accordingly.

IF YOU'RE TRAVELING BY CAR

While you're on the first 4 weeks of the Gluten Solution Program, travel by car gives you the most options. If it's a long car trip, you can freeze food ahead of time and carry it in a cooler to reheat in a motel or hotel microwave. Shorter trips may require only healthy gluten-free snacks.

When you know you'll be dining along the way, research your route ahead of time and locate restaurants and supermarkets using one of the travel Web sites or apps on page 233.

WHERE TO STAY

Today upscale chains like Fairmont, Omni, and Ritz-Carlton have plenty of gluten-free dining options on their restaurant menus. And you can find in-room refrigerators and microwaves in smaller hotels and motels, which means you can keep your own food handy. In addition, some bed-and-breakfasts will accommodate you if they have enough advance notice and understand what you can and can't eat in the morning. Google "gluten-free accommodations" in the town or city where you want to stay and then let the proprietor know what your preferences are. Depending on your level of sensitivity, you may be able to enjoy a piece of whole-wheat toast but not the homemade multigrain granola.

CHAPTER 14

SOUTH BEACH DIET GLUTEN SOLUTION RECIPES

ON THE FOLLOWING PAGES, WE OFFER 20 DELICIOUS SOUTH BEACH Diet–friendly gluten-free recipes from breakfasts to desserts. All were created to show you that you can avoid gluten and still enjoy the dishes you love (though we always recommend you eat baked treats in moderation).

Read through the recipes first to check for ingredients you might not have on hand, like sorghum flour, black bean flour, chickpea flour, almond flour, and xanthan gum (which is often used in gluten-free baking to produce a finer texture). If your local markets don't carry these products, check our list of online resources on page 235 for these ingredients. Also check labels carefully on common supermarket grains like oats and cornmeal, which may have been produced in plants that also manufacture wheat products.

The majority of recipes are for Phase 2, when you will be reintroducing wholesome gluten-free grains into your diet. We also include a Phase 1 "Spaghetti" and Meatballs recipe that uses spaghetti squash instead of wheat pasta along with bread-free meatballs. And our Phase 1 Spice-Rubbed Grilled Pork Chops recipe gives you a homemade gluten-free rub to replace the supermarket rubs you may have on hand that often have gluten additives.

For your convenience, each recipe also features a Hands-On Time (the active time you spend in the kitchen) and Total Time (how long it takes to make a dish from start to finish). You'll see that a number of the recipes can be prepared in 30 minutes or less and that we also provide make-ahead tips when possible. Whether you prefer to do advance prepping or not, pay attention to the "Meanwhiles" in the recipes. Doing two recipe steps at once means quicker meals.

Almond-Pear Quinoa Breakfast Cereal

HANDS-ON TIME: 5 MINUTES · TOTAL TIME: 20 MINUTES

You can make a batch of this cereal (or even a double batch) and store it in the fridge. At breakfast, just scoop out ¾ cup of the cooked quinoa and reheat in the microwave (about 45 seconds) with ¼ cup fat-free milk. (Or take it to the office and reheat there.)

1¼ cups quinoa, rinsed

¼ teaspoon fine sea salt

1 cup unsweetened almond milk

¼ teaspoon ground cinnamon

1 juicy ripe pear

½ teaspoon pure vanilla extract

1 cup fat-free milk, unsweetened almond milk, or unsweetened low-fat soy milk

2 tablespoons sliced almonds (toasted, if desired)

Monk fruit natural no-calorie sweetener, for serving (optional)

In a medium nonstick saucepan, combine the quinoa, salt, and 1 cup water. Bring to a boil, reduce to a high simmer, cover, and cook until partially cooked, about 6 minutes.

Meanwhile, place the almond milk and cinnamon in a small bowl. Core the pear and grate it on the large holes of a box grater into the almond milk. Stir to submerge the pear gratings (this keeps the fruit from turning brown).

Uncover the saucepan and add the almond milk mixture. Return to a simmer, cover, and cook, stirring occasionally, until the quinoa is tender and the milk is mostly absorbed, 9 to 11 minutes.

Remove the pan from the heat and stir in the vanilla. Serve with ¼ cup milk per serving and topped with the almonds (1½ teaspoons per serving) and a sprinkling of monk fruit sweetener, if desired.

MAKES 4 (¾-CUP) SERVINGS

Per serving: 269 calories, 5.5 g fat, 0.5 g saturated fat, 11 g protein, 45 g carbohydrate, 5.5 g fiber, 219 mg sodium

Sausage and Scrambled Egg Breakfast Tostadas

HANDS-ON TIME: 20 MINUTES · TOTAL TIME: 30 MINUTES

Eat these tostadas with a knife and fork or, if the toasted tortillas are not too brittle, fold them in half and eat like a taco. You can toast the tortillas, cook the sausages, and make the tomato salsa well ahead, if you'd like.

¼ cup chopped grape tomatoes

2 scallions, thinly sliced

Coarse kosher salt

Gluten-free chili powder

4 (6-inch) 100% corn tortillas

Olive oil cooking spray

2 gluten-free Italian-style turkey sausage links (3 ounces each)

1 tablespoon extra-virgin olive oil

1 green bell pepper, finely diced

1 small onion, finely diced

2 large eggs

½ cup liquid egg whites (or the whites of 3 large eggs)

¼ cup shredded reduced-fat Mexican-blend cheese

¼ cup nonfat (0%) plain Greek yogurt

In a small bowl, toss together the tomatoes, scallions, and a small pinch each of salt and chili powder. Set the fresh salsa aside.

Preheat the broiler. Place the tortillas on a baking sheet and very lightly coat with olive oil cooking spray. Sprinkle each lightly with a pinch of chili powder. Broil until browned and crisp, 2 to 3 minutes; watch carefully to prevent burning. Set the tortillas aside.

In a large skillet, bring ½ inch of water to a boil. Pierce the sausages in several places, add to the skillet, cover, and cook, turning once, until cooked through, about 7 minutes. Remove the sausages, and when cool enough to handle, dice.

Wipe out the skillet and heat the oil over medium-high heat. Add the bell pepper and onion and cook until the onion is softened and lightly browned, about 7 minutes.

In a small bowl, beat together the whole eggs and egg whites. Add the egg mixture and diced sausage to the skillet and scramble to your preferred doneness. Sprinkle the cheese over the eggs and let sit a minute to melt.

Top each tortilla with eggs (a generous ½ cup each) and a tablespoon each of the yogurt and salsa.

MAKES 4 SERVINGS (1 TOSTADA PER SERVING)

Per serving: 243 calories, 11 g fat, 3 g saturated fat, 20 g protein, 20 g carbohydrate, 2.5 g fiber, 443 mg sodium

Hearty Buttermilk Pancakes with Sautéed Apples

HANDS-ON TIME: 30 MINUTES · TOTAL TIME: 30 MINUTES

Mix up a batch or two of the dry mixture to have on hand; it will keep for several months in the freezer. While the cooking goes pretty quickly, if you're concerned that one batch of pancakes will cool off while you prepare the rest, keep the cooked ones warm in a 200°F oven. Because these pancakes contain chickpea flour, they are higher in protein (with 11 grams per serving) than wheat-based pancakes.

2   large apples (about 8 ounces each), cored, halved, and thinly sliced

1   tablespoon fresh lemon juice

½   cup chickpea flour

½   cup 100% buckwheat flour

2   tablespoons cornmeal

1½   teaspoons gluten-free baking powder

½   teaspoon baking soda

⅛   teaspoon salt

1¼   cups light (1.5%) buttermilk

1   large egg

⅓   cup liquid egg whites (or the whites of 2 large eggs)

1   tablespoon plus 1 teaspoon extra-virgin olive oil

    Olive oil cooking spray

In a large skillet, toss the apple slices with the lemon juice and 3 tablespoons water and cook over medium heat until tender, about 3 minutes. Remove from the heat and cover to keep warm while you make the pancakes.

In a large bowl, whisk together the chickpea flour, buckwheat flour, cornmeal, baking powder, baking soda, and salt. In a separate large bowl or large glass measuring cup, combine the buttermilk, whole egg, egg whites, and oil. Stir the liquid ingredients into the dry ingredients until no lumps remain.

Coat a large nonstick skillet with olive oil cooking spray. Heat the skillet over medium-low heat and ladle a scant ¼ cup batter per pancake into the pan (you should be able to fit about 3 pancakes). Cook until the tops of the pancakes have a few bubbles, about 2 minutes, then flip them over and cook until the undersides are done, about 1 minute. Repeat with the remaining batter.

Serve the pancakes topped with the apple slices and any juice.

MAKES 4 (3-PANCAKE) SERVINGS

Per serving: 268 calories, 8.5 g fat, 2 g saturated fat, 11 g protein, 39 g carbohydrate, 4 g fiber, 530 mg sodium

Orange-Blueberry Breakfast Muffins

HANDS-ON TIME: 15 MINUTES · TOTAL TIME: 45 MINUTES

Xanthan gum is used in gluten-free baking to bind ingredients and help produce a finer texture. But a little xanthan gum goes a long way, so store what you aren't using in the fridge or freezer, where it will keep indefinitely. To have these muffins as part of a complete breakfast, split the muffin and spread each half with some nonfat plain Greek yogurt or serve alongside a poached egg.

- ¾ cup quinoa flakes, toasted
- 1 cup sorghum flour
- 2 tablespoons chia seeds, finely ground
- 2 tablespoons granulated stevia (baking formula)
- 2 teaspoons gluten-free baking powder
- ½ teaspoon baking soda
- ½ teaspoon xanthan gum
- ¼ teaspoon salt
- 1 cup light (1.5%) buttermilk
- 3 tablespoons extra-virgin olive oil
- ⅓ cup liquid egg whites (or the whites of 2 large eggs)
- 2 tablespoons agave nectar
- 2 teaspoons grated orange zest
- 1¼ cups fresh or frozen (no need to thaw) blueberries

Preheat the oven to 375°F. Line a standard 12-cup muffin pan with paper liners. Place the quinoa flakes on a baking sheet and toast until fragrant and crisp, about 15 minutes.

In a large bowl, stir together the sorghum flour, chia seeds, stevia, baking powder, baking soda, xanthan gum, and salt.

In a separate bowl, whisk together the buttermilk, oil, egg whites, agave nectar, and orange zest. Make a well in the center of the dry ingredients, pour in the buttermilk mixture, and stir gently to combine. Fold in the blueberries.

Divide the batter evenly among the muffin cups (this is easily done with a small ice-cream scoop).

Bake until a toothpick inserted in the center of a muffin comes out clean, 17 to 20 minutes. Remove the muffins from the pan and transfer to a rack to cool.

MAKES 12 MUFFINS (1 PER SERVING)

Per muffin: 132 calories, 5 g fat, 1 g saturated fat, 4 g protein, 20 g carbohydrate, 2.5 g fiber, 213 mg sodium

Quiche Lorraine Minis

HANDS-ON TIME: 15 MINUTES · TOTAL TIME: 50 MINUTES

These are a great grab-and-go breakfast. With 19 grams of protein, a single mini quiche is a satisfying and energizing way to start your day. Make a whole batch and refrigerate (they will keep well for at least a week), then reheat them, wrapped in a paper towel, in the microwave for 30 to 45 seconds—take care, though; the cheese will get hot.

Olive oil cooking spray

1 teaspoon extra-virgin olive oil

4 ounces gluten-free Canadian bacon, coarsely chopped

¾ cup chickpea flour

1 can (12 ounces) fat-free evaporated milk

6 tablespoons liquid egg whites

1 whole egg

2 teaspoons Dijon mustard

Pinch each freshly ground black pepper and ground nutmeg

1 cup shredded reduced-fat Swiss cheese (4 ounces)

Preheat the oven to 350°F. If your jumbo muffin pan isn't nonstick, lightly coat the cups with olive oil cooking spray.

In a large nonstick skillet, heat the oil over medium-high heat. Add the Canadian bacon and cook, stirring often, until lightly browned, 4 to 5 minutes.

In a bowl, whisk together the chickpea flour, evaporated milk, egg whites, whole egg, mustard, pepper, and nutmeg until just blended.

Divide the bacon evenly among the muffin cups. Divide the cheese among the cups. Pour the custard mixture over the cheese and bacon (the cups will be about three-fourths full).

Bake until nicely browned on top and cooked through but still moist, 30 to 35 minutes. Transfer to a rack to cool slightly. Serve warm or at room temperature.

MAKES 6 MINI QUICHES (1 PER SERVING)

Per mini quiche: 213 calories, 8 g fat, 3.5 g saturated fat, 19 g protein, 15 g carbohydrate, 1 g fiber, 503 mg sodium

Crispy Fish Fillets with Spicy Mayo

HANDS-ON TIME: 10 MINUTES · TOTAL TIME: 25 MINUTES

Baked fish fillets are often coated with wheat bread crumbs to make them crispy. Here, ground walnuts and chickpea flour are the stand-ins, and a brief turn under the broiler makes the walnut coating extra crunchy. Tomato paste brushed on the fish fillets first not only keeps them moist but also helps keep the walnut topping in place.

- 2 tablespoons no-salt-added tomato paste
- ⅓ cup walnuts, finely ground (use a mini food processor)
- 3 tablespoons chickpea flour
- ¼ teaspoon salt
- 4 fish fillets, such as tilapia, flounder, red snapper, or sea bass (about 6 ounces each)
- 4 teaspoons extra-virgin olive oil
- 2 tablespoons light mayonnaise
- 2 teaspoons fresh lemon juice
- 1 teaspoon smoked paprika
  Pinch cayenne pepper

Preheat the oven to 400°F. In a small bowl, stir together the tomato paste and 2 teaspoons water. In another small bowl, combine the walnuts, chickpea flour, and salt.

Place the fish on a broilerproof baking sheet and brush the tops with the tomato paste mixture.

Sprinkle the walnut mixture over the top of the fish and press to adhere. Drizzle each fillet with 1 teaspoon of the olive oil.

Bake until just cooked through, 10 to 12 minutes. Turn on the broiler and place the fish under the broiler to crisp, 30 to 45 seconds (watch carefully to prevent burning).

Meanwhile, in a small bowl, whisk together the mayonnaise, lemon juice, paprika, and cayenne. Serve the fish with the spicy mayo.

MAKES 4 SERVINGS

Per serving: 308 calories, 17 g fat, 2.5 g saturated fat, 33 g protein, 6 g carbohydrate, 1.5 g fiber, 294 mg sodium

Mushroom and Black Bean Bake

HANDS-ON TIME: 25 MINUTES · TOTAL TIME: 1 HOUR
PLUS 15 MINUTES STANDING TIME

The mushroom-bean mixture can be prepared well ahead and refrigerated. If it seems too dry when you go to use it, stir a spoon or two of the tomato sauce into it to moisten. If you like spice, bump up the chile powder to 1 teaspoon total (½ teaspoon with the mushrooms and ½ teaspoon in the tomato sauce). Leftovers hold up well in the refrigerator for about a week. Reheat briefly in a microwave oven or in a toaster oven set to bake at about 300°F.

  1 can (14.5 ounces) no-salt-added diced tomatoes
  1 can (15 ounces) no-salt-added gluten-free black beans, drained and rinsed
  2 tablespoons no-salt-added tomato paste
  4 teaspoons extra-virgin olive oil
  ½ teaspoon chipotle chile powder
  1 large portobello mushroom cap (6 ounces)
  1 small sweet onion (5 ounces), diced
  2 cloves garlic, minced
  ¼ teaspoon coarse kosher salt
  1 cup nonfat ricotta cheese
  ⅓ cup liquid egg whites (or the whites of 2 large eggs)
  1 large egg
  ¼ cup grated Parmesan cheese
  5 (6-inch) 100% corn tortillas, halved

Preheat the oven to 375°F.

Measure out ½ cup of the diced tomatoes and transfer to a medium bowl. Stir in the beans, lightly crush some of the beans with a fork or potato masher, and set aside.

Transfer the remaining tomatoes to a mini food processor. Add the tomato paste, 2 teaspoons of the oil, and ¼ teaspoon of the chile powder. Purée to a smooth sauce.

With a small spoon, scrape out the black gills from the portobello. Cut the cap into small dice.

In a large nonstick skillet, heat the remaining 2 teaspoons oil over medium-high heat. Add the onion and garlic and cook until beginning to soften, about 2 minutes. Add the mushrooms, sprinkle with the salt and the remaining ¼ teaspoon chile powder, and cook, stirring often, until both the mushrooms and onion are softened, about 4 minutes. Stir in the black bean mixture and cook for 2 minutes to blend the flavors.

Meanwhile, in a small bowl, stir together the ricotta, egg whites, whole egg, and Parmesan.

Spread one-third of the tomato sauce over the bottom of an 8 × 8-inch nonstick baking pan. Top the tomato sauce with 4 tortilla halves, lining up the cut edges with the sides of the pan. Use a fifth tortilla half to cover the hole in the middle. Top with half of the bean mixture and dollop with half of the remaining tomato sauce. Repeat the layering. Spread the ricotta mixture over the top, making sure it goes to the edges of the pan.

Bake until the topping is puffed and golden, 30 to 35 minutes. Let stand for 15 minutes before cutting into quarters and serving.

MAKES 4 SERVINGS

Per serving: 347 calories, 8 g fat, 2 g saturated fat, 24 g protein, 45 g carbohydrate, 9 g fiber, 362 mg sodium

Individual Eggplant Parmesan Stacks

HANDS-ON TIME: 10 MINUTES · TOTAL TIME: 40 MINUTES

Eggplant is often fried before being made into eggplant Parmesan. For this meatless main dish, thick slices are coated in a nut and Parmesan cheese mixture, drizzled with just a little olive oil, and baked until crisp. Once the eggplant is done, it gets topped with tomato slices and a creamy cheese and baked again. It's easy to make, fresh, and light.

- ⅓ cup cornmeal
- ⅓ cup liquid egg whites (or the whites of 2 large eggs)
- ½ cup almond flour
- ⅓ cup grated Parmesan cheese
- ½ teaspoon dried oregano, crumbled
- ¼ teaspoon freshly ground black pepper
- 1 pound eggplant, peeled in stripes (some skin on, some off) and cut crosswise into 8 rounds (¾-inch thick)
- 1 tablespoon extra-virgin olive oil
- ¼ teaspoon salt
- 16 plum tomato slices (from about 3 tomatoes)
- 4 wedges (¾ ounce each) light spreadable cheese, halved horizontally

Preheat the oven to 400°F. Place the cornmeal in a shallow bowl. In another shallow bowl, beat the egg whites with 1 tablespoon water. In a third shallow bowl, mix together the almond flour, Parmesan, oregano, and pepper.

Line a baking sheet with parchment paper. Dip both sides of each eggplant round first in the cornmeal, then in the egg white mixture (letting any excess drip off), and then in the almond flour mixture to coat well. Pat so the almond mixture adheres.

Place the eggplant on the baking sheet and drizzle the oil over the slices. Sprinkle the salt over the top. Bake until the eggplant is tender and the undersides of the slices are golden, about 20 minutes. Turn the eggplant over and top each slice with 2 tomato slices and half of a cheese wedge. Mash the cheese wedge down with a fork.

Bake until the tomato is hot and the cheese has melted slightly, about 10 minutes.

MAKES 4 SERVINGS (2 STACKS PER SERVING)

Per serving: 267 calories, 15 g fat, 3 g saturated fat, 12 g protein, 23 g carbohydrate, 6.5 g fiber, 545 mg sodium

Chicken with Lemon-Scallion Sauce

HANDS-ON TIME: 15 MINUTES · TOTAL TIME: 15 MINUTES

The delicious sauce for this simple chicken dish is thickened with chickpea flour, which, in addition to adding its own hearty flavor, adds protein and fiber. The dish is good all by itself, but it would be great over brown basmati rice or red quinoa (½ cup cooked per serving). To keep the chicken moist and juicy, take care not to overcook it the first time it goes into the pan. It will continue to cook out of the pan from residual heat, and then it gets a second cooking with the sauce.

1¼ cups reduced-sodium gluten-free chicken broth

3 tablespoons chickpea flour

2 teaspoons grated lemon zest

¼ cup fresh lemon juice

¼ teaspoon garlic powder

¼ teaspoon salt

¼ teaspoon freshly ground black pepper

4 teaspoons extra-virgin olive oil

1½ pounds boneless, skinless chicken breasts, very thinly sliced (as for stir-fry)

6 scallions, chopped

2 tablespoons minced fresh cilantro or parsley

In a small bowl, stir ½ cup of the chicken broth into the chickpea flour to make a smooth paste. Then stir in the remaining ¾ cup chicken broth, the lemon zest, lemon juice, garlic powder, salt, and pepper. Stir well to blend. Set aside.

In a large nonstick skillet, heat 2 teaspoons of the oil over medium-high heat. Add the chicken and cook, tossing to separate the pieces, until just opaque, about 2 minutes. (It's okay if they're still a little pink; they will continue to cook later.) With a slotted spoon, transfer the chicken to a plate.

Add the remaining 2 teaspoons oil and the scallions to the pan and stir until beginning to soften, about 1 minute. Stir the chicken broth mixture to recombine and pour the mixture into the pan. Bring to a boil, stirring, then stir the cilantro or parsley into the sauce.

Return the chicken (and the collected juices on the plate) to the pan, toss to coat with the sauce, and cook to heat through, about 45 seconds.

MAKES 4 SERVINGS

Per serving: 263 calories, 9.5 g fat, 1.5 g saturated fat, 38 g protein, 5 g carbohydrate, 1 g fiber, 490 mg sodium

Black Bean "Pizza"
with Tomatoes and Artichokes

HANDS-ON TIME: 10 MINUTES · TOTAL TIME: 35 MINUTES

Black bean flour makes a breadlike base for a vegetarian main-course "pizza." The advantages this crust has over a regular pizza are that, in addition to being gluten free, it is exceptionally high in fiber, protein, and antioxidants (from the black beans). It's best served warm, straight from the oven. But if you want to make the crust ahead, you can. Reheat it in a 325°F oven for about 10 minutes before topping with the tomato-artichoke mixture.

- 1 package (9 ounces) frozen artichoke hearts, thawed and coarsely chopped
- 3 plum tomatoes, diced
- ⅓ cup shredded fresh basil (optional)
- 2 teaspoons balsamic vinegar
- 1½ cups black bean flour
- 1 teaspoon gluten-free baking powder
- ½ teaspoon garlic powder
- ½ teaspoon salt
- ¼ teaspoon freshly ground black pepper
- 6 tablespoons liquid egg whites (or the whites of 2 large eggs)
- 2 tablespoons no-salt-added tomato paste
- 2 teaspoons extra-virgin olive oil
- ¾ cup (3 ounces) shredded reduced-fat cheese, such as Cheddar, Monterey Jack, or Mexican blend

Preheat the oven to 375°F. Line a 10 × 15-inch rimmed baking sheet with parchment paper. Coat the paper lightly with cooking spray (preferably olive oil spray).

In a bowl, toss together the artichoke hearts, tomatoes, basil (if using), and vinegar. Set aside.

In a second bowl, whisk together the black bean flour, baking powder, garlic powder, salt, and pepper. Add the egg whites and ¾ cup plus 3 tablespoons water (if using actual egg whites, add 2 teaspoons more water here) and stir to blend. The batter will resemble a thick cake batter.

Scrape the batter into the lined baking sheet and spread evenly. Bake until the crust is firm on the top, about 10 minutes (don't worry if it cracks).

Meanwhile, in a small bowl, blend together the tomato paste, 2 tablespoons water, and the olive oil.

Remove the crust from the oven and brush all over and all the way to edges with the tomato paste mixture. Sprinkle evenly with the cheese. Return to the oven and bake until the cheese melts and begins to brown, 7 to 9 minutes.

Remove from the oven, top the crust with the artichoke-tomato mixture, and let sit for 5 minutes before cutting into 4 rectangles.

MAKES 4 SERVINGS

Per serving: 321 calories, 8 g fat, 3 g saturated fat, 21 g protein, 44 g carbohydrate, 12 g fiber, 508 mg sodium

"Spaghetti" and Meatballs

HANDS-ON TIME: 15 MINUTES · TOTAL TIME: 40 MINUTES

Spaghetti squash is an oddity of the vegetable world that is a boon to those restricting gluten in their diets. This winter squash, once cooked, has flesh that can be pulled into long pastalike strands that make an exceptionally satisfying stand-in for flour-based noodles. Spaghetti squash even has regular spaghetti beat on the time-saving front, too: It takes only about 10 minutes in the microwave (as opposed to the 20-plus minutes it takes to boil pasta). The meatballs—which are made without any bread crumbs—can be prepared well ahead and frozen. Thaw them in the refrigerator and let them come to room temperature before adding to the simmering sauce. For the bottled marinara, use one that has less than 3 grams of sugar per ½-cup serving.

    1 package (10 ounces) cremini mushrooms
    1 teaspoon extra-virgin olive oil
 2½ cups bottled marinara sauce
  ¾ pound gluten-free lean ground turkey breast
  ⅓ cup plus 4 teaspoons grated Parmesan cheese
    2 tablespoons no-salt-added tomato paste
       Freshly ground black pepper
    1 spaghetti squash (3 pounds)

Measure out about one-third of the mushrooms and very finely mince (this is a good place to use a mini food processor). Thinly slice the remainder of the mushrooms.

In a large nonstick skillet, heat the oil over medium-high heat. Add the sliced mushrooms and cook, without stirring, for 2 minutes. Then stir until softened, about 1 minute longer. Add the marinara sauce and reduce the heat so the sauce simmers while you make the meatballs.

In a medium bowl, combine the turkey, ⅓ cup of the Parmesan, the tomato paste, and a generous pinch of pepper. Form into 24 meatballs, each the size of a large walnut.

Add the meatballs to the simmering sauce, cover, and simmer for 10 minutes. Turn the meatballs over, cover, and cook until cooked through, 10 to 15 minutes longer.

Meanwhile, pierce the spaghetti squash in several places with a knife or kitchen fork. Microwave on high until the squash is firm-tender (but not too soft), about 10 minutes. Test it by piercing it with a sharp knife; there should be a little bit of resistance, but the knife should go in easily. Let stand for 2 minutes.

When just cool enough to handle, use a large sturdy knife to halve the squash lengthwise. Holding it with a potholder, scoop out and discard the seeds from the center, then use a fork to pull the squash flesh into strands, letting them fall into a large bowl. Ladle out about 1 cup of the marinara sauce (just enough to lightly coat) and toss with the spaghetti squash.

To serve, divide the spaghetti squash among 4 pasta bowls and top with the remaining sauce, the meatballs (6 per serving), and Parmesan (1 teaspoon per serving).

MAKES 4 SERVINGS

Per serving: 298 calories, 11 g fat, 4.5 g saturated fat, 23 g protein, 32 g carbohydrate, 7.5 g fiber, 542 mg sodium

Spice-Rubbed Grilled Pork Chops

HANDS-ON TIME: 10 MINUTES · TOTAL TIME: 10 MINUTES

Sometimes store-bought rubs have stabilizers added to keep them from caking, and these can have gluten, so check the label to be sure you're buying a gluten-free product. Better yet, use our gluten-free rub, which features a mix of spices including smoked paprika and garam masala. Garam masala is an Indian blend of hot and sweet spices that can be found on the supermarket spice shelf. The rub is great on pork (as here), but it's equally good on beef or chicken. Make up a big batch so you'll have it on hand. Store in a cool, dry spot in an airtight container for up to 2 months.

1 teaspoon ground coriander

½ teaspoon ground cumin

½ teaspoon garam masala

½ teaspoon smoked paprika

¼ teaspoon dried oregano, crumbled

¼ teaspoon salt

¼ teaspoon freshly ground black pepper

⅛ teaspoon garlic powder

8 boneless pork loin chops (3 ounces each)

1 tablespoon extra-virgin olive oil

In a small bowl, stir together the coriander, cumin, garam masala, paprika, oregano, salt, pepper, and garlic powder.

Lightly coat a grill or grill pan with cooking spray and heat over medium heat.

Sprinkle each side of each pork chop with a little more than ¼ teaspoon of the rub. Rub with oil. Grill the pork until cooked through but still juicy, 1 to 1½ minutes per side.

MAKES 4 SERVINGS (2 CHOPS PER SERVING)

Per serving: 265 calories, 14 g fat, 4.5 g saturated fat, 32 g protein, 0 g carbohydrate, 0.5 g fiber, 216 mg sodium

Tomato-Feta Quinoa Tabbouleh with Pumpkin Seeds

HANDS-ON TIME: 15 MINUTES · TOTAL TIME: 30 MINUTES

Technically, a tabbouleh (a Middle Eastern grain salad) is made with couscous, but in this version, quinoa makes a crunchy, refreshing stand-in. This could also easily be upgraded to a main-dish salad. Just grill chicken or turkey breast cutlets (about 4 ounces per person) and serve atop the quinoa mixture. The salad holds up remarkably well in the refrigerator because the quinoa does not get mushy and would make a good take-along for a lunch at the office.

¾ cup red or white quinoa

¼ teaspoon plus a pinch coarse kosher salt

1 tablespoon fresh lemon juice

1 tablespoon extra-virgin olive oil

¼ teaspoon freshly ground black pepper

1 cup grape tomatoes, quartered

4 scallions, sliced

½ cup chopped fresh flat-leaf parsley

¼ cup crumbled reduced-fat feta cheese

2 tablespoons plus 2 teaspoons pumpkin seeds, toasted and chopped

Cook the quinoa according to package directions, using ¼ teaspoon of the coarse salt in the cooking water.

Meanwhile, in a large bowl, whisk together the lemon juice, oil, and pepper. Add the tomatoes and scallions and sprinkle with a pinch of salt.

Drain the quinoa well and add to the bowl, tossing well to combine. Sprinkle on the feta cheese and toss gently.

Serve at room temperature or chilled, topped with pumpkin seeds (2 teaspoons per serving).

MAKES 4 (SCANT 1-CUP) SERVINGS

Per serving: 138 calories, 5.5 g fat, 1 g saturated fat, 5 g protein, 18 g carbohydrate, 2 g fiber, 72 mg sodium

Turkey and Noodles in Broth

HANDS-ON TIME: 25 MINUTES · TOTAL TIME: 35 MINUTES

This dish is similar to a Vietnamese pho, *which in turn is based on a traditional French dish called pot-au-feu, a one-dish meal of meat and vegetables cooked in a flavorful broth. The Vietnamese spin on the French classic adds noodles and Asian seasonings. For time efficiency, prep the vegetables while the onions are cooking and prep the turkey while the vegetables are cooking in the broth.*

 4 teaspoons extra-virgin olive oil

 1 small red onion (5 ounces), halved and very finely slivered

 3 cloves garlic, thinly sliced

 2 carrots, thinly sliced on an angle

2½ cups reduced-sodium gluten-free chicken broth

 8 ounces snow peas, strings removed, cut crosswise into thirds, on an angle

 2 teaspoons grated lime zest

  Freshly ground black pepper

 1 package (3.75 ounces) cellophane noodles (bean threads)

 1 tablespoon reduced-sodium gluten-free tamari soy sauce

 4 turkey breast cutlets (about 16 ounces total), very thinly sliced across the grain (as for stir-fry)

 1 tablespoon fresh lime juice

In a nonstick Dutch oven, heat 2 teaspoons of the oil over medium-high heat. Add the onion, reduce the heat to medium, and cook, stirring often, until very nicely browned, 7 to 9 minutes. With a slotted spoon, transfer the caramelized onion to a bowl and set aside.

 Add the remaining 2 teaspoons oil to the Dutch oven and heat over medium-high heat. Add the garlic and carrots and cook until the garlic is fragrant, about 1 minute. Add the broth, 1½ cups water, the snow peas, lime zest, and a generous pinch of pepper. Bring to a boil. Reduce to a simmer and cook until the carrots are crisp-tender, about 5 minutes.

 Meanwhile, break the bundles of noodles in half or into thirds (so the noodles won't be so long) and place in a medium bowl. Soften the noodles according to package directions. Drain, return to the bowl, and toss with the tamari soy sauce.

Add the turkey to the simmering broth and cook until just cooked through, 45 seconds to 1 minute. Stir in the lime juice.

To serve, divide the noodles among 4 deep soup bowls. Drizzle in any soy sauce remaining in the bowl. Scoop the turkey and vegetables over the noodles. Ladle one-fourth of the broth (about 1 cup) into each bowl. Top with the caramelized onions.

MAKES 4 SERVINGS

Per serving: 312 calories, 5.5 g fat, 0.5 g saturated fat, 31 g protein, 34 g carbohydrate, 3 g fiber, 553 mg sodium

Toasted Walnut Bread

HANDS-ON TIME: 20 MINUTES · TOTAL TIME: 1 HOUR 15 MINUTES

For the greatest efficiency, measure out the dry ingredients and the wet ingredients (in separate bowls) while the oven preheats and the walnuts toast. If you'd prefer, and to save a little more time, you can toast the walnuts in a toaster oven: 350°F for 3 to 5 minutes. When making a quick bread with wet ingredients (like zucchini), the surest way to tell if the bread is done is with an instant-read thermometer. The center of the bread should register at least 200°F (but not more than 210°F). Enjoy this bread for breakfast (see page 135). Or have a slice as a snack or for dessert with a glass of fat-free or 1% milk.

   3 ounces walnuts (about 1 cup)

1½ cups sorghum flour

 ½ cup nonfat milk powder

 ½ cup gluten-free oat bran

 ¼ cup flaxmeal

  1 tablespoon unsweetened cocoa powder

1½ teaspoons gluten-free baking powder

 ¾ teaspoon fine sea salt

  1 large egg

 ¼ cup liquid egg whites

 ¼ cup extra-virgin olive oil

  2 cups grated zucchini (10 ounces, 1 large or 2 small squash)

Preheat the oven to 350°F. Line the bottom and long sides of a 9 × 5-inch loaf pan with parchment paper, leaving a 1-inch overhang (a piece of parchment about 8½ × 12 inches).

Spread the walnuts on a baking sheet and bake until lightly toasted, 7 to 9 minutes. Transfer to a plate to cool and leave the oven on.

Transfer the walnuts to a mini food processor. Pulse-chop to coarse pieces. Set aside ¼ cup (to stir into the batter). Add about ¼ cup of the sorghum flour to the walnuts remaining in the processor and pulse until ground to the texture of very fine crumbs (take care not to pulse to a paste).

Transfer the ground walnut mixture to the bowl of a stand mixer. Add the rest of the flour, the milk powder, oat bran, flaxmeal, cocoa, baking powder, and salt and blend well.

Beat in the whole egg, egg whites, $\frac{1}{2}$ cup water, and the oil. With a wooden spoon, beat in the zucchini and reserved chopped walnuts (the batter will be very stiff; more like a cookie dough). Scrape into the loaf pan and smooth the top. Bake until a toothpick inserted in the center comes out clean and the center of the bread registers 200°F, 55 minutes to 1 hour.

Let cool in the pan on a rack for 10 minutes. Then using the parchment overhang, pull out of the pan, remove the paper, and set the bread on the rack to cool completely before cutting into $\frac{1}{2}$-inch-thick slices.

MAKES 16 SLICES (1 PER SERVING)

Per slice: 142 calories, 8.5 g fat, 1 g saturated fat, 5 g protein, 15 g carbohydrate, 3 g fiber, 184 mg sodium

Double-Chocolate Cupcakes

HANDS-ON TIME: 15 MINUTES · TOTAL TIME: 35 MINUTES

For these chocolaty treats, choose a high-quality gluten-free dark chocolate with about 70% cacao. This will give you less added sugar and more of the heart-healthy polyphenols found in this type of chocolate. Tapioca starch is added to the brown rice flour here to add body to the cupcakes.

1 cup 1% milk

¼ cup extra-virgin olive oil

1 large egg

2 tablespoons agave nectar

1 teaspoon pure vanilla extract

⅔ cup brown rice flour

½ cup tapioca starch

½ cup granulated stevia (baking formula)

⅓ cup unsweetened cocoa powder

1 teaspoon gluten-free baking powder

½ teaspoon xanthan gum

¼ teaspoon salt

2 ounces gluten-free dark chocolate

Preheat the oven to 350°F. Line 12 cups of a muffin pan with paper liners.

In a small bowl, whisk together the milk, oil, egg, agave nectar, and vanilla.

In a large bowl, whisk together the brown rice flour, tapioca starch, stevia, cocoa, baking powder, xanthan gum, and salt. Add the milk mixture and stir until smooth. Divide the batter evenly among the 12 cups and bake until the tops spring back when lightly touched, about 20 minutes.

Remove the cupcakes from the pan and cool on a rack.

While the cupcakes are cooling, in a microwaveable bowl, heat the chocolate on high power in three or four 20-second increments, stirring well after each, until the chocolate is smooth and melted.

When the cupcakes are cool, spread the melted chocolate over the tops.

MAKES 12 CUPCAKES (1 PER SERVING)

Per cupcake: 183 calories, 12 g fat, 2.5 g saturated fat, 3 g protein, 20 g carbohydrate, 2 g fiber, 110 mg sodium

Lemon Polenta Cake

HANDS-ON TIME: 10 MINUTES · TOTAL TIME: 35 MINUTES

This Italian-style dessert cake, reminiscent of corn bread, is sweet with a hint of lemon and a slight herbal note from the rosemary. Supermarket cornmeal is the cornmeal of choice here (no need to buy cornmeal marketed as "polenta").

   Olive oil cooking spray
½ cup regular cornmeal (not stone-ground), plus more for dusting
¾ cup almond flour
1 teaspoon gluten-free baking powder
¼ teaspoon baking soda
¼ teaspoon salt
1 teaspoon grated lemon zest
1 large egg
⅓ cup liquid egg whites (or the whites of 2 large eggs)
⅓ cup light (1.5%) buttermilk
⅓ cup extra-virgin olive oil
3 tablespoons agave nectar
½ cup granulated stevia (baking formula)
½ teaspoon dried crumbled rosemary

Preheat the oven to 375°F. Coat an 8-inch round cake pan with olive oil cooking spray and dust it with cornmeal. In a large bowl, whisk together the cornmeal, almond flour, baking powder, baking soda, salt, and lemon zest.

In a separate large bowl, whisk together the whole egg, egg whites, buttermilk, oil, agave nectar, stevia, and rosemary. Fold the dry mixture into the egg mixture. Scrape the batter into the pan and bake until a toothpick inserted in the center comes out clean and the sides begin to pull away from the pan, 25 to 30 minutes.

Let cool for 15 minutes in the pan, then run a spatula around the edges of the pan and invert the cake onto a rack. Cut into 10 wedges. Serve warm or at room temperature.

MAKES 10 SERVINGS (1 WEDGE PER SERVING)
Per serving: 175 calories, 12 g fat, 1.5 g saturated fat, 4 g protein, 15 g carbohydrate, 1.5 g fiber, 171 mg sodium

Pistachio Biscotti

HANDS-ON TIME: 10 MINUTES · TOTAL TIME: 40 MINUTES

The flavors of pistachio and lime work really well together, but feel free to experiment with your favorite nut and citrus combo: Try pecan and orange or almond and lemon. Keep the biscotti stored in an airtight container, where they will keep for up to a week. Enjoy one biscotti with a pear or apple and a low-fat or fat-free cappuccino.

1⅓ cups almond flour

¼ cup granulated stevia (baking formula)

½ teaspoon xanthan gum

¼ teaspoon baking soda

¼ teaspoon salt

1 teaspoon grated lime zest

¾ teaspoon ground cinnamon

1 tablespoon plus 1 teaspoon fresh lime juice

⅓ cup liquid egg whites (or the whites of 2 large eggs)

¼ cup pistachios, chopped

Preheat the oven to 350°F. Line a baking sheet with parchment paper.

In a food processor, pulse the almond flour, stevia, xanthan gum, baking soda, salt, lime zest, and cinnamon. Add the lime juice and egg whites and pulse until the dough forms a ball. Transfer to a bowl and knead in the pistachios.

Divide the dough in half and shape each half into a log 6½ inches long, 2½ inches wide, and ½ inch thick. Place the two logs on the baking sheet, spacing them 2 inches apart. Bake until firmed and set, about 20 minutes. Remove from the oven, but leave the oven on and reduce the temperature to 300°F.

Let the logs cool slightly on a rack. Then slice each log crosswise into 10 biscotti. Return the cookies to the baking sheet, laying them flat, and bake until crisp, about 10 minutes. Transfer to a rack to cool.

MAKES 20 BISCOTTI (1 PER SERVING)

Per biscotti: 54 calories, 4.5 g fat, 0.5 g saturated fat, 2 g protein, 3 g carbohydrate, 1 g fiber, 53 mg sodium

Banana-Nut Snack Bars

HANDS-ON TIME: 10 MINUTES · TOTAL TIME: 40 MINUTES

These bars are easily put together and packed full of healthy ingredients. Ideal for an on-the-go snack, they will keep for several days in the fridge in an airtight container. For longer storage, wrap them individually and freeze for up to 3 months.

1   cup gluten-free rolled oats

½   cup pecans

⅓   cup (½ ounce) unsweetened, gluten-free dried apple slices, broken into small bits

3   tablespoons gluten-free dried currants

3   tablespoons ground flaxmeal

¼   teaspoon salt

¾   cup mashed banana (from 2 medium bananas)

3   tablespoons agave nectar

3   tablespoons liquid egg whites (or the white of 1 large egg)

1   teaspoon pure vanilla extract

Preheat the oven to 350°F. Place the oats in a baking pan and bake until fragrant and lightly browned, about 10 minutes. Leave the oven on.

Meanwhile, coat an 8 × 8-inch baking pan with cooking spray. Line the pan with parchment, leaving an overhang on two sides; coat the parchment with cooking spray.

Transfer ½ cup of the toasted oats to a large bowl. Coarsely chop ¼ cup of the pecans and add them to the bowl along with the dried apple, currants, flaxmeal, and salt. In a food processor, finely grind the remaining ½ cup toasted oats and the remaining ¼ cup pecans. Add them to the bowl along with the mashed banana, agave nectar, egg whites, and vanilla. Stir to combine.

Spoon the mixture into the lined baking pan and pat to an even layer. Bake until set, about 20 minutes. Let cool in the pan. Use the parchment overhang to lift it out of the pan, then cut into 10 bars.

MAKES 10 BARS (1 PER SERVING)

Per bar: 150 calories, 6 g fat, 0.5 g saturated fat, 3 g protein, 23 g carbohydrate, 3.5 g fiber, 82 mg sodium

Spiced Carrot Cake

HANDS-ON TIME: 20 MINUTES · TOTAL TIME: 45 MINUTES
PLUS COOLING TIME

A little bit of toasted sesame oil in addition to ground cardamom gives this cake a slightly exotic flavor. If you prefer, you can omit the cardamom and increase the ginger and cinnamon to ¾ teaspoon each. If you do, swap in extra olive oil for the sesame oil. The buckwheat flour (which, despite its name, contains no wheat at all) is high in fiber and protein and adds a slightly nutty flavor to the cake, providing a nice contrast to the sweetness of the carrots.

- ½ cup 100% buckwheat flour
- ½ cup gluten-free oat flour
- ⅓ cup granulated stevia (baking formula)
- 1 teaspoon baking soda
- ½ teaspoon ground cardamom
- ½ teaspoon ground ginger
- ½ teaspoon ground cinnamon
- ¼ teaspoon xanthan gum
- ¼ teaspoon salt
- ⅓ cup plus 1 tablespoon light (1.5%) buttermilk
- 3 tablespoons plus 2 teaspoons agave nectar
- ⅓ cup liquid egg whites (or the whites of 2 large eggs)
- 2 tablespoons extra-virgin olive oil
- 1½ teaspoons dark sesame oil
- 1¼ cups grated carrots
- 4 ounces light cream cheese

Preheat the oven to 350°F. Coat an 8-inch round cake pan with cooking spray. Line the bottom with a round of wax paper and coat the paper with cooking spray.

In a large bowl, whisk together the buckwheat and oat flours, stevia, baking soda, cardamom, ginger, cinnamon, xanthan gum, and salt.

In a separate bowl, whisk together ⅓ cup of the buttermilk, 3 table-spoons of the agave nectar, the egg whites, olive oil, and sesame oil. Stir the liquid ingredients into the flour mixture. Fold in the carrots. Scrape into the cake pan and bake until a toothpick inserted in the center comes out clean and the sides pull away from the pan, about 25 minutes. Cool completely in the pan on a rack. Run a metal spatula around the sides and invert the cake onto a serving platter.

In a medium bowl, with an electric mixer, beat the cream cheese with the remaining 1 tablespoon buttermilk and 2 teaspoons agave nectar. Spread the icing on top of the cake. Cut into 10 wedges.

MAKES 10 SERVINGS (1 WEDGE PER SERVING)

Per serving: 154 calories, 7 g fat, 2 g saturated fat, 5 g protein, 20 g carbohydrate, 2.5 g fiber, 329 mg sodium

RESOURCES

Organizations

AMERICAN CELIAC DISEASE ALLIANCE (ACDA)

2504 Duxbury Place
Alexandria, VA 22308
703-622-3331
americanceliac.org

A national organization devoted to advocating on behalf of the entire celiac community—patients, physicians, researchers, food manufacturers, and other service providers. The site offers the latest on the status of the long-anticipated gluten-free labeling legislation.

CELIAC DISEASE FOUNDATION (CDF)

13251 Ventura Boulevard, #1
Studio City, CA 91604
818-990-2354
celiac.org

Dedicated to celiac awareness, education, advocacy, and research.

CELIAC DISEASE PROGRAM AT BOSTON CHILDREN'S HOSPITAL DIVISION OF GASTROENTEROLOGY AND NUTRITION

300 Longwood Avenue
Boston, MA 02115
617-355-6058
childrenshospital.org

Strives to make life easier for families dealing with celiac disease. Their Celiac Family Health Education program includes online resources and take-home DVDs.

CELIAC SPRUE ASSOCIATION/USA INC.

PO Box 31700
Omaha, NE 68131-0700
877-272-4272
csaceliacs.org

The largest nonprofit celiac support group in America, with chapters and resource units across the country and members worldwide.

CHILDREN'S DIGESTIVE HEALTH AND NUTRITION FOUNDATION: CELIAC (CDHNF)

NASPGHAN
PO Box 6
Flourtown, PA 19031
215-233-0808
cdhnf.org

A professional society of more than 1,400 pediatric gastroenterologists that promotes awareness and research of pediatric digestive and nutritional disorders.

FOOD ALLERGY AND ANAPHYLAXIS NETWORK (FAAN)

11781 Lee Jackson Highway, Suite 160
Fairfax, VA 22033
800-929-4040
www.foodallergy.org

Dedicated to raising public awareness about food allergies and anaphylaxis.

Organizations (*cont.*)

GLUTEN INTOLERANCE GROUP
31214 124 Avenue SE
Auburn, WA 98092-3667
253-218-2956
gluten.net
Oversees the Gluten-Free Certification Program (gfco.org) to assure food integrity and safety of gluten-free packaged products for consumers. The site provides a guide to more than 6,000 products, companies, and manufacturers that have met the group's strict standards confirmed by field inspections. Oversees the Gluten-Free Restaurant Awareness Program (glutenfreerestaurants.org), which helps restaurants establish gluten-free menus and provides a list of certified restaurants for consumers.

NATIONAL FOUNDATION FOR CELIAC AWARENESS (NFCA)
224 South Maple Street
Ambler, PA 19002-0544
215-325-1306
celiaccentral.org
Collaborates with researchers and helps fund research projects designed to find a cure for celiac disease. Works to improve the quality of life for those on a gluten-free diet.

NATIONAL INSTITUTES OF HEALTH (NIH) CELIAC DISEASE AWARENESS CAMPAIGN
c/o National Digestive Diseases Information Clearinghouse
2 Information Way
Bethesda, MD 20892-3570
800-891-5389
celiac.nih.gov
Provides science-based information about the symptoms, diagnosis, and treatment of celiac disease.

Research Centers

The following centers specialize in the expert diagnosis and treatment of people with celiac disease and other forms of gluten sensitivity. Many are involved in ongoing research and clinical trials.

CELIAC CENTER AT BETH ISRAEL DEACONESS MEDICAL CENTER
Harvard Medical School
330 Brookline Avenue
Boston, MA 02215
617-667-7000
bidmc.harvard.edu/celiaccenter

CELIACNOW.ORGCELIAC DISEASE CENTER AT COLUMBIA UNIVERSITY
Harkness Pavilion
180 Fort Washington Avenue, Suite 934
New York, NY 10032
212-342-4529
celiacdiseasecenter.org

CELIAC DISEASE CLINIC AT MAYO CLINIC
507-284-5255 (patients)
507-284-2631 (medical professionals)
mayoclinic.com/health/celiac-disease/ DS00319

UNIVERSITY OF CHICAGO CELIAC DISEASE CENTER
5841 South Maryland Avenue, Mail Code 4069
Chicago, IL 60637
773-702-7593
celiacdisease.net

UNIVERSITY OF MARYLAND CENTER FOR CELIAC RESEARCH
University of Maryland School of Medicine
20 Penn Street, Room S303B
Baltimore, MD 21201
410-328-6749
umm.edu/celiac/

WILLIAM K. WARREN MEDICAL RESEARCH CENTER FOR CELIAC DISEASE
University of California, San Diego
9500 Gilman Drive, MC0623D
La Jolla, CA 92093-0623
858-822-1022
http://celiaccenter.ucsd.edu

Gluten-Aware Dining

See also Apps, below

ALLERGYEATS
allergyeats.com
Helps you locate and rate a restaurant based on its level of "allergy friendliness."

G-FREE FOODIE
gfreefoodie.com
Features recipes, product reviews, articles, blog posts, and restaurants.

GLUTEN FREE REGISTRY
glutenfreeregistry.com
A free, searchable database of more than 28,000 gluten-free-friendly business locations, including bakeries, restaurants, caterers, grocers, and more.

GLUTEN-FREE RESTAURANT AWARE-NESS PROGRAM (GFRAP)
See Gluten Intolerance Group under Organizations, above

GLUTEN-FREE RESTAURANT CARDS FOR CELIACS
celiactravel.com/cards
Offers free printable restaurant cards in 54 languages to help you order gluten free around the world.

TRIUMPH DINING
triumphdining.com
This commercial site sells laminated dining cards in 10 languages tailored to each cuisine; also sells disposable cards for American restaurants and a comprehensive restaurant and grocery guide.

URBAN SPOON
urbanspoon.com
Urban Spoon offers restaurant listings for more than 70 major metropolitan areas and is branching out into Canada and the United Kingdom. To use the site, you choose a metro area and then scroll down and click "Gluten-Free Friendly" in the left-hand menu (along with any other criteria or feature you wish to select, such as a particular type of cuisine). The directory will highlight restaurants that meet your search parameters. Some will note that they have gluten-free menus, or they will have reviews from gluten-free dining patrons. However, it's up to you to research a particular restaurant further, either online or by calling the restaurant, to see if it really can produce a safe gluten-free meal.

Dining Clubs

There are "Meetup" clubs across the United States for gluten-free foodies. Simply go to **meetup.com/celiac**.

Apps for Your Smartphone

More and more apps for the gluten sensitive are being created daily; those included here were popular at the time of publication. To find an app, simply go to the app store feature on your smartphone and type in the name of the application, or Google the name of the app.

Apps for Your Smartphone *(cont.)*

ALLERGYEATS

Has a free AllergyEats app, available only through AllergyEats.com, that's a guide to allergy-friendly restaurants across the United States.

FIND ME GLUTEN FREE

This app helps you find gluten-free-friendly businesses, including restaurants, fast-food franchises, bars, cafes, grocery stores, and more.

GLUTEN FREE NYC

For those with a gluten sensitivity who are living in or visiting New York City, the app provides a complete list of what appetizers, entrées, desserts, brunch items, and pre fixe menu items are safe for consumers to enjoy in restaurants around the city.

GLUTEN FREE REGISTRY

App of some 28,000 gluten-free-friendly business locations, including bakeries, restaurants, caterers, grocers, and more.

GLUTEN-FREE RESTAURANT CARDS

From Celiactravel.com, this app allows you to show restaurant cards in many languages to a waiter or chef, explaining the restrictions for those on a gluten-free diet.

GLUTENFREETRAVELSITE

Offers a free mobile version of their site. It's not technically an app, but it is a more user-friendly web format for use while "on the go." Search GF reviews by city, using an interactive map with markers for places that have been reviewed. Also access the GF Restaurants Menus page, with its growing list of some of the best national and regional restaurant chains offering gluten-free menus.

GLUTEN FREE ULTIMATE SOLUTION

The app from G-Free Foodie provides locations of gluten-free restaurants in the United States near your location via GPS and Search features, and it offers hundreds of gluten-free recipes, many with photos or video.

IS THAT GLUTEN FREE?

This app allows you to search by category or brand to determine whether grocery products are gluten free.

TRIUMPH DINING CARDS

The app version of their printed restaurant cards is for use in communicating your dietary needs to waiters and chefs in various languages.

TRIUMPH DINING GROCERY GUIDE

The app version of their grocery guide. Like the print edition, it lists more than 30,000 gluten-free foods.

Gluten-Aware Travel

BOB AND RUTH'S GLUTEN-FREE DINING AND TRAVEL CLUB
bobandruths.com

A popular gluten-free dining and travel club Web site that can be joined for a fee of approximately $40. Also offers a quarterly newsletter for members.

CELIAC.COM ADVICE ON GLUTEN-FREE TRAVEL
celiac.com/categories/ Gluten%252dFree-Travel

This section of the Celiac.com Web site deals with all aspects of traveling on a gluten-free diet, with reviews of hotels, restaurants, cruise ships, amusement parks, and more. Share your own gluten-free travel experiences here as well.

CRUISE CRITIC
cruisecritic.com
Great site to find cruise reviews, news, deals, and more.

GLUTENFREE PASSPORT
glutenfreepassport.com
A food- and travel-related site from the authors of the *Let's Eat Out* series of books for those with celiac disease, gluten sensitivity, and food allergies. It includes links to buy their book, watch free videos, and more.

GLUTENFREETRAVELSITE
glutenfreetravelsite.com
This site offers thousands of gluten-free dining and travel reviews.

Online Shopping

Always check nutrition labels carefully, if possible, when shopping online to make sure you get the healthiest products.

BEFREEFORME
befreeforme.com
Offers free coupons and samples to consumers with celiac disease, gluten intolerance, or food allergies.

GLUTEN-FREE MALL
glutenfreemall.com
You can shop for more than 1,000 gluten-free products from 130-plus leading brands.

GLUTEN-FREE OATS
glutenfreeoats.com
Offers a variety of gluten-free oats and oat products.

GLUTEN-FREE TRADING COMPANY
gluten-free.net
Gluten-free groceries from suppliers from around the world.

GLUTEN SOLUTIONS
glutensolutions.com
Offers a wide variety of gluten-free foods.

Online Suppliers of Gluten-Free Flours, Grains, and More

BARRY FARM FOODS
barryfarm.com/flours.htm
Offers a large selection of gluten-free flours, including amaranth, sorghum, green pea, cashew, pistachio, and almond, to name just a few.

BOB'S RED MILL
bobsredmill.com
The online source for Bob's Red Mill gluten-free flours, cereals, and other products that you might not be able to find in your local supermarket.

NORTHERN QUINOA CORPORATION
quinoa.com
This Canadian supplier offers a wide variety of quinoa products, including imported.

Other Useful Sites

Celiac.com
A comprehensive, well-written online resource dedicated to the support of those who have celiac disease and gluten sensitivity.

Glutenfreegirl.com
Excellent food blog from celiac sufferer Shauna James Ahern and her chef husband, with recipes, videos, articles, and links.

Other Useful Sites (*cont.*)

Noglutennoproblem.blogspot.com

Musings on the gluten-free life, with recipes, product reviews, sports commentary, and more from runner and author Pete Bronski and his wife, Kelli. Great index of past articles.

Glutenfreediet.ca

Resource center for information about celiac disease, gluten intolerance, and the gluten-free diet from respected nutritionist and author Shelley Case.

Simplygluten-free.com

Television chef, freelance writer, and cookbook author Carol Kicinski's gluten-free blog. Recipes, recommendations for gluten-free products, and lots more.

Glutenfreedietitian.com

How to follow a nutritious gluten-free diet from respected nutritionist, dietitian, and author Tricia Thompson.

Glutenfreedrugs.com

Authored and maintained by a clinical pharmacist, this nonprofit Web site features the latest news on medications, food labeling, celiac research, and more.

Publications for the Gluten Aware

DELICIOUS LIVING

deliciousliving.com

A complimentary publication distributed by natural-food stores. It began as a food magazine for the natural-foods industry but now covers a wide range of natural health topics. Search on "gluten" or "gluten-free" for recipes and articles.

DELIGHT GLUTEN-FREE MAGAZINE

delightglutenfree.com

A bimonthly international food and lifestyle publication for people living with food allergies and sensitivities.

EASY EATS

easyeats.com

An all-digital food and lifestyle magazine that challenges the traditional approach of what it means to be gluten free, looking at life through a positive lens.

GLUTEN-FREE LIVING

glutenfreeliving.com

This magazine provides practical information about the gluten-free diet.

LIVING WITHOUT

livingwithout.com

A magazine for people with food allergies and sensitivities.

SELECT BIBLIOGRAPHY

CHAPTER 1: THE ACCIDENTAL GLUTEN DOCTOR

Agarwal S, Morgan T, et al. Coronary calcium score and prediction of all-cause mortality in diabetes. *Diabetes Care* 2011;34:1219–1224.

Agatston AS, Janowitz WR, et al. Quantification of coronary artery calcium using ultrafast CT. *J Am Coll Cardiol* 1990;15:827–832.

————. Ultrafast computed tomography-detected coronary calcium reflects the angiographic extent of coronary arterial atherosclerosis. *Am J Cardiol* 1994;74: 1272–1274.

Akram K, O'Donnell RE, Agatston AS, et al. Influence of symptomatic status on the prevalence of obstructive coronary artery disease in patients with zero calcium score. *Atherosclerosis* 2009;3:533–537.

Blaha, MJ, Budoff, MJ, Agatston A, et al. Associations between C-reactive protein, coronary artery calcium, and cardiovascular events: Implications for the JUPITER population from MESA, a population-based cohort study. *Lancet* 2011;378:684–692.

Blaha MJ, DeFilippis AP, Agatston A, et al. The relationship between insulin resistance and incidence and progression of coronary artery calcification: The Multi-Ethnic Study of Atherosclerosis (MESA). *Diabetes Care* 2011;34:749–751.

Janowitz WR, Agatston AS, et al. Comparison of serial quantitative evaluation of calcified coronary artery plaque by ultrafast CT in persons with and without obstructive CAD. *Am J Cardiol* 1991;68:1–6.

Rubin J, Nasir K, Agatston AS, et al. Coronary calcium score and outcomes. *Curr Cardiovasc Imaging Rep* 2010;3:342–349.

Rubio-Tapia A, Kyle RA, et al. Increased prevalence and mortality in undiagnosed celiac disease. *Gastroenterology* 2009;137:88–93.

CHAPTER 2: MY JOURNEY TO GLUTEN AWARENESS

Aude YW, Agatston AS, Almon M, et al. The national cholesterol education program diet vs a diet lower in carbohydrates and higher in protein and monounsaturated fat: A randomized trial. *Arch Intern Med* 2004;164(19):2141–2146.

Beunza JJ, Toledo E, et al. Adherence to the Mediterranean diet, long-term weight change, and incident overweight or obesity: The Seguimiento Universidad de Navarra (SUN) cohort. *Am J Clin Nutr* 2010;92:1484–1493.

Hayes MR, Miller CK, et al. A carbohydrate-restricted diet alters gut peptides and adiposity signals in men and women with metabolic syndrome. *J Nutr* 2007;137:1944–1950.

Jakobsen MU, Dethlefsen C, et al. Intake of carbohydrates compared with intake of saturated fatty acids and risk of myocardial infarction: Importance of the glycemic index. *Am J Clin Nutr* 2010;91:1764–1768.

Leidy HJ, Tang M, et al. The effects of consuming frequent, higher protein meals on appetite and satiety during weight loss in overweight/obese men. *Obesity* 2011;19:818–824.

Maki KC, Rains TM, et al. Effects of a reduced-glycemic-load diet on body weight, body composition, and cardiovascular disease risk markers in overweight and obese adults. *Am J Clin Nutr* 2007;85:724–734.

McKeown NM, Troy LM, et al. Whole- and refined-grain intakes are differentially associated with abdominal visceral and subcutaneous adiposity in healthy adults: The Framingham Heart Study. *Am J Clin Nutr* 2010;92:1165–1171.

Miller M, Beach V, et al. Comparative effects of three popular diets on lipids, endothelial function, and C-reactive protein during weight maintenance. *J Am Diet Assoc* 2009;109:713–717.

Oh K, Hu FB, et al. Dietary fat intake and risk of coronary heart disease in women: 20 years of follow-up of the Nurses' Health Study. *Am J Epidemiol* 2005;161:672–679.

O'Neil CE, Nicklas TA, et al. Whole-grain consumption is associated with diet quality and nutrient intake in adults: The National Health and Nutrition Examination Survey, 1999–2004. *J Am Diet Assoc* 2010;110:1461–1468.

Park Y, Subar AF, et al. Dietary fiber intake and mortality in the NIH-AARP Diet and Health Study. *Arch Intern Med* 2011;171:1061–1068.

Salas-Salvadó J, Bulló M, et al. Reduction in the incidence of type 2 diabetes with the Mediterranean diet: Results of the PREDIMED-Reus nutrition intervention randomized trial. *Diabetes Care* 2011;34:14–19.

CHAPTER 3: CELIAC DISEASE OR GLUTEN SENSITIVITY?

Barbeau WE. What is the key environmental trigger in type 1 diabetes—Is it viruses, or wheat gluten, or both? *Autoimmun Rev* 2012;12:295–299.

Bizzaro N, Tozzoli R, et al. Cutting-edge issues in celiac disease and in gluten intolerance. *Clinic Rev Allerg Immunol* 2012;42:279–287.

Brar P, Kwon GY, et al. Change in lipid profile in celiac disease: Beneficial effect of gluten-free diet. *Am J Med* 2006;119:786–790.

Briani C, Samaroo D, et al. Celiac disease: From gluten to autoimmunity. *Autoimmun Rev* 2008;7:644–650.

Brown AC. Gluten sensitivity: problems of an emerging condition separate from celiac disease. *Expert Rev Gastroenterol Hepatol* 2012;6:43–55.

Carroccio A, Mansueto P, et al. Non-celiac wheat sensitivity diagnosed by double-blind placebo-controlled challenge: Exploring a new clinical entity. *Am J Gastroen* 2012;107:1898–1906.

Castillo-Ortiz JD, Durán-Barragán S, et al. Anti-transglutaminase, antigladin and ultra purified anti-gladin antibodies in patients with a diagnosis of rheumatoid arthritis. *Reumatol Clin* 2011;7:27–29.

Catassi C, Fabiani E, et al. A prospective, double-blind, placebo-controlled trial to establish a safe gluten threshold for patients with celiac disease. *Am J Clin Nutr* 2007;85:160–166.

Catassi C, Kryszak D, et al. Detection of celiac disease in primary care: A multicenter case-finding study in North America. *Am J Gastroenterol* 2007;102:1454–1460.

———. Natural history of celiac disease autoimmunity in a USA cohort followed since 1974. *Ann Med* 2010;42:530–538.

Di Sabatino A, Corazza GR. Nonceliac gluten sensitivity: Sense or sensibility? *Ann Intern Med* 2012;156:309–311.

El-Chammas K, Danner E. Gluten-free diet in nonceliac disease. *Nutr Clin Pract* 2011;26:294–299.

Fasano A, Berti I, et al. Prevalence of celiac disease in at-risk and not-at-risk groups in the United States: A large multicenter study. *Arch Intern Med* 2003;163:286–292.

Ferch CC, Chey WD. Irritable bowel syndrome and gluten sensitivity without celiac disease: Separating the wheat from the chaff. *Gastroenterology* 2012;142:664–666.

Ford, RPK. The gluten syndrome: A neurological disease. *Med Hypotheses* 2009;73:438–440.

Green, PHR. *Celiac Disease: A Hidden Epidemic*. New York: William Morrow, 2010.

———. Where are all those patients with Celiac disease? *Am J Gastroenterol* 2007;102:1461–1463.

Hadjivassiliou M, Sanders DS, et al. Gluten sensitivity: From gut to brain. *Lancet Neurol* 2010;9:318–330.

Jackson JR, Eaton WW, et al. Neurologic and psychiatric manifestations of celiac disease and gluten sensitivity. *Psychiatr Q* 2012;83:91–102.

Jordá FC, López Vivancos J. Fatigue as a determinant of health in patients with celiac disease. *J Clin Gastroenterol* 2010;44:423–427.

Newnham ED. Does gluten cause gastrointestinal symptoms in subjects without coeliac disease? *J Gastroenterol Hepatol* 2011;26 Suppl3:132–134.

Passananti V, Santonicola A, et al. Bone mass in women with celiac disease: Role of exercise and gluten-free diet. *Dig Liver Dis* 2012;44:379–383.

Riddle MS, Murray JA, et al. The incidence and risk of celiac disease in a healthy US adult population. *Am J Gastroenterol* 2012;107:1248–1255.

Rubio-Tapia A, Ludvigsson JF, et al. The prevalence of celiac disease in the United States. *Am J Gastroenterol* 2012;107:1538–1544.

Sapone A, Bai J, et al. Spectrum of gluten-related disorders: Consensus on new nomenclature and classification. *BMC Med* 2012;10:13.

Sapone A, Lammers KM, et al. Divergence of gut permeability and mucosal immune gene expression in two gluten-associated conditions: Celiac disease and gluten sensitivity. *BMC Med* 2011;9:23.

Tursi A, Brandimarte G. The symptomatic and histologic response to a gluten-free diet in patients with borderline enteropathy. *J Clin Gastroenterol* 2003;36:13–17.

Lionetti E, Catassi C. New clues in celiac disease epidemiology, pathogenesis, clinical manifestations, and treatment. *Int Rev Immunol* 2011;30:219–231.

Pietzak M. Celiac disease, wheat allergy, and gluten sensitivity: When gluten free is not a fad. *JPEN J Parenter Enteral Nutr* 2012;36 Suppl1:68S–75S.

Vande Voort JL, Murray JA, et al. Lymphocytic duodenosis and the spectrum of celiac disease. *Am J Gastroenterol* 2009;104:142–148.

Verdu EF. Editorial: Can gluten contribute to irritable bowel syndrome? *Am J Gastroenterol* 2011;106:516–518.

Verdu EF, Armstrong D, et al. Between celiac disease and irritable bowel syndrome: The "no man's land" of gluten sensitivity. *Am J Gastroenterol* 2009;104:1587–1594.

Volta U, De Giorgio R. New understanding of gluten sensitivity. *Nat Rev Gastroenterol Hepatol* 2012;9:295–299.

CHAPTER 4: WHY NOW?

Atchison J, Head L, et al. Wheat as food, wheat as industrial substance; comparative geographies of transformation and mobility. *Geoforum* 2010;41:236–246.

Day L, Augustin MA, et al. Wheat-gluten uses and industry needs. *Trends in Food Science & Technology* 2006;17:82–90.

Delcour JA, Joye IJ, et al. Wheat gluten functionality as a quality determinant in cereal-based food products. *Annu Rev Food Sci Technol* 2012;3:469–492.

Fasano A. Leaky gut and autoimmune diseases. *Clin Rev Allergy Immunol* 2012;42: 71–78.

Fortun PJ, Hawkey CJ. Nonsteroidal antiinflammatory drugs and the small intestine. *Curr Opin Gastroenterol* 2005,21:169–175.

Hotz C, Gibson RS. Traditional food-processing and preparation practices to enhance the bioavailability of micronutrients in plant-based diets. *J Nutr* 2007;137: 1097–1100.

Lohi S, Mustaalahti K, et al. Increasing prevalence of coeliac disease over time. *Aliment Pharmacol Ther* 2001;26:1217–1225.

Molberg Ø, Uhlen AK, et al. Mapping of gluten T-cell epitopes in the bread wheat ancestors: Implications for celiac disease. *Gastroenterology* 2005;128:393–401.

Sigthorsson G, Tibble J, et al. Intestinal permeability and inflammation in patients on NSAIDs. *Gut* 1998;43:506–511.

van den Broeck HC, de Jong HC, et al. Presence of celiac disease epitopes in modern and old hexaploid wheat varieties: Wheat breeding may have contributed to increased prevalence of celiac disease. *Theor Appl Genet* 2010;121:1527–1539.

Zannini E, Pontonio E, et al. Applications of microbial fermentations for production of gluten-free products and perspectives. *Appl Microbiol Biotechnol* 2012;93:473–485.

CHAPTER 5: FRIENDLY BACTERIA (YOUR NEW BFF)

Arendt EK, Moroni A, et al. Medical nutrition therapy: Use of sourdough lactic acid bacteria as a cell factory for delivering functional biomolecules and food ingredients in gluten free bread. *Microb Cell Fact* 2011;10 Suppl1:S15.

Arora T, Sharma R. Fermentation potential of the gut microbiome: Implications for energy homeostasis and weight management. *Nutr Rev* 2011;69:99–106.

Blaser MJ, Atherton JC. Helicobacter pylori persistence: Biology and disease. *J Clin Invest* 2004;113:321–333.

Blaser MJ, Chen Y, et al. Does Heliobacter pylori protect against asthma and allergy? *Gut* 2008;57:561–567.

Blaser MJ, Falkow S. What are the consequences of the disappearing human microbiota? *Nat Rev Microbiol* 2009;7:887–894.

Blaser MJ, Kirschner D. The equilibria that allow bacterial persistence in human hosts. *Nature* 2007;449:843–849.

Boskey ER, Cone RA, et al. Origins of vaginal acidity: High D/L lactate ratio is consistent with bacteria being the primary source. *Hum Reprod* 2001;16:1809–1813.

Calasso M, Vincentini O, et al. The sourdough fermentation may enhance the recovery from intestinal inflammation of coeliac patients at the early stage of the gluten-free diet. *Eur J Nutr* 2012;51:507–512.

Cho I, Blaser MJ. The human microbiome: At the interface of health and disease. *Nat Rev Genet* 2012;13:260–270.

Cho I, Yamanishi S, et al. Antibiotics in early life alter the murine colonic microbiome and adiposity. *Nature* 2012;488:621–626.

Crow JM. That healthy gut feeling. *Nature* 2011;480(7378):S88–S89.

Deplancke B, Gaskins HR. Microbial modulation of innate defense: Goblet cells and the intestinal mucus layer. *Am J Clin Nutr* 2001;73 Suppl:1131S–1141S.

Di Cagno R, De Angelis M, et al. Pasta made from durum wheat semolina fermented with selected lactobacilli as a tool for a potential decrease of the gluten intolerance. *J Agric Food Chem* 2005;53:4393–4402.

———. Proteolysis by sourdough lactic acid bacteria: Effects on wheat flour protein fractions and gliadin peptides involved in human cereal intolerance. *Appl Environ Microbiol* 2002;68:623–633.

———. Sourdough bread made from wheat and nontoxic flours and started with selected lactobacilli is tolerated in celiac sprue patients. *Appl Environ Microbiol* 2004;70:1088–1096.

Fasano, A. Novel therapeutic/integrative approaches for celiac disease and dermatitis herpetiformis. *Clin Devel Immunol* 2012;2012:959061.

Gianfrani C, Siciliano RA, et al. Transamidation of wheat flour inhibits the response to gliadin of intestinal T cells in celiac disease. *Gastroenterology* 2007;133: 780–789.

Gobbetti M, Rizzello CG, et al. Sourdough lactobacilli and celiac disease. *Food Microbiol* 2007;24:187–196.

Greco L, Gobbetti M, et al. Safety for patients with celiac disease of baked goods made of wheat flour hydrolyzed during food processing. *Clin Gastroenterol Hepatol* 2011;9:24–29.

Hatakka K, Savilahti E, et al. Effect of long term consumption of probiotic milk on infections in children attending day care centres: Double blind, randomised trial. *British Med J* 2001;322:1–5.

Ichinohe T, Panga IK, et al. Microbiota regulates immune defense against respiratory tract influenza A virus infection. *PNAS* 2011;108:5354–5359.

Karlsson CLJ, Önnerfält J, et al. The microbiota of the gut in preschool children with normal and excessive body weight. *Obesity* 2012;20:2257–2261.

Kau AL, Ahern PP, et al. Human nutrition, the gut microbiome, and immune system: Envisioning the future. *Nature* 2011;474:327–336.

Ley RE, Bäckhed F, et al. Obesity alters gut microbial ecology. *PNAS* 2005;102: 11070–11075.

Ludviggson JF, Fasano A. Timing of introduction of gluten and celiac disease risk. *Ann Nutr Metab* 2012;60 Suppl2:22–29.

Natividad JM, Huang X, et al. Host responses to intestinal microbial antigens in gluten-sensitive mice. *PLoS One* 2009;4(7):e6472

Neyrinck AM, Delzenne NM. Potential interest of gut microbial changes induced by non-digestible carbohydrates of wheat in the management of obesity and related disorders. *Curr Opin Clin Nutr Metab Care* 2010;13:722–728.

Nistal E, Caminero A, et al. Differences of small intestinal bacteria populations in adults and children with/without celiac disease: Effect of age, gluten diet, and disease. *Inflamm Bowel Dis* 2012;18:649–656.

Penders J, Thijs C, et al. Factors influencing the composition of the intestinal microbiota in early infancy. *Pediatrics* 2006;118:511–521.

Ray K. Microbiota: Tolerating gluten—A role for gut microbiota in celiac disease? *Nat Rev Gastroenterol Hepatol* 2012;9:242.

Reid G. How science will help shape future clinical applications of probiotics. *Clinical Infectious Diseases* 2008;46:S62–66.

Reid G, Dols J, et al. Targeting the vaginal microbiota with probiotics as a means to counteract infections. *Curr Opin Clin Nutr Metab Care* 2009;12:583–587.

Schippa S, Iebba V, et al. A distinctive "microbial signature" in celiac pediatric patients. *BMC Microbiol* 2010;10:175.

Sellitto M, Bai G, et al. Proof of concept of microbiome-metabolome analysis and delayed gluten exposure on celiac disease autoimmunity in genetically at-risk infants. *PLoS One* 2012;7(3):e33387.

Sonnenburg JL. Genetic pot luck. *Nature* 2010;464:837–838.

Stepniak D, Spaenij-Dekking L, et al. Highly efficient gluten degradation with a newly identified prolylendoprotease: Implications for celiac disease. *Am J Physiol Gastrointest Liver Physiol* 2006;291:G621–G629.

Thakkar K, Boatright RO, et al. Gastroesophageal reflux and asthma in children: A systematic review. *Pediatrics* 2010;125;e925–e930.

Thum C, Cookson AL, et al. Can nutritional modulation of maternal intestinal microbiota influence the development of the infant gastrointestinal tract? *J Nutr* 2012;142:1921–1928.

Tilg H. Obesity, metabolic syndrome, and microbiota: Multiple interactions. *J Clin Gastroenterol* 2010; 44 Suppl1:S16–S18.

Trasande L, Blustein J, et al. Infant antibiotic exposures and early-life body mass. *Int J Obes* (Lond) 2012 Aug 21. [Epub ahead of print]

Turnbaugh, PJ, Hamady M, et al. A core gut microbiome in obese and lean twins. *Nature* 2009;457:480–485.

Turnbaugh PJ, Ley RE, et al. An obesity-associated gut microbiome with increased capacity for energy harvest. *Nature* 2006;444:1027–1031.

Wen L, Ley RE, et al. Innate immunity and intestinal microbiota in the development of Type 1 diabetes. *Nature* 2008;455:1109–1113.

Yatsunenko T, Rey FE, et al. Human gut microbiome viewed across age and geography. *Nature* 2012;486:222–228.

CHAPTER 6: GLUTEN-RELATED DISORDERS: THE GREAT IMITATORS

Barton SH, Kelly DG, et al. Nutritional deficiencies in celiac disease. *Gastroenterol Clin North Am* 2007;36:93–108, vi.

Bruno PP, Carpino F, et al. An overview on immune system and migraine. *Eur Rev Med Pharmacol Sci* 2007;11:245–248.

Caro, RA. *The Passage of Power: The Years of Lyndon Johnson.* New York: Knopf, 2012.

Cosnes J, Cellier C. Incidence of autoimmune diseases in celiac disease: Protective effect of the gluten-free diet. *Clin Gastroenterol Hepatol* 2008;6:753–758.

Dallek R. "The Medical Ordeals of JFK." *Atlantic Monthly,* December 2002.

Dicke WK, Weijers HA, et al. Coeliac disease. II. The presence in wheat of a factor having deleterious effects in cases of celiac disease. *Acta Paediatr* 1953;42:34–42.

Fasano A. "Surprises from Celiac Disease." *Scientific American,* August 2009.

Green, PH. "Was JFK the Victim of an Undiagnosed Disease Common to the Irish?" George Mason University History News Network, 20 January 2004. http://hnn.us/articles/1125.html

Hernandez L, Green PH. Extraintestinal manifestations of celiac disease. *Curr Gastroenterol Rep* 2006;8:383–389.

Lea ME, Harbord M, et al. Bilateral occipital calcification associated with celiac disease, folate deficiency, and epilepsy. *AJNR* 1995;16:1498–1500.

Mandel LR. Endocrine and autoimmune aspects of the health history of John F. Kennedy. *Ann Intern Med* 2009;151:350–354.

Meloni A, Mandas C, et al. Prevalence of autoimmune thyroiditis in children with celiac disease and effect of gluten withdrawal. *J Pediatr* 2009;155:51–55.

Rampertab SD, Nakechand Pooran N, et al. Trends in the presentation of celiac disease. *Am J Med* 2006;119:355.

Rashtak S, Pittelkow MR. Skin involvement in systemic autoimmune diseases. *Curr Dir Autoimmun* 2008;10:344–358.

Smyth DJ, Plagnol V, et al. Shared and distinct genetic variants in type 1 diabetes and celiac disease. *N Engl J Med* 2008;359:2767–2777.

Tilg H. Diet and intestinal immunity. *N Engl J Med* 2012;366:181–183.

Ventura A, Magazzù G, et al. Duration of exposure to gluten and risk for autoimmune disorders in patients with celiac disease. SIGEP Study Group for Autoimmune Disorders in Celiac Disease. *Gastroenterology* 1999;117:297–303.

CHAPTER 7: THE NOT-SO-PLACEBO EFFECT

Biesiekierski JR, Newnham ED, et al. Gluten causes gastrointestinal symptoms in subjects without celiac disease: A double-blind randomized placebo-controlled trial. *Am J Gastroenterol* 2011;106:508–514.

Brottveit M, Vandvik PO, et al. Absence of somatization in non-coeliac gluten sensitivity. *Scand J Gastroenterol* 2012;47:770–777.

Turner JA, Deyo RA, et al. The importance of placebo effects in pain treatment and research. *JAMA* 1994;271:1609–1614.

CHAPTER 8: IT STARTS EARLY

Anderson SE, Whitaker RC. Household routines and obesity in US preschool-aged children. *Pediatrics* 2010;125:420–428.

Collins CE, Okely AD, et al. Parent diet modification, child activity, or both in obese children: An RCT. *Pediatrics* 2011;127:619–627.

Gahagan S. Development of eating behavior: Biology and context. *J Dev Behav Pediatr* 2012;33:261–271.

Geary N, Garcia O. *The Food Cure for Kids: A Nutritional Approach to Your Child's Wellness.* Guilford, CT: Lyons Press, 2010.

Gupta RS, Springston EE, et al. The prevalence, severity, and distribution of childhood food allergy in the United States. *Pediatrics* 2011;128:e9–e17.

Hammons AJ, Fiese BH. Is frequency of shared family meals related to the nutritional health of children and adolescents? *Pediatrics* 2011;127:e1565–e1574.

Hogen Esch CE, Wolters VM, et al. Specific celiac disease antibodies in children on a gluten-free diet. *Pediatrics* 2011;128:547–552.

Hollar D, Messiah SE, Agatston AS, et al. Healthier options for public schoolchildren program improves weight and blood pressure in 6- to 13-year-olds. *J Am Diet Assoc* 2010;110:261–267.

Jadresin O, Misak Z, et al. Compliance with gluten-free diet in children with coeliac disease. *J Pediatr Gastroenterol Nutr* 2008;47:344–348.

Mazzone L, Reale L, et al. Compliant gluten-free children with celiac disease: An evaluation of psychological distress. *BMC Pediatr* 2011;11:46.

Roma E, Roubani A, et al. Dietary compliance and life style of children with coeliac disease. *J Hum Nutr Diet* 2010;23:176–182.s

Tanpowpong P, Broder-Fingert S, et al. Predictors of gluten avoidance and implementation of a gluten-free diet in children and adolescents without confirmed celiac disease. *J Pediatr* 2012;161:471–475.

Waters E, de Silva-Sanigorski A, et al. Interventions for preventing obesity in children. *Cochrane Database Syst Rev* 2011 Dec 7;(12):CD001871.

CHAPTER 9: JUNK FOOD BY ANOTHER NAME

Bergamo P, Maurano F, et al. Immunological evaluation of the alcohol-soluble protein fraction from gluten-free grains in relation to celiac disease. *Mol Nutr Food Res* 2011;55:1266–1270.

Gaesser GA, Angadi SS. Gluten-free diet: Imprudent dietary advice for the general population? *J Acad Nutr Diet* 2012;112:1330–1333.

Gobbetti M, Cagno RD, et al. Functional microorganisms for functional food quality. *Crit Rev Food Sci Nutr* 2010;50:716–727.

Papista C, Gerakopoulos V, et al. Gluten induces coeliac-like disease in sensitised mice involving IgA, CD71 and transglutaminase 2 interactions that are prevented by probiotics. *Lab Invest* 2012;92:625–635.

Yan F, Polk DB. Probiotics: Progress toward novel therapies for intestinal diseases. *Curr Opin Gastroenterol* 2010;26:95–101.

PART II

See also citations for earlier chapters.

Agatston A. *The South Beach Diet Supercharged.* Emmaus, PA: Rodale, 2008.

———. *The South Beach Wake-Up Call.* Emmaus, PA: Rodale, 2011.

Bronski P, McLean Jory M. *The Gluten-Free Edge: A Nutrition and Training Guide for Peak Athletic Performance and an Active Gluten-Free Life.* New York: Experiment, 2012.

Brown, M. *Gluten-Free, Hassle-Free.* New York: Demos Health, 2009.

Case, S. *Gluten-Free Diet: A Comprehensive Guide.* Regina, SK: Case Nutrition Consulting, 2010.

Gibala MJ, Little JP, et al. Short-term sprint interval versus traditional endurance training: Similar initial adaptations in human skeletal muscle and exercise performance. *J Physiol* 2006;575:901–911.

Gibala MJ, McGee SL. Metabolic adaptations to short-term high-intensity interval training: A little pain for a lot of gain? *Exerc Sport Sci Rev* 2008;36:58–63.

Leidy HJ, Tang M, et al. The effects of consuming frequent, higher protein meals on appetite and satiety during weight loss in overweight/obese men. *Obesity* 2011;19:818–824.

Lieberman, S. *The Gluten Connection.* Emmaus, PA: Rodale, 2007.

Mahoney CR, Taylor HA. Effect of breakfast composition on cognitive processes in elementary school children. *Physiol Behav* 2005;85:635–645.

Sedlock DA, Fissinger JA, et al. Effect of exercise intensity and duration on postexercise energy expenditure. *Med Sci Sports Exerc* 1989;21:662–666.

Talanian JL, Galloway SD, et al. Two weeks of high-intensity aerobic interval training increases the capacity for fat oxidation during exercise in women. *J Appl Physiol* 2007;102:1439–1447.

Thompson, T. *The Gluten-Free Nutrition Guide.* New York: McGraw-Hill, 2008.

Thornton MK, Potteiger JA. Effects of resistance exercise bouts of different intensities but equal work on EPOC. *Med Sci Sports Exerc* 2002;34:715–722.

Treuth MS, Hunter GR, et al. Effects of exercise intensity on 24-h energy expenditure and substrate oxidation. *Med Sci Sports Exerc* 1996;28:1138–1143.

PART III

See citations for earlier chapters.

INDEX

Underscored page references indicate boxed text.

Visit SOUTHBEACHDIET.COM

For more health and weight loss tools, great recipes, customized meal plans, and
support from registered dietitians and a vibrant community of South Beach Diet
followers, visit SouthBeachDiet.com.

DELIVERING QUALITY SERVICE

DELIVERING QUALITY SERVICE

◇ ◇ ◇

Balancing Customer Perceptions and Expectations

Valarie A. Zeithaml
A. Parasuraman
Leonard L. Berry

THE FREE PRESS
A Division of Macmillan, Inc.
NEW YORK

Collier Macmillan Publishers
LONDON

The Free Press
A Division of Macmillan, Inc.
866 Third Avenue, New York, N.Y. 10022

Collier Macmillan Canada, Inc.

Printed in the United States of America

printing number
4 5 6 7 8 9 10

Library of Congress Cataloging-in-Publication Data

Zeithaml, Valarie A.
   Delivering quality service : balancing customer perceptions and
expectations / Valarie A. Zeithaml, A. Parasuraman, Leonard L.
Berry.
      p.   cm.
   Includes bibliographical references.
   ISBN 0–02–935701–2
   1. Customer service.   2. Service industries—Quality control—
Mathematical models.   I. Parasuraman, A.   II. Berry, Leonard L.
III. Title.
HF5415.5.Z45   1990
658.8'12—dc20   89–23592
                                                              CIP

To the Marketing Science Institute for encouraging and supporting the research stream on which this book is based.

To my father, John McKinley Hoyle,
for thinking the big thought.

—V. Z.

To my mother, and in memory of my father.

—A. P.

To Lester Gold, a special uncle,
who taught me to touch all of the bases.

—L. B.

CONTENTS

PREFACE

IN 1983 WE SUBMITTED OUR FIRST PROPOSAL to the Marketing Science Institute (MSI) for funds to do an exploratory research study on the subject of service quality. Little did we know at the time that we were embarking on a research *journey* as infinite as the subject itself.

As we prepare this preface we are six months away from the new decade of the 1990's. And we are still on our research journey under the auspices of MSI, soon to do the fieldwork for phase IV. Phase I was an extensive qualitative study of service customers and service-company executives that resulted in our developing a model of service quality. Phase II was a large-scale empirical study that focused on the customer side of our service-quality model. From this phase we developed a methodology for measuring service quality that we call SERVQUAL and we refined our conclusions concerning the dimensions customers use to judge service quality.

Phase III was an empirical study that focused on the service provider half of our model and our most complex and ambitious effort to date. Phase III alone involved research in 89 separate field offices of five national service companies. The three research phases together have included customer focus-group interviews, employee focus-group interviews, in-depth executive interviews, customer surveys, manager surveys, and first-line employee surveys. We have studied six service sectors thus far: appliance repair, credit cards, insurance, long-distance telephone, retail banking and securities brokerage.

Phase IV centers on the topic of customer service expectations: how customers form their expectations and the key influences that affect this process. Our research protocol has been to explore through qualitative research, model what we find, and then test relationships within the model quantitatively. We will follow this protocol with our expectations research, doing a large number of customer focus groups in phase IV. In phase IV we will also add services we have not yet studied (automobile service, business equipment service, hotels, and truck rental) to some of the services included in the earlier phases.

In this book we present the fruits of our research journey to date. Using our model as the central framework, we seek to demonstrate that service quality is a subject that one can grab hold of, understand, and do something about. It *is* a subject that lends itself to research insight and managerial application.

From the very beginning of our research effort in 1983 we have been interested in three central questions:

- What is service quality?
- What causes service-quality problems?
- What can organizations do to solve these problems and improve their service?

With three phases of research complete, we believe we have something to say about each of these questions and we have written this book to say it. Although we have published a series of journal articles and research monographs on various facets of our research, this is our first attempt to bring everything together in one volume—our model, our methodologies, our findings, and our conclusions. We also go beyond our formal research findings and present many ideas, quotes, and company case histories that we have picked up on our journey. Having devoted a significant portion of the last seven years living the quality of service issue—reading everything we could get our hands on, talking to anyone who would talk to us, doing our formal studies, becoming the toughest of service critics in our own lives as customers—we have the patterns and nuances of our internal thoughts to share on this subject, too.

Our objectives for this book can be distilled quite simply:

- to attack head-on the mystique, mush, and myths that surround the service-quality issue and limit progress;
- to offer a framework that managers can actually use to understand and improve service quality;
- to offer specific and practical guidelines for improving service; and
- to convey the sense of urgency that we feel about improving service quality in America.

Our book is for senior and middle mangers in all types of service organizations. It is decidedly for *line* executives, not just for staff executives. Although we use the terms *company* or *firm* as a writing convenience, we believe strongly that managers in not-for-profit organizations can gain from this volume and we hope they will give it a try.

All of our formal research has been done in the United States and thus we focus on the United States as the setting for our discussion. We do not wish to imply that our findings necessarily apply to other countries as we have no empirical basis for making such an inference. We can say, however, that scholars throughout the world are using our research as a basis for their own studies, a very pleasing development that became evident to us at the International Research Seminar in Marketing held in the South of France during May 1988 and the Symposium on Quality in Services held in Karlstad, Sweden, during August 1988.

We have many people to thank who have supported our research financially and intellectually. First and foremost, we wish to express our deep appreciation to the Marketing Science Institute in Cambridge, Massachusetts, a one-of-a-kind jewel of an organization that funds leading-edge academic research of interest to its company sponsors. We know of no other research organization in America that has done more to build a bridge between the academic and business communities, and to advance marketing knowledge, than MSI.

We owe a great debt to Diane Schmalensee, head of research operations at MSI through phases I-III and the start-up of phase IV; she worked tirelessly to help us succeed in our work. Katherine Jocz, manager of research operations, has also been tremendously helpful, as have John Farley and Frederick Webster who served as MSI executive directors during our research. Alden Clayton, a past president of MSI, was very supportive of us during the crucial early days of our research journey.

Including phase IV, more than 15 major U.S. companies have been directly involved in the research. Hoping that we shall not offend anyone through omission, we wish to single out several executives who have been major sources of help and inspiration to us: Mike English, John Falzon, Tom Gillett, Donald Hughes, Linda Kanner, Dawn Lesh, Mary Lo-Sardo, Claudia Marshall, David Richardson, and Fred Thiemann. We also wish to thank Allen Paison and Jeffrey Marr from Walker Research in Indianapolis who provided significant logistical assistance to us in managing our massive data collection effort for phase III.

Last but not least, we thank Bob Wallace, senior editor at The Free Press, who believed in this book project from the outset, and Glenda Bessler, an incredibly good secretary and friend to the Texas members of the team. Glenda spent many late hours hovering over her computer typing and retyping our chapter drafts. She did a wonderful job, as did

Michael Guiry, a graduate student, and Bridget Clayton, a secretary, at Duke University. Michael and Bridget contributed significantly to the completion of the chapters prepared in North Carolina. Their diligence, attention to detail, and responsiveness were excellent examples of service quality in action.

As for the three of us, we take great pleasure in bringing to you the product of our collaboration. We three have been intellectual partners and friends for many years and it is personally satisfying to us to publish this work. We shared equally in the book's preparation.

Valarie Zeithaml
A. Parasuraman
Leonard L. Berry

1

◇ ◇ ◇

SERVICE LEADERSHIP SPELLS PROFITS

S ERVICE QUALITY is a central issue in America today. In a recent Gallup survey, executives ranked the improvement of service and tangible product quality as the single most critical challenge facing U.S. business.

One reason service quality has become such an important issue is that America's economy has become a service economy. Services account for approximately three-fourths of the gross national product and nine out of ten new jobs the economy creates. As David Birch writes:

> It used to be that we were good at growing things. We still are, but with virtually no people involved. Agricultural employment has gone from well over half of all jobs to about 2% of them.
>
> It used to be that we were good at making things. We still are, but with very few people involved. . . . Today, only 9% of Ameri-can workers actually labor in factories.
>
> Yet, we have created millions of jobs. . . . It's not surprising that what these people are doing instead of making things is providing services.[1]

Virtually all organizations compete to some degree on the basis of service. It is difficult to name even one industry for which service matters are unimportant. Study the strategies of manufacturing companies such as Ford Motor Company or Corning Glass Works and what you find is a paramount role for service. Indeed, as the decade of the 1990's unfolds, more and more executives in manufacturing firms will be as keenly in-terested in *service quality* as executives in banking, health-care, and trans-portation businesses are today. As manufacturing executives find it increasingly difficult to establish sustainable, technology-based compet-itive advantages, they will direct added attention and resources to value-

1

added service as a truer source of superiority. And as manufacturers compete more on service, there will be less distinction between manufacturing and service businesses.

Services are also crucial to America's future as a worldwide competitor. The U.S. government is counting on significant growth in net service exports in the 1990's to play a key role in addressing the country's balance of trade problems. And yet, America's net positive trade balance in services fell steadily throughout the 1980's, prompting some observers to suggest that the United States is on the verge of taking the same international beating in services that it has already endured in manufacturing. The principal culprit is seen as mediocre service quality. As Quinn and Gagnon write:

> It will take hard and dedicated work not to dissipate our broad-based lead in services, as we did in manufacturing. Many of the same causes of lost position are beginning to appear. Daily we encounter the same inattention to quality, emphasis on scale economies rather than customers' concerns, and short-term financial orientation that earlier injured manufacturing.[2]

The central role for services in the American economy is a key factor behind service quality's rising prominence as an institutional and societal issue. Services are so much a part of what we produce, consume, and export in this nation that it would be surprising if we weren't concerned about quality.

A second factor behind service quality's rising prominence is that superior quality is proving to be a winning competitive strategy. McDonald's. Federal Express. Nordstrom. American Airlines. American Express. L. L. Bean. Domino's Pizza. Disney World. Club Med. Deluxe Corporation. Marriott. IBM. In every nook and cranny of the service economy, the leading companies are obsessed with service excellence. They use service to be different; they use service to increase productivity; they use service to earn the customers' loyalty; they use service to fan positive word-of-mouth advertising; they use service to seek some shelter from price competition.

Service excellence pays off richly for reasons we develop in more detail later in this chapter. With service excellence, everyone wins. Customers win. Employees win. Management wins. Stockholders win. Communities win. The country wins.

THE URGENT NEED FOR SERVICE LEADERSHIP

How do we explain the incongruity that service excellence pays off and yet is in such short supply? The signs of indifferent, careless, and incompetent service in America are everywhere.

In a national banking study, three out of ten consumers recall a service problem at their current or former financial institution, typically an error of one kind or another. More than half of those recalling problems deemed them serious enough to switch financial institutions or to close accounts.[3]

In an *Atlanta Journal* and *Atlanta Constitution* survey of readers, 91 percent of the respondents said that quality of service had declined over the previous 20 years. Wrote one reader: "The animals are running the zoo."[4]

Time magazine recently devoted a cover story to the service problem, claiming that "Personal service has become a maddeningly rare commodity in the American marketplace."[5]

The *Wall Street Journal*, in a story about health-care service, stated: "The problems are manifold: Bad diagnoses. Unnecessary surgery. Over prescribing or misrepresenting drugs. High rates of hospital infection. Lab-test errors. Faulty medical devices. Alcoholic or drug-addicted doctors."[6] Lowell Levin of Yale University's medical school advises surgery patients to use a magic marker to indicate just where on their bodies the surgery is to be done, claiming his advice wouldn't sound ridiculous if people only knew how often mistakes do occur.[7]

Stanley Marcus, retired chairman of Neiman-Marcus, admonishes specialty and department store retailers for forgetting their sales-service heritage. Marcus writes:

> Poor selling saved me $48,373 in 1983. That year, I decided I would not buy anything I didn't need unless someone sold it to me. Whenever I found something I wanted, but didn't encounter sales persuasiveness, I did not buy. By the end of the year, my savings total was $48,373.[8]

MANAGING IS NOT ENOUGH

The research that we present in this book documents the central role that leadership plays in delivering excellent service. We have seen firsthand how strong management commitment to service quality energizes and stimulates an organization to improved service performance. We have seen firsthand how role ambiguity, poor teamwork, and other negatives fester in a rudderless, leaderless environment, sapping an organization's service quality.

True service leadership builds a climate for excellence that prevails over operational complexities, external market pressures, or any other impediments to quality service that might exist. Mediocre service in America is common, but it is not a given. In every single industry we have examples of companies delivering superb service. Excellent service is not a pipe dream; it is possible to overcome the conditions that foster service mediocrity. *The key is genuine service leadership at all levels of an organization—leadership that offers the direction and inspiration to sustain committed servers.*

Managing is not enough. Service work can be difficult and demoralizing. Customers can be rude. Company policies can be suffocating. Sheer numbers of customers to serve can be overwhelming. End-of-the-day fatigue can be desensitizing. Over time many service employees get "beat up" by the service role and become less effective with customers even as they gain technical experience that should produce the opposite result.

Listen to psychologist James Carr as he describes how a novel he read about the circus made him recognize the transformation he himself underwent in service roles:

> It was not the story line . . . that left its mark on me. It was the description of the social atmosphere through which the characters moved. All who lived under the big top—the freaks, the acrobats, even the animals—were real to each other. Everyone else—specifically anyone in the audience—was a "flatty."
>
> . . . I recalled how I had despaired, during a brief stint as a ticket agent during World War II, over the futility of trying to give individual attention to the masses of rail travelers clamoring to get somewhere . . . and I remembered the irritation I had felt when the crowds became unmanageable at several counter jobs I had held in my youth. There had been times when it seemed the only salvation was to retreat from involvement with individuals and to devote my attention exclusively to the specifics of the job at hand. When I did this, the customers became two-dimensional nonentities without personality or feelings. . . . At the time I had not referred to them as flatties but oh how descriptive was the term when I encountered it. . . . Even though I had treated people that way—often considering it businesslike—I realized that I had always resented being treated as a flatty![9]

Few of us, like Carr, wish to be treated as a flatty by service providers. Few service providers, again like Carr, begin a new job treating customers in this way. Robotlike service traits almost always develop on the job.

People in service work need a vision in which they can believe, an achievement culture that challenges them to be the best they can be, a sense of team that nurtures and supports them, and role models that show them the way. This is the stuff of leadership.

In their book, *Leaders: The Strategies for Taking Charge*, Bennis and Nanus point out that the principal distinction between leaders and managers is that leaders emphasize the emotional and spiritual resources of an organization, its values, and aspirations, whereas managers emphasize the physical resources of the organization, such as raw materials, technology, and capital.[10]

The root cause of our quality malaise in America today—the reason service isn't better than it is despite the fruits of excellent service—is the insufficiency of service leadership. Too many service workers are overmanaged and underled. Thick policy manuals rule management's belief in good judgment of frontline servers. Memoranda from above supersede face-to-face, give-and-take dialogue with employees. The goal of profit takes precedence over the goal of providing a service good enough that people will pay a profit to have it.[11]

To materially improve service, we must devote more energy and attention in our businesses and business schools to the development of leadership values and capabilities. Otherwise, the temptation of service mediocrity will continue to win out over the promise of service excellence.

CHARACTERISTICS OF SERVICE LEADERS

Service leaders come in all shapes and sizes. They do not come from some kind of magical service cookie cutter. Having said this, there are some characteristics of service leadership about which it is useful to generalize. Here are some of the most important characteristics:

1. *Service vision.* Service leaders see service quality as a success key. They see service as integral to the organization's future, not as a peripheral issue. They believe fundamentally that superior service is a winning strategy, a profit strategy.

Regardless of the markets targeted, the menu of services offered, or the pricing policies followed, service leaders see quality of service as the foundation for competing. Whatever the specifics of the vision, the idea of service excellence is a central part.

Service leaders never waver in their commitment to service quality. They see service excellence as a never-ending journey in which the only effective option is to plug away toward better quality every day of every week of every month of every year. They understand that service quality is not a program; that there are no quick fixes, no magic formulas, no quality pills to swallow.

Service leaders understand that service excellence requires a full-court press—all of the time.* They understand that a company cannot turn the service issue on and off like a water faucet. As L. L. Bean, Inc., President Leon Gorman states: "A lot of people have fancy things to say about customer service, including me. But it's just a day-in, day-out, ongoing, never-ending, unremitting, persevering . . . type of activity."[12]

2. *High standards.* True service leaders aspire to legendary service; they realize that good service may not be good enough to differentiate their organization from other organizations.

Service leaders are interested in the details and nuances of service, seeing opportunities in small actions that competitors might consider trivial. They believe that how an organization handles the little things sets the tone for how it handles the big things. They also believe that the little things add up for the customer and make a difference. This is why Jim Daniel, CEO of the Friendly Bank in Oklahoma City has the bank's lobby floor polished daily. And why Robert Onstead, CEO of Randall's Food and Drugs in Houston, insists on lighting his parking lots so brightly that "customers could read newspapers in the parking lots at midnight if they wished to do so."[13]

Service leaders are zealous about doing the service right the first time. They value the goal of zero defects, striving continually to improve the reliability of service. They recognize the flip side of a 98 percent reliability rate, which is 2 percent unreliability. This is why Will Potter, CEO of Maryland-based Preston Trucking Company, has each employee agree in writing to abide by the company's service philosophy which states, in part:

> Once I make a commitment to a customer or another associate, I promise to fulfill it on time. I will do what I say when I say I will do it. . . . I understand that one claim or one mistake is one error too many. I promise to do my job right the first time and to continually seek performance improvement.

* For readers who are not basketball fans, we are using the phrase "full-court press" to mean unremitting vigilance.

3. In-the-field leadership style. Service leaders lead in the field, where the action is, rather than from their desks. They are visible to their people, endlessly coaching, praising, correcting, cajoling, sermonizing, observing, questioning, and listening. They emphasize two-way, personal communications because they know this is the best way to give shape, substance, and credibility to the service vision and the best way to learn what is really going on in the field.

Service leaders also employ their hands-on approach to build a climate of teamwork within the organization. They challenge the organizational unit to be excellent in service, not just the individual employee, using the influence of their offices to bring the team together frequently for meetings, rallies, and celebrations.

Sam Walton, the founder and chairman of retailing giant Wal-Mart Stores, Inc., practices in-the-field leadership as well as any senior executive in America today. Walton and other top Wal-Mart executives spend most of their time each week visiting stores, spreading the gospel, and listening to the sounds of the business. Each Friday the Wal-Mart management team reassembles in the Bentonville, Arkansas, headquarters for mandatory meetings in which they share insights from the field. On the next day several hundred headquarters personnel and managers visiting from the field come together in Wal-Mart's famous Saturday morning meeting, a potpourri of results reporting, plans presentations, cheers, hoopla, homespun philosophy, recognition of outstanding performers, bantering, and exhortations for improvement personally led by Sam Walton himself. With its own communications satellite, Wal-Mart has the capability to broadcast the Saturday meeting directly to its stores. As securities analyst Joseph Ellis once remarked in a speech: "Wal-Mart operates like a small company in terms of how it communicates with its people."[14]

4. Integrity. One of the essential characteristics of service leaders is personal integrity. The best leaders value doing the right thing—even when inconvenient or costly. They place a premium on being fair, consistent, and truthful—and, as a result, earn the trust of associates. As Peter Drucker writes: "The final requirement of effective leadership is to earn trust. Otherwise there won't be any followers—and the only definition of a leader is someone who has followers."[15]

Service leaders recognize the impossibility of building a service-minded attitude in an organization whose management lacks integrity. They recognize the interconnection between service excellence and employees' pride and understand that employees' pride is shaped in part by their perceptions of management fairness.

When executives buy and sell companies as though they were cattle, demonstrating scant interest in what happens to employees and customers as a result; when they inflate prices and then quickly mark the prices down so they can use the term *sale*, when they train and script salespeople to use bait-and-switch, scare, and other unethical tactics to pressure customers to buy what they don't need—these executives completely undermine their own credibility on the subject of service quality. Employees see for themselves that management cares not at all about servicing and satisfying customers. And most employees eventually ask themselves: "Why give my all to a company that lacks integrity? Why bust my chops for a company in which I do not believe?"[16]

Quality and integrity are inseparable, a point powerfully made in an essay entitled "The Quest for Quality":

> As the phrase "the honest workman" suggests, workmanship is founded in personal integrity. Those imbued with it have nothing but scorn for sloppiness, shabbiness, cheapness, sharp dealing or false fronts. Thus if the instinct of workmanship could be stimulated throughout the population, it would affect far more than the economy. In a "quality society," honesty, excellence, and the principle of giving full value for what we receive would become the rule of conduct both in business and personal relationships. What began as an effort to improve quality could end in a revolutionary improvement in the overall quality of life.[17]

THE PAYOFF OF QUALITY

Service leaders, as we have just noted, fundamentally believe that high quality pays off on the bottom line. Many executives, however, are not so sure. Many executives are not yet convinced that hard-dollar investments to improve service will come back as profit gains.

And these executives may be right. Investments to improve service may not come back as profit gains. Indeed, a lot of money is wasted in organizations every year in the name of quality improvement. From adding costly service features that are unimportant to customers to spending training money unwisely, it is quite common for organizations to throw money away pursuing better service quality. As a car-rental agent confesses: "The computer training was real good. I know how to do all this technical stuff, but nobody prepared me for dealing with all these different types of people."[18]

Actually improving service in the eyes of customers is what pays off. When service improvement investments lead to *perceived* service improvement, quality becomes a profit strategy.

The positive relationship between perceived quality and profitability is documented empirically. The massive data base from the Profit Impact of Market Strategy (PIMS) program shows this relationship unequivocally. In *The PIMS Principles*, Buzzell and Gale make the point about as clearly as it can be made:

> In the long run, the most important single factor affecting a business unit's performance is the quality of its products and services, relative to those of competitors. A quality edge boosts performance in two ways:
>
> - In the short run, superior quality yields increased profits via premium prices. As Frank Perdue, the well-known chicken grower, put it: "Customers will go out of their way to buy a superior product, and you can charge them a toll for the trip." Consistent with Perdue's theory, PIMS businesses that ranked in the top third on relative quality sold their products or services, on average, at prices 5–6% higher (relative to competition) than those in the bottom third.
> - In the longer term, superior and/or improving relative quality is the more effective way for a business to grow. Quality leads to both market expansion and gains in market share. The resulting growth in volume means that a superior-quality competitor gains scale advantages over rivals. As a result, even when there are short-run costs connected with improving quality, over a period of time these costs are usually offset by scale economies. Evidence of this is the fact that, on average, businesses with superior quality products have costs about equal to those of their leading competitors. As long as their selling prices are not out of line, they continue to grow while still earning superior profit margins.[19]

Exhibit 1–1, from the PIMS data base, graphically shows the positive relationship between relative perceived quality and return on sales or return on investment.

QUALITY CREATES TRUE CUSTOMERS

Excellent service pays off because it creates true customers—customers who are glad they selected a firm after the service experience, customers who will use the firm again and sing the firm's praises to others.

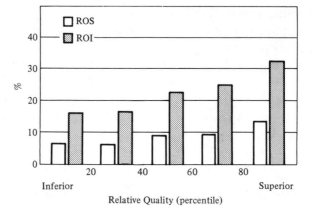

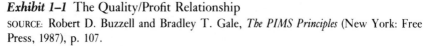

Exhibit 1–1 The Quality/Profit Relationship
SOURCE: Robert D. Buzzell and Bradley T. Gale, *The PIMS Principles* (New York: Free Press, 1987), p. 107.

True customers are like annuities—they keep pumping revenue into the firm's coffers. Stew Leonard, the much-heralded retailer whose Norwalk, Connecticut, food store annually does $3,000 in business per square foot, understands the annuity analogy as well as anyone:

> We should never let a customer leave the store unhappy because we look at each customer as a potential $50,000 asset. An average customer spends $100 a week on food shopping. That's more than $5,000 a year, and more than $50,000 over ten years. Customer service is big business when you look at the long-term picture.[20]

The essence of services marketing is service. Whereas the marketing textbooks stress the four Ps of marketing—product, place, promotion, and price—in a service business the most important competitive weapon is the fifth P of *performance*. It is the performance of the service that separates one service firm from others; it is the performance of the service that creates true customers who buy more, are more loyal, pay Frank Perdue's "toll for the trip," and who spread favorable word of mouth.

Excellent service differentiates otherwise similar competitors in a way that is important to customers. Whereas competing service firms often look the same with similar facilities, equipment, and menus of services, these firms do not feel the same to customers. A genuinely warm greeting from a service provider or the graceful handling of a special request can help one firm seem very different to its customers than other suppliers of similar services.

Thus, it is critical to make the distinction between services and service. *Competitors commonly offer the same services and different service.* That is why James Robinson, CEO of American Express Company, says: "Quality is our only form of patent protection."[21]

In effect, excellent service companies perform better on the bottom line because they perform better for their customers. Customers respond to these firms because they perceive more value in their offers than in competitive offerings. Value is the customer's "overall assessment of the utility of a product based on perceptions of what is received and what is given."[22] The concept of value helps explain how companies with strong service reputations are often able to charge higher prices than their competitors. Customers have to expend more than money to use a service; they also have to bear nonmonetary prices, for example, time and psychic cost.[23] These customers may be quite willing to assume more monetary cost to reduce nonmonetary cost and/or to obtain an otherwise stronger service.

QUALITY LEADS TO EFFICIENCIES

The PIMS data base shows that companies with high relative perceived quality have a cost of doing business that is similar to their main competitors. This is so even though quality improvement frequently involves increased investment in technology, marketing research, employee training, performance measurement, reward systems, and so forth.

What drives down costs most significantly is market share growth. Companies with high market shares benefit costwise from scale economies. Companies with high market shares built through high quality benefit from these scale economies *and from higher revenues due to heavy sales volume and premium prices.*

Quality improvement also leads to operational efficiencies beyond those associated with scale economies. The reality is that service errors and foul-ups add cost to the service delivery system. From computer time to fix account errors to more telephone lines to handle customer problems, service sloppiness steals from the bottom line.

In the early 1980s, a Merrill Lynch & Company, Inc. task force concluded that the firm's direct cost of service snafus was $210 million a year. This included the costs involved in staffing departments dedicated to correcting problems and errors.[24] Audits by Technical Assistance Research Programs, Inc. (TARP) at over a dozen financial service firms show that poor service and ineffective customer communications cause up to one-third of the total workload.[25]

Raymond Larkin, executive vice-president of operations at American Express, makes the point:

> I can't emphasize enough that quality is as bottom line as a company can get. This is as true in a service business as it is in manufacturing. For example, in our Card business, there is rework if errors are made in the first place—if remittances are not processed, if billings are incorrect, if establishments are not paid on time, if Cardmember benefits are not properly communicated. All this generates inquiries and additional processing—or what we call "avoidable input." Reducing avoidable input is the service equivalent to reducing rejects in manufacturing.[26]

The potential payoff from service excellence is considerable. Quality does pay. We know this from the PIMS research. We know this from the TARP research. We know this from the many companies we have worked with and observed closely over the years. And we know it from our own empirical research in service quality that we have written this book to share.

OVERVIEW OF THE BOOK

This book integrates the concepts, ideas, and findings that have emerged from an ongoing, multiphase study of service quality which we started in 1983. From this research, sponsored by the Marketing Science Institute in Cambridge, Massachusetts, we have developed a conceptual model of service quality and a methodology for measuring customer perceptions of service quality. We also have developed many ideas about what companies need to do to improve service quality.

We use our model as a framework for the book as it provides a structure for understanding service quality, measuring it, diagnosing service-quality problems, and deriving solutions to the problems—the very subjects an executive wishing to improve quality needs to entertain. We refer to the model as the *gaps model* because it features discrepancies or gaps that need to be closed to offer excellent service.

In chapter 2 we develop the customer part of our model, defining the concept and dimensions of service quality. In chapter 3 we present the managerial part of the model, focusing on four gaps that cause service-quality problems. In chapters 4 through 7 we take a closer look at these four gaps; in each chapter we focus on the underlying reasons for a gap and make suggestions for closing it. In chapter 8 we offer suggestions on how to get started in a service-improvement effort, a challenge that often appears to be overwhelming. And in chapter 9, the final chapter, we discuss emerging service quality issues and challenges for the decade of the 1990's. The book's appendixes include descriptions of our research methods and our survey instruments.

2

◇ ◇ ◇

THE CUSTOMERS' VIEW
OF SERVICE QUALITY

W HEN WE STARTED our research program in service quality, we expected to find a varied and rich literature that would guide us. We
found nothing of the kind! Instead we found a literature almost exclusively devoted to tangible goods quality, defined in terms of conformance
to manufacturers' specifications.[1] As a result, quality control principles
and practices that we uncovered, while pertinent to evaluating and ensuring goods quality, were inadequate for understanding service quality.
This inadequacy stems from the three fundamental ways services differ
from goods in terms of how they are produced, consumed, and evaluated.

First, services are basically *intangible*. Because they are performances
and experiences rather than objects, precise manufacturing specifications
concerning uniform quality can rarely be set. Unlike automobiles and
audiocassettes, airline transportation and aerobic exercises cannot be measured, tested, and verified in advance of sale to assure quality. Moreover,
when what is being sold is purely a performance, the criteria customers
use to evaluate it may be complex and difficult to capture precisely.

Second, services—especially those with a high labor content—are *het-
erogeneous*: their performance often varies from producer to producer,
from customer to customer, and from day to day. The quality of the
interactions that bank tellers, flight attendants, and insurance agents have
with customers can rarely be standardized to ensure uniformity the way
quality of goods produced in a manufacturing plant can.

Third, production and consumption of many services are *inseparable*.
Quality in services often occurs during service delivery, usually in an
interaction between the customer and the provider, rather than being
engineered at the manufacturing plant and delivered intact to the customer. Unlike goods producers, service providers do not have the benefit

15

of a factory serving as a buffer between production and consumption. Service customers are often in the service factory, observing and evaluating the production process as they experience the service.

While the literature on quality has been predominantly goods-oriented, a few contributions have focused on service quality.[2] From these writings emerge the following themes:

- Service quality is more difficult for customers to evaluate than goods quality. Therefore, the criteria customers use to evaluate service quality may be more difficult for the marketer to comprehend. How customers evaluate investment services offered by a stockbroker is more complicated and varied than how they evaluate insulation materials. Customers' assessment of the quality of health-care services is more complex and difficult than their assessment of the quality of automobiles.
- Customers do not evaluate service quality solely on the outcome of a service (e.g., how a customer's hair looks after a hair cut); they also consider the process of service delivery (e.g., how involved, responsive, and friendly the hair stylist is during the hair cut).
- The only criteria that count in evaluating service quality are defined by customers. Only customers judge quality; all other judgments are essentially irrelevant. Specifically, service-quality perceptions stem from how well a provider performs vis-à-vis customers' expectations about how the provider should perform.

EXPLORATORY CUSTOMER STUDY

The sparse literature on service quality provided us with several general insights. Clearly, it was not rich enough to develop a comprehensive conceptual foundation for understanding and improving service quality. A number of key questions remained unanswered: How exactly do customers evaluate the quality of a service? Do they directly make a global evaluation or do they assess specific facets of a service in arriving at an overall evaluation? If the latter, what are the multiple facets or dimensions on which they evaluate the service? Do those dimensions vary across services and different customer segments? If customers' expectations play a crucial role in the assessment of service quality, which factors shape and influence those expectations?

To seek answers to these and related questions we undertook an exploratory study consisting of 12 customer focus-group interviews, 3 in each of four service sectors: retail banking, credit cards, securities brokerage, and product repair and maintenance. These service businesses vary along key attributes used to categorize services.[3] For example, retail banking and credit-card services provide immediate customer benefits, while securities-brokerage and product-repair services provide more enduring benefits. Although product repair and maintenance services concern customers' tangible possessions, the other three services pertain to customers' intangible (financial) assets. Banking and securities-brokerage services are more labor intensive and interactive than the other two.

We purposely selected a broad spectrum of consumer services to study in this first phase of our research because we were looking for service-quality insights that would transcend the boundaries of specific industries. We also varied the composition of the focus groups to ensure that our findings would be generalizable to a variety of settings. Additional details concerning the composition and conduct of the focus groups are outlined in "Focus-Group Interviews."

FOCUS-GROUP INTERVIEWS

We controlled the composition of the 12 focus groups (3 groups per service sector) in accordance with guidelines traditionally followed in the marketing research field. Specifically, we screened respondents to ensure that they had engaged in one or more transactions pertaining to the service in question within the previous three months. Thus each focus group consisted of recent users of one of the four services. Between 8 and 12 respondents participated in each focus group. To maintain similarity among members and assure maximum participation, we assigned respondents to groups on the basis of sex and age. Six of the 12 groups included only males and 6 included only females. However, we interviewed at least one male group and one female group for each of the four services. Respondents in each group were roughly in the same age bracket; but the three focus groups for each service category covered different age brackets to ascertain the viewpoints of a broad cross section of customers.

We conducted eight focus groups in a metropolitan area in southwestern United States. We distributed the remaining four groups—one on the West Coast, one in the Midwest, and two in the East—to achieve geographic diversity.

A nationally recognized company from each of the four service sectors sponsored and participated in our study. We did not, however,

reveal the identities of these firms to the focus-group participants because our interest was in customers' quality evaluations in a service
category in general, as opposed to their assessment of the participating firm in that category.

One member of the research team served as the moderator for each
of the focus groups. The questions we asked to stimulate discussion
covered topics such as instances of, and reasons for, satisfaction and
dissatisfaction with the service; descriptions of an ideal service (e.g.,
ideal bank or ideal credit card); the meaning of service quality; factors
important in evaluating service quality; and performance expectations
concerning the service.

FOCUS-GROUP FINDINGS

Through the focus-group interviews we learned a great deal about how
customers view service quality. Customers talked about many things—
their expectations, their priorities, their experiences. They told us about
high quality and low quality. They talked about many different attributes, some dealing with the service itself; others dealing with the person
delivering the service.

Even though the specific examples and experiences the respondents
shared with us were unique to the service category being discussed, we
detected a number of underlying patterns in the responses—patterns
remarkably consistent across all four sets of focus-group interviews.
These common patterns offered us valuable insights about how customers define and evaluate service quality.

Definition of Service Quality. The focus groups unambiguously supported the notion that the key to ensuring good service quality is meeting
or exceeding what customers expect from the service. One female participant described a situation when a repairman not only fixed her broken
appliance but also explained what had gone wrong and how she could fix
it herself if a similar problem occurred in the future. She rated the quality
of this service excellent because it exceeded her expectations. A male
respondent in a banking-services focus group described the frustration he
felt when his bank would not cash his payroll check from a nationally
known employer because it was postdated by one day. When someone
else in the group pointed out legal constraints preventing the bank from
cashing his check, he responded, "Well, nobody in the bank explained
that to me!" Not receiving an explanation in the bank, this respondent

perceived that the bank was unwilling, rather than unable, to cash the check. This in turn resulted in a perception of poor service quality.

Similar experiences, both positive and negative, were described by customers in every focus group. It was clear to us that judgments of high and low service quality depend on how customers perceive the actual service performance in the context of what they expected. Therefore service quality, as perceived by customers, can be defined as *the extent of discrepancy between customers' expectations or desires and their perceptions*.

Factors Influencing Expectations. The common themes emerging from the focus groups suggested several key factors that might shape customers' expectations. First, what customers hear from other customers—*word-of-mouth communications*—is a potential determinant of expectations. For instance, several respondents in our product-repair focus groups indicated that the high quality of service they expected from the repair firms they chose stemmed from the recommendations of their friends and neighbors.

Second, in each of the four sets of focus groups, respondents' expectations appeared to vary somewhat depending on their individual characteristics and circumstances, suggesting thereby that *personal needs* of customers might moderate their expectations to a certain degree. For example, in the credit-card focus groups, while some customers expected credit-card companies to provide them with the maximum possible credit limits, other customers wished that their credit-card companies were more stringent than they then were.

Third, the extent of *past experience* with using a service could also influence customers' expectation levels. More experienced participants in the securities-brokerage focus groups, for instance, seemed to have somewhat lower expectations regarding brokers' behavioral attributes such as friendliness and politeness; however, they appeared to be more demanding with respect to brokers' technical competence and effectiveness.

Fourth, *external communications* from service providers play a key role in shaping customers' expectations. Under external communications we include a variety of direct and indirect messages conveyed by service firms to customers: a bank's print advertisement promising the friendliest tellers in town, a television commercial for a credit card touting its acceptability around the world, a repair firm's receptionist guaranteeing the arrival of a service representative at an appointed time, or a brokerage firm's glossy brochures implying a promise of superior service.

One factor whose influence on expectations is subsumed under the general influence of external communications is price. This factor plays an important role in shaping expectations, particularly those of prospective customers of a service. To illustrate, for customers contemplating the purchase of brokerage services for the first time, price is likely to influence their choice of a certain type of broker (e.g. a full-service versus a discount broker) as well as their expectations from the chosen broker. The securities-brokerage focus groups we conducted, while consisting of respondents who were already using brokerage services, did reveal differences in expectations between users of full-service and discount brokers, implying a link between price levels and expectation levels.

Dimensions of Service Quality. Perhaps the most revealing and most unique insights emerging from our focus groups concern the criteria used by customers in judging service quality. The numerous examples and experiences that respondents shared with us in the 12 focus groups provided us with a rich reservoir of customers' expectations as reflected by specific questions that customers apparently ask, and answer, in assessing service quality. After we sifted through these questions several times, it was clear that the same general criteria underlay sets of service-specific questions spanning the four sectors. We identified ten general criteria or dimensions and labeled them tangibles, reliability, responsiveness, competence, courtesy, credibility, security, access, communication, and understanding the customer. Exhibit 2–1 contains concise definitions of these dimensions and illustrates each dimension with service-specific evaluative questions emerging from the focus groups.

The ten dimensions defined and illustrated in exhibit 2–1 are not necessarily independent of one another. For instance, facets of credibility and security may indeed overlap somewhat. Because our focus-group research was exploratory and qualitative, measurement of possible overlap across the ten dimensions had to await a subsequent quantitative phase of research (described in the next section). We are confident that the set of ten general dimensions of service quality is exhaustive and appropriate for assessing quality in a broad variety of services. Even though the *specific* evaluative criteria may vary from service to service, the general dimensions underlying those criteria are captured by our set of ten.

In summary, from our exploratory study we were able to (1) define service quality as the discrepancy between customers' expectations and perceptions; (2) suggest key factors—word-of-mouth communications, personal needs, past experience, and external communications—that influence customers' expectations; and (3) identify ten general dimensions that represent the evaluative criteria customers use to assess service quality. Exhibit 2–2 provides a pictorial summary of these findings.

Dimension and Definition	Examples of Specific Questions Raised by Customers
Tangibles: Appearance of physical facilities, equipment, personnel, and communication materials.	• Are the bank's facilities attractive? • Is my stockbroker dressed appropriately? • Is my credit card statement easy to understand? . Do the tools used by the repair person look modern?
Reliability: Ability to perform the promised service dependably and accurately.	• When a loan officer says she will call me back in 15 minutes, does she do so? • Does the stockbroker follow my exact instructions to buy or sell? . Is my credit card statement free of errors? • Is my washing machine repaired right the first time?
Responsiveness: Willingness to help customers and provide prompt service.	• When there is a problem with my bank statement, does the bank resolve the problem quickly? • Is my stockbroker willing to answer my questions? • Are charges for returned merchandise credited to my account promptly? • Is the repair firm willing to give me a specific time when the repair person will show up?
Competence: Possession of the required skills and knowledge to perform the service.	• Is the bank teller able to process my transactions without fumbling around? . Does my brokerage firm have the research capabilities to accurately track market developments? • When I call my credit card company, is the person at the other end able to answer my questions? • Does the repair person appear to know what he is doing?
Courtesy: Politeness, respect, consideration, and friendliness of contact personnel.	. Does the bank teller have a pleasant demeanor? . Does my broker refrain from acting busy or being rude when I ask questions? • Are the telephone operators in the credit card company consistently polite when answering my calls? • Does the repair person take off his muddy shoes before stepping on my carpet?

(continued)

Exhibit 2–1 Ten Dimensions of Service Quality

Dimension and Definition	Examples of Specific Questions Raised by Customers
Credibility: Trustworthiness, believability, honesty of the service provider.	• Does the bank have a good reputation? • Does my broker refrain from pressuring me to buy? • Are the interest rates/fees charged by my credit card company consistent with the services provided? • Does the repair firm guarantee its services?
Security: Freedom from danger, risk, or doubt.	• Is it safe for me to use the bank's automatic teller machines? • Does my brokerage firm know where my stock certificate is? • Is my credit card safe from unauthorized use? • Can I be confident that the repair job was done properly?
Access: Approachability and ease of contact.	• How easy is it for me to talk to senior bank officials when I have a problem? • Is it easy to get through to my broker over the telephone? • Does the credit card company have a 24-hour, toll-free telephone number? • Is the repair service facility conveniently located?
Communication: Keeping customers informed in language they can understand and listening to them.	• Can the loan officer explain clearly the various charges related to the mortgage loan? • Does my broker avoid using technical jargon? • When I call my credit card company, are they willing to listen to me? • Does the repair firm call when they are unable to keep a scheduled repair appointment?
Understanding the Customer: Making the effort to know customers and their needs.	• Does someone in my bank recognize me as a regular customer? • Does my broker try to determine what my specific financial objectives are? • Is the credit limit set by my credit card company consistent with what I can afford (i.e., neither too high nor too low)? • Is the repair firm willing to be flexible enough to accommodate *my* schedule?

Exhibit 2-1 Continued

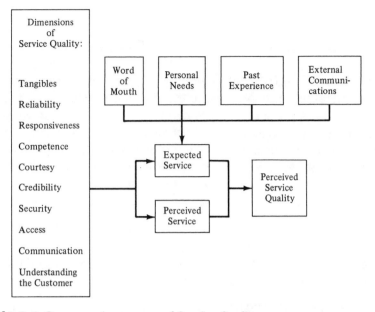

Exhibit 2-2 Customer Assessment of Service Quality

SERVQUAL: AN INSTRUMENT
FOR MEASURING SERVICE QUALITY

Building on the conceptual definition of service quality and the ten evaluative dimensions from our exploratory research, we embarked on a quantitative research phase to develop an instrument for measuring customers' perceptions of service quality. To ensure that our instrument would have sound statistical properties and broad acceptability, this phase of our research involved customer surveys in five different service sectors: product repair and maintenance, retail banking, long-distance telephone, securities brokerage, and credit cards. Details of these surveys are summarized in "Development of SERVQUAL."

Our quantitative research phase resulted in a parsimonious instrument (SERVQUAL) consisting of two sections: (1) An expectations section containing 22 statements to ascertain the general expectations of customers concerning a service, and (2) a perceptions section containing a matching set of 22 statements to measure customers' assessments of a specific firm within the service category. The instructions and statements for the two sections of SERVQUAL are presented in appendix A.[4]

DEVELOPMENT OF SERVQUAL

In developing SERVQUAL—our instrument for measuring customers' perceptions of service quality—we followed well-established procedures for designing scales to measure constructs that are not directly observable. We developed 97 items capturing the 10 dimensions of service quality identified in our exploratory phase. We then recast each item into a pair of statements—one to measure expectations about firms in general within the service category being investigated, and the other to measure perceptions about the particular firm whose service quality was being assessed.

> *Sample expectation statement:* "When these firms promise to do something by a certain time, they should do so."

> *Sample perception statement:* "When XYZ promises to do something by a certain time, it does so."

A seven-point scale ranging from 7 (strongly agree) to 1 (strongly disagree) accompanied each statement.

We refined and condensed the 97-item instrument through a series of repeated data-collection and -analysis steps. We performed this instrument purification to eliminate items that failed to discriminate well among respondents with differing quality perceptions about firms. We gathered data for the initial refinement of the 97-item instrument from a quota sample of 200 customers, divided equally between males and females. Included in the sample were recent users of one of the following five services: appliance repair and maintenance, retail banking, long-distance telephone, securities brokerage, and credit cards. We converted the raw questionnaire data into perception-minus-expectation scores for the various items. These difference scores could range from $+6$ to -6, with more positive scores representing higher perceived service quality. We analyzed the difference scores using several statistical analyses. These analyses resulted in the elimination of roughly two-thirds of the original items and the consolidation of several overlapping quality dimensions into new, combined dimensions. To verify the reliability and validity of the condensed scale, we administered it to four independent samples of approximately 190 customers each. We gathered data on the service quality of four nationally known firms: a bank, a credit-card issuer, an appliance repair-and-maintenance firm, and a long-distance telephone company. Analysis of data from the four samples led to additional refinement of the instrument and confirmed its reliability and validity. The final instrument consists of 22 items, spanning the five dimensions of service quality described in the chapter: tangibles, reliability, responsiveness, assurance, and empathy.

The various statistical analyses conducted in constructing SERV-QUAL revealed considerable correlation among items representing several of the original ten dimensions. In particular, the correlations suggested consolidation of the last seven dimensions listed in exhibits 2–1 and 2–2 into two broader dimensions labeled *assurance* and *empathy*. The remaining dimensions—*tangibles, reliability*, and *responsiveness*—remained intact throughout the scale development and refinement process. Exhibit 2–3 shows the correspondence between the original ten dimensions and SERVQUAL's five dimensions.

When we examined the content of the final items making up the two new dimensions (assurance and empathy), we found that the items still

SERVQUAL Dimensions

Original Ten Dimensions for Evaluating Service Quality	Tangibles	Reliability	Responsiveness	Assurance	Empathy
Tangibles	//////				
Reliability		//////			
Responsiveness			//////		
Competence				//////	
Courtesy				//////	
Credibility				//////	
Security				//////	
Access					//////
Communication					//////
Understanding the Customer					//////

Exhibit 2–3 Correspondence between SERVQUAL Dimensions and Original Ten Dimensions for Evaluating Service Quality

represented key features of the seven dimensions that were consolidated. Therefore, although SERVQUAL had only five distinct dimensions, they captured facets of all of the ten originally conceptualized dimensions. The items making up the consolidated dimensions also suggested concise definitions for them. These definitions, along with the definitions of the three original dimensions that remained intact, follow:

Tangibles	Appearance of physical facilities, equipment, personnel, and communication materials
Reliability	Ability to perform the promised service dependably and accurately
Responsiveness:	Willingness to help customers and provide prompt service
Assurance:	Knowledge and courtesy of employees and their ability to convey trust and confidence
Empathy:	Caring, individualized attention the firm provides its customers

RELATIVE IMPORTANCE OF THE SERVQUAL DIMENSIONS

The five SERVQUAL dimensions, by virtue of being derived from systematic analysis of customers' ratings from hundreds of interviews in several service sectors, are a concise representation of the core criteria that customers employ in evaluating service quality. As such, it is reasonable to speculate that customers would consider all five criteria to be quite important. In fact, when we asked users of credit-card, repair-and-maintenance, long-distance telephone, and retail banking services to rate the importance of each SERVQUAL dimension on a scale of 1 (not all important) to 10 (extremely important), we found that all five dimensions were considered critical. As exhibit 2–4 reveals, the mean importance ratings for reliability, responsiveness, assurance, and empathy are above 9 for all four services; the mean ratings for tangibles, while somewhat low by comparison, are still in the upper end of the 10-point scale, ranging from 7.14 to 8.56.

Anticipating that the mean importance ratings may not reveal a clear picture of the relative importance of the five dimensions, we also asked

Exhibit 2–4 Importance of SERVQUAL Dimensions in Four Service Sectors

	Mean Importance Rating on 10- Point Scale*	Percentage of Respondents Indicating Dimension Is Most Important
Credit-Card Customers (n = 187)		
Tangibles	7.43	0.6
Reliability	9.45	48.6
Responsiveness	9.37	19.8
Assurance	9.25	17.5
Empathy	9.09	13.6
Repair-and-Maintenance Customers (n = 183)		
Tangibles	8.48	1.2
Reliability	9.64	57.2
Responsiveness	9.54	19.9
Assurance	9.62	12.0
Empathy	9.30	9.6
Long-Distance Telephone Customers (n = 184)		
Tangibles	7.14	0.6
Reliability	9.67	60.6
Responsiveness	9.57	16.0
Assurance	9.29	12.6
Empathy	9.25	10.3
Bank Customers (n = 177)		
Tangibles	8.56	1.1
Reliability	9.44	42.1
Responsiveness	9.34	18.0
Assurance	9.18	13.6
Empathy	9.30	25.1

* Scale ranges from 1 (not at all important) to 10 (extremely important).

the respondents which one dimension they would choose as being the most critical in their assessment of service quality. The respondents' choices, summarized in exhibit 2–4, clearly show that reliability is the most critical dimension, *regardless of the service being studied.* The results contained in exhibit 2–4, when considered collectively, imply an important message from customers to service providers: Appear neat and organized, be responsive, be reassuring, be empathetic, and most of all, be reliable—*do what you say you are going to do.*

We have used the SERVQUAL instrument in many different studies since we initially developed and tested it. Results from those studies have consistently shown reliability to be the most important dimension, and tangibles the least important. Most recently, we asked samples averaging about four hundred customers of each of five nationally known companies (two banks, two insurance companies, and a long-distance telephone company) to allocate a total of 100 points across the five dimensions according to how important they perceived each dimension to be. Based on responses from 1,936 customers, the average allocations received by the five dimensions are as shown in exhibit 2–5. The patterns of point-allocations by customers of each of the five companies were essentially similar to the consolidated pie chart (exhibit 2–5). Even though it is possible that the relative rankings of the dimensions as perceived by customers might change in the future, we are confident that the number one concern of customers today, regardless of type of service, is reliability; and the facet that matters the least to current customers in assessing quality of service is tangibles (the importance of tangibles as a quality cue to *potential* customers may be higher, however).

PERFORMANCE ALONG THE SERVQUAL DIMENSIONS

As perceived by customers, how well are service companies doing along the SERVQUAL dimensions? Results from our five-company

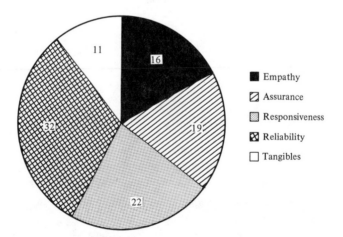

Exhibit 2–5 Relative Importance of SERVQUAL Dimensions when Customers Allocate 100 Points

study are very revealing. Exhibit 2–6 shows the mean SERVQUAL scores (i.e., perception-expectation scores) by dimension for the total customer sample. In this exhibit, the more negative the SERVQUAL score, the more serious the service-quality shortfall in the eyes of customers. Notice how the single most important dimension of service, reliability, has the most negative SERVQUAL score. And the second most important dimension, responsiveness, has the second most negative SERVQUAL score. The least important dimension, tangibles, has a slightly positive SERVQUAL score, implying that the companies in our study on average exceeded customers' expectations on this dimension! Clearly, there is a mismatch between the priorities expressed by customers and the levels of quality delivered by the companies.

Exhibit 2–7 shows the average SERVQUAL scores (aggregated across all five dimensions) for each company in our study. Two scores are shown for each company: an unweighted score, which is the simple average of the scores on the five dimensions, and a weighted score, which is an average that takes into account the relative weights assigned by customers when they allocated 100 points to the five dimensions. (Procedures for computing the unweighted and weighted scores, as well as other potential applications of the SERVQUAL scale and data, are given in appendix A.)

The negative SERVQUAL scores (both unweighted and weighted) across the board clearly show that there is room for service-quality im-

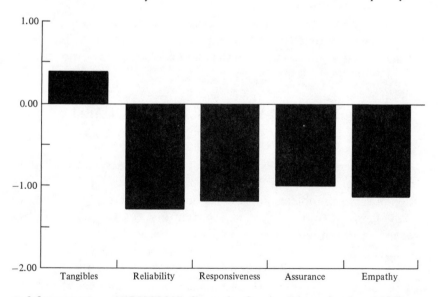

Exhibit 2–6 Mean SERVQUAL Scores by Service Dimension (n = 1,936)

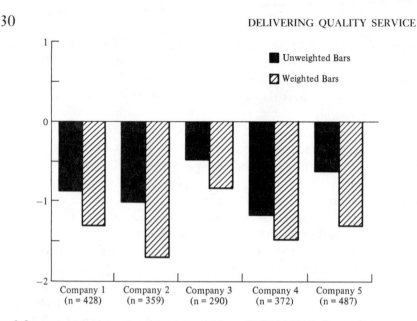

Exhibit 2–7 Unweighted and Weighted Mean SERVQUAL Scores by Company

provement in every company in our study. Even more significant is that the weighted scores are more negative than the unweighted scores in all five companies! This indicates that each company is performing most poorly on facets that are most critical to customers. The discrepancy between the unweighted and weighted scores in each company suggests the potential opportunity for improving quality of service perceptions by shifting emphasis and resources to the more critical facets of the service.

IMPACT OF SERVICE PROBLEMS ON QUALITY PERCEPTIONS

Are customers' perceptions of quality of service influenced by whether or not they experienced a recent service problem? Does satisfactory resolution of service problems improve service quality perceptions? We explored these questions in our five-company study. The results, summarized in exhibit 2–8, are revealing.

Exhibit 2–8 shows the average SERVQUAL scores (aggregated across all five dimensions and all five companies), broken out by the following pairs of customer subgroups: (1) customers who had experienced a recent service problem and those who had not; and (2) among customers who

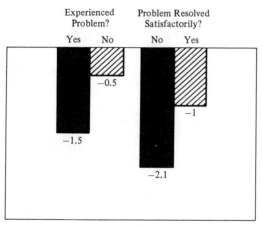

Exhibit 2–8 SERVQUAL Scores for Different Sample Groups

had experienced service problems, those who felt their problems were satisfactorily resolved and those who did not feel that way.[5] Clearly, when customers experience a service problem their perceptions of service quality are adversely affected. Moreover, companies fare best when they prevent service problems altogether and fare worst when service problems occur and are not resolved to the customers' satisfaction.

The implications of the findings summarized in exhibit 2–8 are clear: The most important thing a service company can do is *be reliable*—that is, perform the service dependably and accurately . . . do it right the first time. When a service problem does crop up, however, all is not lost . . . unless the company ignores it. In other words, by resolving the problem to the customer's satisfaction—by performing the service *very* right the second time—the company can significantly improve customer-retention rates.

At a time when many service companies view complaining customers with disdain—in the words of a focus-group participant in our exploratory research: "When you have a problem with their service they treat you like you have a disease!"—those companies that are truly dedicated to satisfactory problem resolution can reap handsome dividends. Research conducted by Technical Assistance Research Programs, Inc. (TARP), a consulting firm specializing in the study of customers' complaints, has shown that the average return from investments made to satisfactorily handle customers' complaints and inquiries ranges from 100 percent (for marketers of durable goods such as washing machines and refrigerators) to 170 percent (for banks).[6] Companies that epitomize exemplary quality of service are well aware of the excellent returns from resolving customers' problems to their satisfaction. Maryanne Rasmussen, vice-president of worldwide quality at one such company, American Express, nicely sums up the benefits of proper problem resolution: "The formula I use is: Better complaint handling equals higher customer satisfaction equals higher brand loyalty equals higher profitability."[7]

IMPACT OF QUALITY PERCEPTIONS
ON WILLINGNESS TO RECOMMEND

Word-of-mouth recommendations (i.e., recommendations from friends and relatives) play a much greater role in customers' purchases of services than in their purchases of goods.[8] In light of the importance of word-of-mouth communications, we examined the association between customers' perceptions of the quality of service rendered by a company and their willingness to recommend the company to their friends. The results (aggregated across all five companies) are summarized in exhibit 2–9.

As the SERVQUAL scores represented by the bar chart in exhibit 2–9 show, there is a dramatic difference between the quality perceptions of customers who would and those who would not recommend their service companies to their friends. Clearly, a substantial improvement in customers' perceptions of a company's quality of service is required before they become positive spokespersons for it. Alternatively, striving to perform all facets of a service flawlessly the first time—and satisfactorily resolving any flaws that may occur—not only enhances a customer's

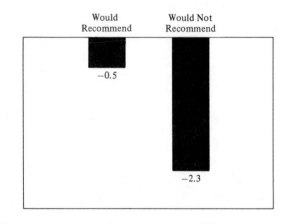

Exhibit 2–9 SERVQUAL Scores for Customers Who Would and Would Not Recommend the Company to a Friend

service-quality perceptions but also greatly increases his or her likelihood of recommending the company to prospective customers.

SUMMARY

In this chapter we reviewed a stream of customer research consisting of a series of qualitative studies (focus groups) followed by a series of quantitative studies (customer surveys). The qualitative phase of the research yielded a definition of service quality (i.e., discrepancy between customers' expectations and perceptions), identified the factors that influence customers' expectations (word of mouth, personal needs, past experience, and external communications from service providers), and revealed ten general dimensions or evaluative criteria that customers use in assessing service quality. A major outcome of the quantitative phase of our research was SERVQUAL—the 22-item instrument for measuring customers' expectations and perceptions along five quality dimensions (tangibles, reliability, responsiveness, assurance, and empathy). Studies conducted in the quantitative phase also illuminated the relative importance of the five dimensions (reliability most important; tangibles least important) and indicated how well service companies are performing along those dimensions. The collective findings from these studies suggest key opportunities for companies to improve their quality of service as perceived by customers. The findings also emphasize the significant benefits that companies can reap by providing superior service quality.

As revealed by our customer research described in this chapter, the key to delivering high-quality service is to balance customers' expectations and perceptions and close the gaps between the two. The SERV-QUAL methodology can help determine where and how serious the gaps are. In attempting to close SERVQUAL gaps, a company would benefit from an understanding of internal (i.e., within-company) shortfalls or gaps that might be responsible for the external (i.e., customer-perceived) shortfalls. A major component of our multiphase study focused on identifying such internal gaps and relating them to customers' perceptions of service quality. The findings from this component of our study are the focus of the next chapter.

3

◇ ◇ ◇

POTENTIAL CAUSES OF SERVICE-QUALITY SHORTFALLS

EXECUTIVES STRIVING TO ACHIEVE a distinctive position and a sustainable advantage in today's increasingly competitive business world no doubt realize the importance of delivering superior quality service by meeting or exceeding customers' expectations. However, simply believing in the importance of providing excellent service quality is not enough. Executives who are truly dedicated to service quality must put in motion a continuous process for: (1) monitoring customers' perceptions of service quality; (2) identifying the causes of service-quality shortfalls; and (3) taking appropriate action to improve the quality of service.

The SERVQUAL approach discussed in the preceding chapter focused on assessing and understanding customers' perceptions of service quality. This chapter focuses on deficiencies within companies that contribute to poor service-quality perceptions by customers. Based on findings from the exploratory phase of our research, it develops a conceptual model linking customer-perceived quality deficiencies to within-company deficiencies or gaps. After discussing the conceptual model, the chapter outlines two additional research phases focusing on within-company gaps. Subsequent chapters discuss the findings from these two research phases and suggest remedial actions for closing the gaps.

EXPLORATORY EXECUTIVE STUDY

To gain insights about executives' views on what constitutes quality of service, we conducted a series of in-depth, face-to-face interviews as part of our exploratory research phase that included the customer focus-group interviews discussed in chapter 2. We interviewed executives from four nationally recognized companies chosen from the same four service sectors in which we conducted our customer focus group interviews; retail banking, credit cards, securities brokerage, and product repair and maintenance. The individuals we interviewed came from marketing, operations, customer relations, and senior management—areas in which executives should have a keen interest in service quality.

Our focus in the interviews was wide ranging. What did the executives perceive to be service-quality from the customers' perspective? Which key criteria did they believe their customers used in judging the quality of service provided by their companies? Which problems did they face in consistently delivering high-quality service? Which steps did they take to control or improve the quality of their services? Our dialogue with the executives provided us with a wealth of information concerning potential causes of service-quality shortfalls.

EXECUTIVE STUDY FINDINGS

As was true of the customer focus-group interviews, remarkably consistent patterns emerged from the four sets of executive interviews. Although some of the responses were specific to the companies and industries selected, most of the responses revealed common themes that cut across company and industry boundaries. These themes, which offer critical clues for achieving effective service-quality control, can be cast in the form of four key discrepancies or gaps pertaining to executive perceptions of service quality and the tasks associated with service delivery to customers. *These four gaps, which we define and discuss shortly, are the major causes of the service-quality gap customers may perceive* (i.e., the discrepancy between their expectations and perceptions as discussed in chapter 2).

To facilitate discussion of the various gaps, we denote the service-quality shortfall perceived by customers as Gap 5 and the shortfalls within the service provider's organization as Gaps 1 through 4. Because an aim of this chapter is to link the customer and provider gaps in the form of a conceptual framework for understanding and improving service quality, let us first review the diagram in exhibit 3–1 which represents Gap 5. (Exhibit 3–1 is an abbreviated version of exhibit 2–2.) As exhibit 3–1 shows, Gap 5 represents the potential discrepancy between the expected and perceived service from the customers' standpoint. Key determinants of the service expected by customers include word-of-mouth

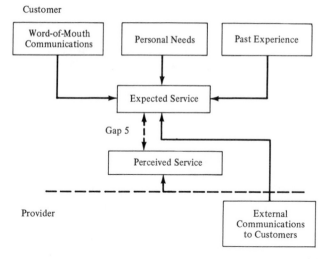

Exhibit 3–1 Gap 5: Between Customers' Expectations and Perceived Service

communications, personal needs, past experience, and external communications from the service provider. Next, we define and discuss each of the four service-provider gaps that contribute to Gap 5.

GAP 1: CUSTOMERS' EXPECTATIONS—MANAGEMENT-PERCEPTIONS GAP

In each of the four service sectors examined in our exploratory research, many of the executives' perceptions about what customers expect from superior quality service were congruent with the expectations expressed by customers themselves in the focus groups. Examples of attributes of quality service mentioned by both executives and customers include friendly and efficient bank tellers, error-free credit-card statements, honest securities brokers who have their customers' best interests at heart, and prompt repair of broken appliances. However, a number of discrepancies were also evident between expectations expressed by customers and executives' understanding of those expectations.

For example, privacy or confidentiality during transactions emerged as a pivotal quality attribute in every banking and securities-brokerage focus group we conducted. Customers in our focus groups expressed concern that their sensitive discussions with bank personnel or stockbrokers could easily be overheard by others because the service provider's physical facilities were not designed to ensure privacy. Yet the bank and securities brokerage executives we talked to were apparently oblivious to the importance attached by customers to transaction privacy. Not once did customers' concern for privacy surface in the executive interviews as a key ingredient of service quality.

A second illustration concerns the physical and security features of credit cards (e.g., the likelihood that unauthorized people could use the cards) which generated substantial discussion in the customer focus-group interviews but did not surface as a critical quality attribute in the executive interviews. Likewise, several customers in the credit-card focus groups expressed a preference for lower credit limits and higher minimum payments, implying a desire for disincentives to spend. Yet the executive interviews did not evidence cognizance of the fact that not all credit-card customers desire high credit limits. In fact, when asked to list in order of importance the most critical dimensions of service quality from the customers' perspective, one executive named credit availability first and stated that it would be a "great disservice" if customers are not given a "big enough limit."

In the product-repair-and-maintenance sector, focus-group participants indicated that they were unlikely to view large, nationally known repair service firms as high-quality firms. They consistently touted the quality of small, independent repair firms as being exemplary because such firms were much more reliable and responsive to customers' concerns. In contrast, most executive comments indicated that the size of their company and their national network of repair facilities would signal strength from a quality standpoint. Ironically, even though we did not reveal the identity of the repair company participating in our research to focus-group participants, several of them brought its name up and stated that they would not like to do business with it because it was too big, uncaring, and impersonal.

As demonstrated by the preceding illustrations, service-firm executives may not always be completely aware of which characteristics connote high quality to customers. Managers may not know about certain service features critical to meeting customers' desires; or, even when aware of such features, they may not know which levels of performance customers desire along those features.

When senior executives with the authority and responsibility for setting priorities do not fully understand customers' service expectations, they may trigger a chain of bad decisions and suboptimal resource allocations that result in perceptions of poor service quality. One example of misplaced priorities stemming from an inaccurate understanding of customers' expectations is spending far too much money on sprucing up the appearance of a company's physical facilities when customers may be much more concerned with how convenient, comfortable, and functional the facilities are. Another example is focusing training programs for contact personnel almost exclusively on the internal aspects of their jobs (e.g., filling out paperwork, following company rules and regulations) with little or no emphasis on aspects likely to be of greater concern to customers (e.g., answering customers' questions patiently and reassuringly, explaining the service to customers). The upshot is that senior managers' inaccurate understanding of what customers expect and what really matters to them, diagrammed as Gap 1 exhibit 3–2, is likely to result in service-delivery performance that is perceived by customers as falling short of their expectations (Gap 5). The necessary first step in improving quality of service (i.e., narrowing Gap 5) is for management to acquire accurate information about customers' expectations (i.e., close Gap 1).

Gap 2: Management's Perceptions–Service-Quality Specifications Gap

Management's correct perceptions of customers' expectations is necessary, but not sufficient, for achieving superior quality service. Another prerequisite for providing high service quality is the presence of performance standards mirroring management's perceptions of customers' expectations. However, a recurring theme that emerged from our executive interviews was the difficulty the executives experienced in translating their understanding of customers' expectations into service-quality specifications.

As we mentioned earlier, our exploratory research revealed a number

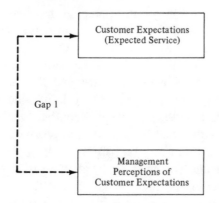

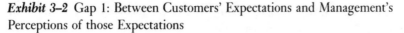

Exhibit 3–2 Gap 1: Between Customers' Expectations and Management's Perceptions of those Expectations

of areas of congruence between characteristics customers considered as indicators of high-quality service and those executives believed were critical to customers. In most of these instances, the executives had not converted their knowledge of customers' expectations into concrete performance standards. They cited a variety of constraints they believed to be insurmountable hurdles in setting service specifications consistent with customers' expectations. For instance, all the repair firm executives we interviewed were acutely aware that customers view rapid response to appliance breakdowns as a vital ingredient of high-quality service. Nonetheless, they found it difficult to establish precise performance standards for response time because of a lack of trained service personnel and wide fluctuations in customers' demand for service. As one executive observed, peak demand for repairing air conditioners and lawn mowers occurs during summer months, just as most service personnel want to go on vacations.

The apparent sense of frustration evident in the preceding example is also likely to be experienced by executives in other companies who believe that setting standards to deliver to certain customers' expectations is simply impossible. Their belief may stem from a variety of assumptions; for example, customers' expectations are unreasonable, the degree of variability inherent in the service defies standardization, the demand for the service is too hard to predict, the way the company and its personnel operate cannot be changed. Although some of these assumptions may be valid in some situations, whether they are legitimate long-term constraints that are impossible to overcome is questionable. Such assumptions may merely be rationalizations for management's reluctance to tackle head-on the difficult challenge of setting service standards.

In fact, the real reason for the potential gap between awareness of customers' expectations and the translation of that awareness into appropriate service standards may be the absence of wholehearted management commitment to service quality. David Garvin, after completing an extensive field study on goods quality, observed: "the seriousness management attached to quality problems [varies]. It's one thing to say you believe in defect-free products, but quite another to take time out from a busy schedule to act on that belief and stay informed."[1] Garvin's observations about good-producing companies clearly apply to service companies as well, particularly in view of the greater difficulty associated with achieving effective service-quality control.

While many service executives believe that it is impossible to set precise service specifications, a few companies have shown such a belief to be erroneous. National Westminster Bank USA is a case in point. Nat West set performance standards for its employees and also communicated those standards to customers in the form of performance guarantees in a series of creative television commercials called Raising the Standards of Banking. One commercial promised customers an immediate payment of $5 if they were displeased with the way they were greeted by a Nat West employee. Another commercial promised to pay customers $50 if their personal loan applications were not responded to by 5:00 P.M. the following day. Impressively, Nat West had to pay just two customer claims in the first six months of the campaign. According to Howard Deutsch, senior vice president/division head for quality improvement at Nat West, "By setting high service standards and putting our money where our mouth is, we're doing more than simply talking quality service. . . . We're guaranteeing it."[2]

Although perceived resource and market constraints, coupled with management indifference, may lead to Gap 2 (diagrammed in exhibit 3–3), this is a gap that can be closed effectively as demonstrated by Nat West. The quality of service delivered by customer-contact personnel is critically influenced by the standards against which they are evaluated and compensated. Standards signal to contact personnel what management's priorities are and which types of performance really count. When service standards are absent or when the standards in place do not reflect customers' expectations (e.g., when directory-assistance telephone operators are judged solely on the number of calls they handle per day) quality of service as perceived by customers is likely to suffer. In contrast, when

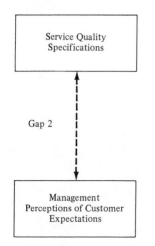

Exhibit 3–3 Gap 2: Between Management's Perceptions of Customers' Expectations and Service Quality Specifications

there are standards reflecting what customers expect (e.g., courteous treatment, quick response, and fulfilled promises as in the case of Nat West) the quality of service they receive is likely to be enhanced. Therefore, closing Gap 2—by setting performance standards that reflect customers' expectations—should have a favorable impact on customers' service-quality perceptions (Gap 5).

GAP 3: SERVICE-QUALITY SPECIFICATIONS—SERVICE-DELIVERY GAP

Each of the four companies that we examined did have some specifications for maintaining high service quality. The securities brokerage company, for example, required its customer-contact personnel to answer 90 percent of the phone calls from customers within ten seconds. This company also had a standard for keeping error rates in transactions within 1 percent. However, the executives we interviewed in this company (as well as in the other three companies) invariably expressed frustration at the inability of their employees to meet these service-performance standards.

Executives mentioned a variety of reasons for the discrepancy between service-performance standards and actual service delivery (i.e., Gap 3 depicted in exhibit 3–4). Most of these reasons pertain to the unwillingness and/or inability to contact personnel to meet the standards. When asked what caused service-quality problems in their companies, executives consistently mentioned the pivotal role of contact personnel. In the

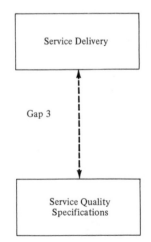

Exhibit 3–4 Gap 3: Between Service-Quality Specifications and Service Delivery

repair and maintenance company, for instance, one executive's immediate response to the source of service-quality problems was "Everything involves a person—a repair person. It's so hard to maintain standardized quality."

A stock-brokerage executive, anguishing over his company's inability to keep transaction error rates within the specified 1 percent, lamented: "I can handle 1 percent of 1,000 transactions but 1 percent of 300,000 transactions is another matter . . . [because] *blowout*—when the system stops working—may be close." In this instance, even though a performance standard was in place, meeting the standard was no longer possible because the volume of transactions had far outstripped existing capacity to process them accurately. Executives in the other companies also gave similar examples of service-performance shortfalls due to sheer increases in service loads without commensurate increases in capacity to serve.

Clearly then, even when guidelines exist for performing services well and treating customers correctly, high-quality service performance is not a certainty. A service-performance gap (Gap 3) is still likely due to a number of constraints (e.g., poorly qualified employees, inadequate internal systems to support contact personnel, insufficient capacity to serve). To be effective, service standards must not only reflect customers' expectations but also be backed up by adequate and appropriate resources (people, systems, technology). Standards must also be enforced to be effective—that is, employees must be measured and compensated on the basis of performance along those standards. Thus, even when standards accurately reflect customers' expectations, if management fails to "give teeth" to them—if it does not facilitate, encourage, and require their achievement—standards do no good. When the level of service-delivery performance falls short of the standards (Gap 3), it falls short of what customers expect as well (Gap 5). The implied direct association between Gaps 3 and 5 suggests that narrowing Gap 3—by ensuring that all the resources needed to achieve the standards are in place—should also reduce Gap 5.

Gap 4: Service Delivery—External Communications Gap

As we mentioned earlier, a key determinant of customers' expectations is the service provider's external communications (see exhibit 3–1). Promises made by a service company through its media advertising, sales force, and other communications raise expectations which serve as the standard against which customers assess service quality. A discrepancy between the actual service and the promised service (i.e., Gap 4 depicted in exhibit

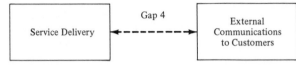

Exhibit 3–5 Gap 4: Between Service Delivery and External Communications to Customers about Service Delivery

3–5) therefore has an adverse effect on customers' perceptions of service quality (i.e., Gap 5). Customers who participated in our focus groups described many instances of poor service quality because of broken promises. A case in point is the following experience of a repair focus-group participant in her own words: "When I called [the repair company] for an appointment to come fix my washing machine they said that mine would be first call the next morning. . . . I took the next morning off from work and waited . . . and waited. . . . Finally at noon *I* called *them* and asked when their day began!"

Several of the executives we interviewed also described instances of broken promises because of inadequate coordination between operations and marketing. For instance, when the bank participating in our study introduced a new student-loan program, the marketing arm of the bank sold too many of the loans too fast without verifying in advance whether the operations group was geared up to mail out the loan checks as promised. Not surprisingly, broken promises and irate customers were the result. During the month following the introduction of the loan service the bank received over five hundred complaint letters from frustrated customers asking, "Where's my check?"

In addition to unduly elevating expectations through exaggerated claims, the executive interviews suggested another less obvious way in which external communications could influence customers' service-quality assessments. Some of the executives suggested that customers are not always aware of everything done behind the scenes to serve them well. By neglecting to inform customers of such behind-the-scenes efforts, companies may be forgoing an opportunity to favorably influence customers' service *perceptions*.

For instance, the securities-brokerage company had a "48-hour-rule" prohibiting its account executives from buying or selling securities for their personal accounts for the first 48 hours after information about the securities was supplied by the company. The brokers could advise clients and buy or sell on their behalf right away but they had to wait 48 hours before buying or selling for their own accounts. The company did not communicate this information to its customers, perhaps contributing to a perception that "all the good deals are probably made by the brokers for themselves" (a perception which surfaced in the securities-brokerage focus groups). One bank executive indicated that customers were unaware of the bank's behind-the-counter, on-line teller terminals which would "translate into visible effects on customer service." Making customers aware of hidden evidence of a company's commitment to quality service could improve customers' service perceptions. Customers who are aware that a company is taking concrete steps to serve their best interests are likely to perceive a delivered service in a more favorable way.

Customers' service perceptions may also be enhanced by educating customers to be better users of the service (e.g., telling brokerage customers the best times to call to check on their account status) and by adequately explaining to customers facets of the service process which they may consider to be irksome (e.g., why a customer ID is needed for certain bank transactions). Service companies frequently fail to capitalize on such opportunities to improve customers' perceptions. As one bank executive observed, "We don't teach our customers how to use us well and why we do the things we do."

In short, external communications can affect not only customers' expectations about a service but also customers' perceptions of the delivered service. Discrepancies between service delivery and external communications about it (Gap 4) adversely affect customers' assessment of service quality (Gap 5). Gap 4 essentially reflects an underlying breakdown in coordination between those responsible for delivering the service and those in charge of describing and/or promoting the service to customers. When the latter group of individuals do not fully understand the reality of the actual service delivery, they are likely to make exaggerated promises or fail to communicate to customers aspects of the service intended to serve them well. The result is poor service-quality perceptions. Effectively coordinating actual service delivery with external communications, therefore, narrows Gap 4 and hence favorably affects Gap 5 as well.

A SERVICE-QUALITY MODEL

The various gaps discussed thus far are the key ingredients in a recipe for gaining a good understanding of service quality and its determinants. Exhibit 3–6 shows how these ingredients can be combined to parsimoniously portray the provider's and customer's sides of the service-quality equation and the linkage between the two. The conceptual model in exhibit 3–6 conveys a clear message to managers wishing to improve

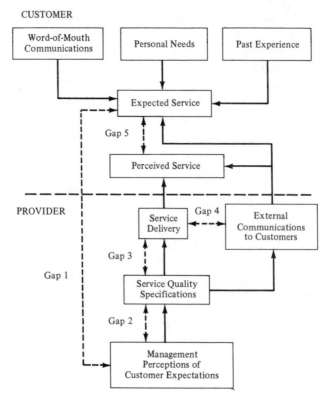

Exhibit 3–6 Conceptual Model of Service Quality

quality of service: The key to closing Gap 5 is to close Gaps 1 through 4 and keep them closed. To the extent that one or more of Gaps 1 through 4 exist, customers perceive service-quality shortfalls.

The conceptual model in exhibit 3–6 also implies a logical process which companies can employ to measure and improve quality of service. This process is diagrammed in exhibit 3–7. The sequence of questions in the five boxes on the left side of exhibit 3–7 correspond to the five gaps embedded in the conceptual model in exhibit 3–6. Specifically, the process begins with gaining an understanding of the nature and extent of Gap 5 and then successively searching for evidence of Gaps 1 through 4, taking corrective action wherever necessary.

Which factors are potential causes underlying the internal gaps (Gaps 1 through 4)? Which corrective actions are available to eliminate those causal factors? How can a company quantify the size of each gap and the extent to which the causal factors are contributing to it? To address these and other related issues, we undertook two additional research studies:

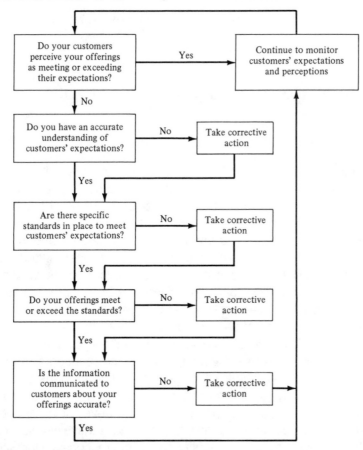

Exhibit 3-7 Process Model for Continuous Measurement and Improvement of Service Quality

(1) an in-depth study to uncover and understand potential antecedents of the four gaps; and (2) an empirical study to measure the relative sizes of the gaps and their antecedents. A description of these studies is given in "Additional Studies on Gaps 1–4." Findings from these studies and their implications are the focus of chapters 4 through 7.

SUMMARY

In this chapter we discussed our findings from exploratory qualitative research with senior executives; these findings were instrumental in our development of the service-quality-gap model. The findings revealed four key internal shortfalls or gaps that could contribute to poor quality of service as perceived by customers:

ADDITIONAL STUDIES ON GAPS 1 THROUGH 4

In-Depth Study

Building on what we had learned about the four internal gaps from our exploratory executive study, we conducted a comprehensive case study of a nationally known bank. We selected three of the bank's regions (each of which had at least 12 branches) and interviewed managers and employees at various levels individually and in focus groups. Top and middle managers responded to open-ended questions about their perceptions of customers' expectations of service quality (Gap 1), service-quality standards set by the organization to deliver quality (Gap 2), and differences between standards set by management and the level of service actually delivered (Gap 3). We conducted seven focus-group interviews with tellers, customer-service representatives, lending personnel, and branch managers from the three regions to help identify factors contributing to Gaps 3 and 4. Finally, we interviewed bank managers whose responsibilities included customer communications (bank marketing, advertising, and consumer affairs executives) and the president and creative director of the bank's advertising agency to identify the factors responsible for Gap 4.

We next conducted a systematic group interview with 11 senior managers of six nationally known service firms (two full-service banks, two national insurance companies, and two national telephone companies) to verify and generalize the factors we identified as contributing to Gaps 1 through 4. We presented our conceptual model, explained the four gaps, and questioned the managers about the factors responsible for the gaps in their firms. We also presented and discussed lists of factors derived from the preceding stage of our study. The managers augmented the lists and evaluated the factors on the basis of experience in their industries and organizations.

We then combined insights gained from the various stages with those from relevant marketing and organizational behavior literature and developed a classification of the main factors responsible for each of the four gaps. Chapters 4 through 7 are organized around the key factors pertaining to each gap.

Empirical Study

To measure Gaps 1 through 4 and the extent to which their antecedents were contributing to them, we conducted a major empirical study. In this study we used mail surveys to collect data from customers, contact personnel, and managers of five nationally known service companies (two insurance companies, two banks, and one long-distance telephone company). In all, 1,936 customers, 728 contact personnel, and 231 managers responded to our surveys.

The customer survey included the SERVQUAL instrument and questions to measure the relative importance of the five service-quality dimensions. Appendix A contains the SERVQUAL instrument and outlines the procedure for computing SERVQUAL scores. The manager and contact personnel surveys included the expectations section of SERVQUAL and the questions to measure the relative importance of the five service-quality dimensions. (Respondents completed both these sections *the way they thought their customers would complete them.*) A comparison of managers' and contact personnel's responses to these sections with customers' responses to the matching sections on the customer survey yielded measures of Gap 1 (appendix B gives further details on the measurement of Gap 1). The manager and contact personnel surveys also included questions to directly assess the extent of Gaps 2 through 4 and to measure the factors identified by the in-depth study as contributing to the four internal gaps. Appendix B contains the questions used to measure the gaps and their antecedents and outlines the corresponding scoring procedures.

Gap 1, the discrepancy between customers' expectations and managements' perceptions of those expectations; Gap 2, the discrepancy between managements' perceptions of customers' expectations and service-quality specifications; Gap 3, the discrepancy between service-quality specifications and actual service delivery; and Gap 4, the discrepancy between actual service delivery and what is communicated to customers about it. We linked customer-perceived quality shortfalls (Gap 5) to these four gaps in the form of a conceptual model of service quality. The conceptual model serves as a concise framework for understanding, measuring, and improving service quality. This chapter also outlined additional studies that we conducted to identify potential causes of the four internal gaps and to empirically examine the association between the gaps and their proposed antecedents. These studies' findings form the basis for chapters 4 through 7.

4

◊ ◊ ◊

GAP 1:
NOT KNOWING WHAT
CUSTOMERS EXPECT

K NOWING WHAT CUSTOMERS EXPECT is the first and possibly most crit-ical step in delivering quality service. Stated simply, providing ser-vices that customers perceive as excellent requires that a firm know what customers expect. Being a little bit wrong about what customers want can mean losing a customer's business when another company hits the target exactly. Being a little bit wrong can mean expending money, time, and other resources on things that don't count to customers. Being a little bit wrong can even mean not surviving in a fiercely competitive market.

This chapter details the first gap in the service-quality model: the dif-ference between what customers expect and what management perceives they expect. Sometimes this gap occurs because companies overlook or underestimate the need to fully understand customers' expectations. De-spite a genuine interest in providing service quality, many companies miss the mark by thinking inside out—they know what customers should want and deliver that—rather than outside in. When this happens, companies provide services that do not match customers' expectations: important fea-tures are left out and the levels of performance on features that are provided are inadequate. Because services have few clearly defined and tangible cues, Gap 1 may be considerably larger in service companies than it is in man-ufacturing firms.[1]

KEY REASONS FOR GAP 1

Our research focusing on the provider's side of the gaps model indi-cates that three conceptual factors contribute to Gap 1. These factors, illustrated in exhibit 4–1, are (1) *lack of marketing research orientation*, evidenced by insufficient marketing research, inadequate use of research findings, and lack of interaction between management and customers; (2) *inadequate upward communication* from contact personnel to management; and (3) *too many levels of management* separating contact personnel from top managers. Exhibit 4–2 defines these factors and presents several specific issues pertaining to them. In this chapter, we describe the problems stemming from these factors and offer suggestions for dealing with them to close Gap 1. We then discuss empirical findings from our research pertaining to Gap 1 and the organizational factors contributing to it.

GAP 1 PROBLEM: INSUFFICIENT MARKETING RESEARCH

Many service firms are new to marketing research. In fact, many service organizations are new to everything about marketing, believing that the operations function is more critical to success in the business.[2] Banks that close their branch lobbies in midafternoon to facilitate balancing the day's transactions and that issue monthly statements designed without input from customers exemplify an operations orientation. An

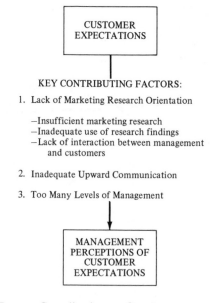

Exhibit 4–1 Key Factors Contributing to Gap 1

Factor and Definition	Specific Illustrative Issues
Marketing Research Orientation: Extent to which managers make an effort to understand customers' needs and expectations through formal and informal information-gathering activities.	• Is research conducted regularly to generate information about what customers want? • Does the marketing research a company conducts focus on quality of service delivered by it? • Do managers understand and utilize the research findings? • Do managers mingle with customers to learn what is on their minds?
Upward Communication: Extent to which top management seeks, stimulates, and facilitates the flow of information from employees at lower levels.	• Do managers encourage suggestions from customer contact personnel concerning quality of service? • Are there formal or informal opportunities for customer contact personnel to communicate with management? • How frequently do managers have face-to-face contact with customer contact personnel?
Levels of Management: Number of managerial levels between the topmost and bottommost positions.	• Do too many managerial levels separate top managers from those responsible for dealing with and serving customers?

Exhibit 4–2 Conceptual Factors Pertaining to Gap 1

operations orientation diverts focus from customers and reduces efforts to understand their needs and expectations.

Because marketing research is a key vehicle for understanding customers' expectations and perceptions of services, a firm that does not collect this information is more than likely to have a large Gap 1. A firm that does marketing research, but not on the topic of customers' expectations, may also have a large Gap 1. To close this gap, marketing research must focus on service quality issues such as which features are most important to customers, which levels of these features customers expect, and what customers think the company can and should do when problems occur in service delivery.

CLOSING GAP 1: RESEARCHING
CUSTOMERS' EXPECTATIONS

Finding out what customers expect is essential to providing service quality. Even when a service firm is small and has limited resources to conduct research, avenues are open to explore what customers expect. In exhibit 4–3 and in the discussion that follows, we present selected methods of researching customers' expectations beginning with the simplest (and least expensive) and ending with the most comprehensive (and often most costly) marketing research strategies.

Using Complaints Strategically

Many companies depend solely on customers' complaints to stay in touch. Unfortunately, research conducted by TARP, a Washington, D. C., research organization has provided convincing evidence that customers' complaints are a woefully inadequate source of information: only 4 percent of customers with problems actually complain to companies. The other 96 percent stay dissatisfied, telling an average of nine to ten other people of their dissatisfaction.[3]

Even though listening to complaints is rarely sufficient to understand customers' expectations, complaints can become part of a larger process of staying in touch with customers. In particular, they can provide important information about the failures or breakdowns in the service system. If compiled, analyzed, and fed back to employees who can correct the problems, complaints can become an inexpensive and continuous source of adjustment for the service process.

L. L. Bean, for example, tracks complaints by product, tallying and summarizing them daily, and places them in a problem file accessible to all employees. The approach allows top management to review the key areas of customers' dissatisfaction on a regular basis, and to make changes swiftly to meet customers' expectations. Customer-service representatives are also able to act knowledgeably and helpfully when providing service to customers.[4]

Complaints also offer opportunities for managers and contact personnel to interact with customers, thereby learning detailed and rich information about products and services. Although a goods firm, Procter & Gamble Company recognizes the strategic advantages of providing service in the form of an 800-number that customers can call with problems. Through the telephone interaction, customer-service personnel ask specific questions, get to the heart of customers' problems, and learn more

Exhibit 4–3 Selected Methods for Understanding Customers' Expectations

	Investment of Money	Investment of Time	Primary Uses
Strategic use of complaints	Low	Low	Identifying problems in the service process
Customers' desires in similar industries	Low	Low	Developing an initial framework for customers' expectations in focal industry
Research on intermediate customers	Moderate	Moderate	Efficient way to gain in-depth information on end customers
Key client studies	Moderate	Moderate	In-depth information on most important customers
Customer panels	Moderate to high	Moderate to high	Continuous source of information on changing customers' expectations
Transaction-based studies	Moderate	Moderate	Provides feedback on service-quality performance of each component of service quality.
Comprehensive customers' expectations studies	High	High	Establishes measures that are customer-based; provides foundation for tracking studies which provide a dynamic view of customers' expectations and perceptions

about the company's products. This information is then summarized and given to management as input when planning product or marketing changes.[5] Senior vice-presidents also spend three hours a week answering the phone, hearing customers' firsthand, answering questions, and addressing problems that are raised. Describing the value of the experience, one executive said, "I can't tell you what I do differently as a result of answering the phone, but I can tell you that no decision is made quite the same way."[6]

To truly understand customers' needs, companies can encourage and facilitate customers' feedback about problems. British Airways, for example, installed customer-complaint booths at Heathrow Airport where disgruntled passengers could air their grievances on videotape. Besides giving customers immediate relief from their annoyances, British Air found that the complaint videotapes gave vivid information to management about customers' problems and expectations.[7]

RESEARCHING WHAT CUSTOMERS WANT IN SIMILAR INDUSTRIES

As we discussed in chapter 2, our research revealed that customers have service expectations on dimensions that are similar across many industries. The five dimensions of quality service are the same across industries, and sometimes the way these dimensions are manifest is also similar across industries. Hospital patients and customers of hotels, for example, expect many of the same features when using these two services. Besides expert medical care, patients in hospitals expect comfortable rooms, courteous staff, and food that tastes good—the same features salient to hotel customers. In these and other industries that share common customers' expectations, managers may find it helpful to seek knowledge from executives in these other service industries. Because hotels have used marketing and marketing research longer than hospitals have, insights about hotel guests' expectations can inform about patients' expectations. Hospital administrators at Albert Einstein Medical Center in Philadelphia, for example, asked a group of nine local hotel executives for advice in understanding and handling patients. Many improvements resulted, including better food, easier-to-read name tags, more prominent information desks, and radios in many rooms.[8]

RESEARCHING INTERMEDIATE CUSTOMERS

Intermediate customers, such as contact employees, dealers, distributors, agents, or brokers, are people the company serves who serve the end customers. Researching the needs and expectations of these customers can be a useful and efficient way to obtain information about end users.

One way to research intermediate customers is to provide a service to them, such as education or training, then learn about their customers (and your own end customers) in the process. The interaction with intermediate customers provides opportunities for understanding end customers' expectations and problems. It can also help the company learn about and satisfy the service expectations of intermediate customers, a process critical in their providing quality service to end customers.

CONDUCTING KEY-CLIENT STUDIES

When the firm sells to businesses or to intermediate customers, rather than to end customers, some clients are large and important enough to study individually and in depth. To General Electric Company's (GE) aerospace group, for example, key clients included the Army, Navy, Air Force, and several airframe and electronics companies. To fully understand these clients' needs, as well as the strengths and weaknesses of the aerospace group vis-à-vis its competitors, the GE group interviewed 600 customers at all management levels of these key clients.[9] In a similar but more extensive effort, IBM Corporation created a customer council comprised of its top 50 clients. The company and the council meet regularly to determine where IBM will go in configuring and redesigning computer architecture.

These in-depth research studies can also be appropriate for end customers when key clients, who are larger or more important than others, can be identified. Law firms, for example, could focus on clients involved in major cases, banks could study their top depositors or borrowers, and airlines could research key corporate clients.

CREATING CUSTOMER PANELS

Firms can use customer panels to represent large segments of end customers. J. Bildner and Son's, a company that owns specialty food stores in Manhattan, keeps in touch through a customer advisory panel composed of 15–20 customers randomly selected in the stores. The panel meets three or four times a year to talk about products and services.[10] Similarly, New York State Electric and Gas Corporation formed a customer advisory panel of 15–21 members to represent a cross section of its small user customers (e.g., farmers, homemakers, consumer education people, the elderly) to test and assess their needs.[11] These panels allow the company to receive regular and timely information from customers.

TRACKING SATISFACTION WITH INDIVIDUAL TRANSACTIONS

A research trend gaining in popularity in service businesses involves transaction-based customer surveys. In this method, customers are surveyed immediately after a particular transaction about their satisfaction with the contact personnel with whom they interacted. Immediately after Sears, Roebuck & Company employees deliver furniture to homes—after they assemble the products, if necessary—they ask customers to complete five-item surveys measuring helpfulness, friendliness, and professionalism. Immediately after American Express customer-service representatives handle billing problems, they mail customers surveys that measure employees' courtesy and competence, and the customers' overall satisfaction. This type of research is simple, fresh, and provides management with current information about interactions with customers. Further, the research allows management to associate service-quality performance with individual contact personnel so that high performance can be rewarded and low performance corrected. It also serves as an incentive for employees to provide better service because they understand how and when they are being evaluated.

ENGAGING IN COMPREHENSIVE CUSTOMER-EXPECTATION STUDIES

Metropolitan Life Insurance Company of New York markets personal insurance to policyholders, group health and life coverage to corporations, and pension plans to both groups. The company developed a comprehensive program of measuring the expectations of all its customers, including both external and internal (employee) customers. According to John Falzon, senior vice-president of quality and planning, the importance of measuring service quality "applies equally across the board, not excluding internal customers. Maybe only 25 percent of our people are servicing an outside customer."[12]

Using companywide employee surveys, focus group interviews, and SERVQUAL, Met Life regularly monitors the expectations and perceptions of their customers. The 22-item generic SERVQUAL questionnaire, customized by adding questions covering specific aspects of service they wanted to track, formed the foundation for the comprehensive customer-expectation study.

The research strategy that American Express used to improve its service quality is another illustration of a comprehensive approach to understanding the needs and expectations of customers. The company sought and used input from as many sources as possible: customer research studies, customer complaints, employee surveys, and retailer studies. They found that customers were most concerned with *timeliness* (statements arriving at about the same time each month; address change corrections appearing quickly); *accuracy* (their names and addresses spelled correctly and bills accurate); and *responsiveness* (charges or payments reflected on their next statement). Through additional research, the company was able to establish the exact number of days that customers defined as responsive for the various company processes (e.g., two days for reissuing lost cards, 15 days for deciding on an application). Using this in-depth information, the company changed processes in the organization and tracked the changes in customers' perceptions that resulted.[13]

A comprehensive program works best when top management is dedicated to finding the truth about the company's customers. As an example, at Milliken and Company, the textiles company lauded for its customer service, the chairman spends 80 percent of his time "fathoming the needs of the customer." To support this mind-set, as he calls his dedication to customers, the company conducts extensive and detailed surveys to find whether and in which ways Milliken is responsive to them, researching all interactions including phone courtesy and billing.[14]

Customers' expectations change over time. As competition increases, as tastes change, and as customers become more knowledgeable, companies must continue to update their information and strategies. To stay in touch, New York State Electric and Gas Corporation continually monitors customers' desires through surveys, complaint analysis, focus groups, roundtables, customer panels, and face-to-face discussions with people in the organization.[15]

Recognizing that customers' expectations were dynamic, Merrill Lynch created a customer profiling and information system for "identifying client needs, updating these needs, and enabling account executives to match products to these needs."[16] Similarly, American Airlines Inc. used an ongoing in-flight survey to "ask our customers about their impressions of the ticket-buying process, the flight attendants, the gate agents—even the type of airplane they flew on."[17]

As shown in exhibit 4–3, the types of marketing research that we discuss in this section require different levels of investment and are appropriate for meeting slightly different service-quality objectives. We recommend a portfolio of these approaches designed to match each company's resources and to address the key areas needed to understand its customers. In chapter 8, we discuss this portfolio research approach in more detail.

GAP 1 PROBLEM: INADEQUATE USE OF MARKETING RESEARCH FINDINGS

Conducting marketing research is only the first part of understanding the customer. A service firm must also use the research findings in a meaningful way. The misuse or nonuse of research data can lead to a large gap in understanding customers' expectations. When managers do not read research reports because they are too busy dealing with the day-to-day challenges of the business, when they do not understand how to interpret the data because the research is too complex and technical, or when they lack confidence in the research, companies fail to use the resources available to them and Gap 1 widens. Understanding how to make the best use of research—to apply what they have learned to the business—is a key way to close Gap 1.

CLOSING GAP 1: USING MARKETING RESEARCH FINDINGS EFFECTIVELY

Managers must learn to turn research information and insights into action. The most comprehensive research does not help a company stay in touch unless the information gets to the right people in the firm in a timely manner. Consider the following examples of firms that have developed actionable research programs:

- Stew Leonard, of the much-acclaimed dairy store in Connecticut, believes that the suggestion box is the "pulse of the business." He empties it every day, compiles the list of recommendations, and distributes it to managers and employees. "Criticism and approval are taken to heart," says Leonard.[18]
- Goodyear Tire & Rubber Company conducts enough telephone interviews each week to obtain reliable information on customers' satisfaction with each of its 1,200 retail stores. When dissatisfied customers are identified, they are asked if they would like to be contacted by the store or district manager to address unresolved

complaints or problems. The company also follows some buyers up to two years to track their experiences, attitudes, and satisfaction. These results are compiled and regularly reported back to managers in marketing, production, and product development.[19]

- J. C. Penney Company, Inc., helps store managers understand and use research through a how-to bulletin. The bulletin advises them to ask shoppers leaving without packages questions to help them understand important service issues. The brochure also suggests guidelines about the optimal number (a minimum of 15 per week) and place (main entrance and within the store) for customer interviews. Ways to use customer feedback are emphasized.[20]

These examples illustrate creative and effective ways to use marketing research findings to improve quality of service. When management uses information, data, and findings from market research to understand customers' expectations, Gap 1 decreases.

GAP 1 PROBLEM: LACK OF INTERACTION BETWEEN MANAGEMENT AND CUSTOMERS

In some service firms, especially ones that are small and localized, owners or managers may be in constant contact with customers, thereby gaining firsthand knowledge of customers' expectations and perceptions. But in large service organizations, managers do not always get the opportunity to experience firsthand what their customers want. This problem is illustrated in a comment from a bank's customer-service representative interviewed in an early stage of our research:

CUSTOMER-SERVICE REPRESENTATIVE: "We have three floors. Our manager, when he first got here, sat on the second floor. Now he is on the third floor in his enclosed office. He told us he doesn't want to be with the public. He needs time for himself. What are his priorities? He doesn't know what's going on on the first floor. I've had lots of customers ask for the manager. I say, 'I'm sorry, he's on a month's vacation.' "

The larger a company is, the more difficult it may be for managers to interact directly with customers and the less firsthand information they have about customers' expectations. Even when they read and digest research reports, managers can lose the reality of customers if they never get the opportunity to experience actual service. A theoretical view of how things are supposed to work cannot provide the richness of the service encounter. To truly understand customers' needs, management benefits from hands-on knowledge of what really happens in stores, on customer-service telephone lines, in service queues, and in face-to-face service encounters. If Gap 1 is to be closed, managers in large firms need some form of customer contact.

CLOSING GAP 1: INCREASING INTERACTION BETWEEN MANAGEMENT AND CUSTOMERS

Robert Crandall, CEO of American Airlines, illustrates the value in experiencing service firsthand.

> Commitment and dedication on the part of your people only happens when there's the same commitment and dedication on the part of the boss. Top management must confront the realities of the marketplace daily. I don't sit on some mountaintop, telling the American Airlines passenger service department how to deal with problems. I get out there and watch them work. I take regular trips on American—not because I have to go somewhere, but because I want to see for myself how we're doing.[21]

Managers can spend time on the line, interacting with customers and experiencing service delivery. A formal program for encouraging informal interaction is often the best way to ensure that the contact takes place. Radio Shack, for example, has a program called Adopt a Store through which senior managers spend time in stores collecting information and interacting with the staff.[22] Weinstock, a retailer in Sacramento, California, requires the entire headquarters staff to work the selling floor—in the trenches—seven times a year. "The plan was to give headquarters personnel hands-on knowledge of what really happens in stores, and not just a front office theoretical view of how things are supposed to work. What better way, the company reasoned, than to put central staff right in the trenches of selling?"[23]

The marketing director at Milliken called his experience working the swing shift "naive listening," and he described its benefits as follows:

> Getting close to the customer is a winner! . . . I worked the second shift (3:00 P.M. to midnight) and actually cleaned carpeting as well as hard-surface floors. I operated all the machinery they used daily, plus handled the same housekeeping problems. . . . Now I can put together my trade advertising as well as my entire merchandising

program based directly upon the needs of my customers as I observed them . . . I'm learning—from new-product introduction to maintenance of existing products—exactly what our health care customers require.[24]

As this example illustrates, direct interaction with customers adds clarity and depth to the manager's understanding of customers' expectations and needs.

GAP 1 PROBLEM: INSUFFICIENT UPWARD COMMUNICATION FROM CONTACT PERSONNEL TO MANAGEMENT

Customer-contact personnel are in regular contact with customers. Through this interaction, they come to understand a great deal about customers' expectations and perceptions. If the information they know can be passed on to top management, top managers' understanding of their customers may improve. In fact, it could be said that in many companies, top management's understanding of their customers depends largely on the extent and types of communication received from customer-contact personnel and from noncompany-contact personnel (e.g., independent insurance agents, retailers) who represent the company and its services. When these channels of communication are closed, management may not get feedback about problems encountered in service delivery and about how customers' expectations are changing.

In focus-group interviews conducted in one of our studies, several bank employees clearly illustrated the lack of effective upward communication.

BRANCH MANAGER: "I've been in this bank for 27 years and this is the first time I have had a regional VP that has never been in the branch."

ANOTHER: "He never will."

ANOTHER: "I haven't seen the man in a year and a half. That has a lot to do with our attitude. We're getting orders from someone we never see."

CLOSING GAP 1: IMPROVING UPWARD COMMUNICATION FROM CONTACT PERSONNEL TO MANAGEMENT

Sam Walton, founder of Wal-Mart, the highly successful discount retailer, once remarked, "Our best ideas come from delivery and stock boys."[25] To be sure he stays in touch with the source of new ideas, he spends considerable time in his stores working the floor, helping clerks or approving personal checks, even showing up at the loading dock with a bag of doughnuts for a surprised crew of workers.[26] "He would have his plane drop him next to a wheat field where he would meet a Wal-Mart truck driver. Giving his pilot instructions to meet him at another landing strip 200 miles down the road, he would make the trip with the Wal-Mart driver, listening to what he has to say about the company."[27]

Upward communication of this sort provides information to upper-level managers about activities and performances throughout the organization. Specific types of communication that may be relevant are formal (e.g., reports of problems and exceptions in service delivery) and informal (e.g., discussions between contact personnel and upper-level managers). Managers who stay close to their contact people benefit not only by keeping their employees happy but also by learning more about their customers.

Companies can use a variety of approaches for successfully achieving upward communication. For instance, Richard Rogers, president of Syntex Corporation, eats breakfast in the employee cafeteria every morning so he can be available to employees who want to see him.[28] Each year, Bill Marriott, Jr., visits 80 percent of the company's hotels, inspects a third of the flight kitchens, and eats at company restaurants as often as five times a week.[29] He is known for walking around his hotels at all hours, surveying breakfast preparations at 6: 15 A.M., or looking over rooms for the slightest imperfection.[30] Staying close to the customer is part of the Marriott tradition. William Marriott, Bill's father and Marriott's founder, is said to have read almost all of the customer comment cards for the entire 56 years of his leadership.[31]

Jim Kuhn, vice-president for individuality at McDonald's Corporation, sums up one reason why the fast-food company has been so successful: "We can never lose sight of the fact that this organization is run from the counter. A big part of the job is listening to the crew people."[32]

Companies such as McDonald's, Marriott, and Syntex encourage, appreciate, and reward upward communication from contact people. Through this important channel, management learns about customers' expectations from those employees in regular contact with customers and can thereby reduce the size of Gap 1.

GAP 1 PROBLEM: TOO MANY LEVELS BETWEEN CONTACT PERSONNEL AND MANAGEMENT

The number of managerial levels separating customer-contact personnel from top managers can affect the size of Gap 1. Multiple levels of management inhibit communication and understanding because they place barriers between top managers, who set standards for service quality, and contact people, who actually deliver quality to customers. As discussed in the previous section, Gap 1 can be reduced through upward communication from customer-contact personnel; this channel of communication becomes less effective the greater the number of levels because information is likely to be lost or misinterpreted in each translation from level to level. The greater the number of levels, the less likely that information employees possess about customers' expectations actually reaches managers. Therefore, the greater the number of levels between customer-contact personnel and top managers, the larger Gap 1 is likely to be.

CLOSING GAP 1: REDUCE THE NUMBER OF LEVELS BETWEEN CONTACT PERSONNEL AND MANAGEMENT

Many large organizations today are recognizing the value of reducing management levels that make companies sluggish and slow to adapt. IBM Corporation is removing managers from the middle and putting them in contact with customers, believing that the company must learn to react quickly and flexibly if it is to remain the leader in an increasingly competitive and dynamic computer market. IBM uses an approach it calls Best of Breed in which each area of the company identifies the competitor that best satisfies the expectations of a group of customers; then they set out to find out how to perform to that level. Only by eliminating unnecessary layers and teaching managers to focus on the outside—on customers and competitors—can the industry giant behave like a nimble, flexible company in all the markets it serves. Eliminating levels of management allows managers to be closer to customers, to understand their needs and expectations.

Milliken prides itself on having reduced the number of middle managers (called management associates) from 52,000 in 1981 to 31,000 in 1988. John Rampey, a senior executive and frequent spokesman for the company, claims that the more layers eliminated, the better the company understands the expectations of customers. He explains that remaining associates benefit from self-management and the creativity and problem solving that result from more direct interaction with the company. While removing the layers can be a painful process in the short term for employees, the long-term benefits of knowledge of customers, flexibility, and creativity make it worth the effort.

EMPIRICAL FINDINGS ABOUT GAP 1

A common piece of folk wisdom, and one that we implicitly invoked in discussing the importance of upward communication earlier in this chapter, holds that contact personnel, by virtue of their proximity to customers, understand customers' expectations better than managers understand them. In our empirical study of the five large service companies, we had an opportunity to evaluate the soundness of this folk wisdom. As described in our technical appendix B at the end of the book, we had customers complete the Servqual scale. Then we had contact personnel and managers fill out the expectations and dimensional-importance sections of Servqual as they perceived their customers would complete it.

Results of the comparison of these scores provides evidence that partially contradicts the folk wisdom. Exhibit 4–4 shows customers' expectations and contact personnel and managers' predictions of those expectations on the five dimensions of service quality. Reading across the rows, averages with similar letters indicate perceptions that are the same in a statistical sense. Different letters show that perceptions are statistically different.

On the dimension of tangibles, contact people were more accurate than managers in predicting customers' expectations. But in reliability, responsiveness, assurance, and the overall level of expectations, managers were significantly more accurate than contact personnel in predicting customers' expectations. These results suggest that managers understand customers' expectations better than contact personnel in the companies

Exhibit 4–4 Comparison of Customers' Expectations with Managers' and Contact Personnel's Perceptions of Those Expectations

	Customers	Contact Personnel	Managers
Tangibles	5.29[a]	5.50[b]	5.54[b]
Reliability	6.48[a]	6.09[b]	6.39[a]
Responsiveness	6.40[a]	6.12[b]	6.32[a]
Assurance	6.47[a]	6.27[b]	6.43[a]
Empathy	6.25[a]	5.96[b]	6.06[b]
Total	6.19[a]	6.00[b]	6.15[a]

* Reading across the rows, numbers with similar letters indicate perceptions that are statistically the same. Numbers with different letters indicate perceptions that are statistically different.

we studied. Whether or not these results would occur in other companies would depend on their managers' and contact personnel's understanding of customers' expectations and hence the size of Gap 1 for the two groups of employees. Procedures for measuring the status of Gap 1—as well as Gaps 2 through 4—in any company are discussed in appendix B.

As the preceding discussion and the evidence in exhibit 4–4 indicate, Gap 1 as defined in our service-quality model (i.e., the difference between customers' expectations and managers' perceptions of those expectations) was not a serious shortfall in the companies we studied. In fact, the *weighted expectation* scores—scores that capture not only the expectation levels along the SERVQUAL dimensions but also the relative importance of the dimensions themselves—for managers and customers were similar for all five companies. (The procedure for computing the weighted expectation scores is described in appendix B.) On the scale of 1 to 7 that we used to measure expectations, the weighted scores for the two groups were as follows:

	Managers	Customers
Company 1	6.4	6.3
Company 2	6.3	6.3
Company 3	6.3	6.3
Company 4	6.1	6.4
Company 5	6.0	6.4

Despite the relatively small Gap 1 in each of the five companies, our findings about the factors that could potentially result in Gap 1 revealed opportunities for improvement in each company. Exhibit 4–5 reports the average scores for the five companies on marketing research orientation, upward communication, and levels of management. These scores are on seven-point scales on which higher scores represent more favorable levels (further details about how these factors are measured are in appendix B). The discrepancy between each average score and a score of 7 (the highest possible score) represents the potential for improvement. The results for the five firms we studied imply that improvements can be made along all these factors. However, the perception that too many levels of management separate contact personnel from top management is a more significant problem than either a lack of marketing research orientation or

Exhibit 4–5 Scores on Factors Pertaining to Gap 1*

	Marketing Research Orientation	Upward Communication	Levels of Management
Company 1	5.3	4.7	3.3
Company 2	4.2	4.7	3.6
Company 3	4.3	4.4	3.8
Company 4	5.0	5.0	2.2
Company 5	4.7	4.4	2.3
All companies	4.7	4.6	3.0

* Scores are average values on a seven-point scale on which higher numbers represent more favorable scores.

inadequate upward communication. Indeed, the consistency of this finding across all five of our sample companies, coupled with our finding that top managers had a more accurate view of customers' expectations, suggest an intriguing hypothesis: In large companies, too many levels of management may be inhibiting *downward communication* from top management to contact personnel. The managerial sophistication and market knowledge of top decision makers in large companies apparently give them an accurate understanding of customers' expectations. Ironically, the multiple levels of management characteristic of many large companies may be significant hurdles in conveying top management knowledge about what customers expect down to the customer-contact personnel responsible for meeting customers' expectations. A rich reservoir of knowledge about customers' expectations does a company little good if it is blocked at the upper echelons of management. Top management must disseminate that knowledge to the lower levels by breaking down or working around intermediate barriers to effective downward communication.

SUMMARY

This chapter identified the key problems which result in Gap 1, a discrepancy between what customers expect and what management perceives that they expect. These problems include insufficient marketing research, inadequate use of marketing research findings, lack of interaction between management and customers, insufficient upward communication from contact employees to managers, and too many managerial levels between contact personnel and top management. We described each of these problems and discussed specific strategies and tactics for closing Gap 1. Finally, we presented empirical findings from our research pertaining to Gap 1 and its antecedents and explored the implications of these findings.

5

◊ ◊ ◊

GAP 2:
THE WRONG SERVICE-
QUALITY STANDARDS

A s DISCUSSED IN CHAPTER 4, understanding customers' expectations is
the first step in delivering high service quality. Once managers
accurately understand what customers expect, they face a second critical
challenge: using this knowledge to set service-quality standards for the
organization. Management may not be willing (or able) to put the systems
in place to match or exceed customers' expectations. A variety of factors—
including resource constraints, short-term profit orientation, market conditions, or management indifference—may account for Gap 2, the
discrepancy between managers' perceptions of customers' expectations
and the actual specifications they establish for service delivery.

Gap 2 is a wide gap in many companies. A recurring theme in the
executive interviews in our research was the difficulty experienced in
attempting to match or exceed customers' expectations. Many executives
cannot or will not change company systems of service delivery to enhance
customers' perceptions. Doing so often requires altering the very process
by which work is accomplished. At other times, change requires new
equipment or technology. Change also necessitates aligning executives
from different parts of the firm to collectively understand the big picture
of service quality from the customer's point of view. And almost always
change requires a willingness to be open to different ways of structuring,
calibrating, and monitoring the way service is provided.

In our extensive research on the gap constructs and measures (see
chapter 3 for details), we identified the four conceptual factors (shown in
exhibit 5–1 and described in exhibit 5–2 which result in the following
major reasons for Gap 2: (1) *inadequate commitment to service quality*, (2) *lack*

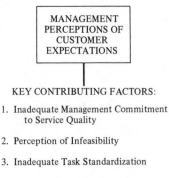

KEY CONTRIBUTING FACTORS:

1. Inadequate Management Commitment
   to Service Quality

2. Perception of Infeasibility

3. Inadequate Task Standardization

4. Absence of Goal Setting

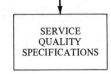

Exhibit 5–1 Key Factors Contributing to Gap 2

of perception of feasibility, (3) *inadequate task standardization*, and (4) *absence of goal setting*. In this chapter, we discuss these reasons and offer suggestions on ways to overcome them. We conclude with a description of the empirical results from our research relating to Gap 2.

GAP 2 PROBLEM: INADEQUATE MANAGEMENT COMMITMENT TO SERVICE QUALITY

The absence of total management commitment to service quality virtually guarantees a wide Gap 2. Emphasis on other company performance objectives, such as cost reduction and short-term profit, is easier to measure and track; therefore it may supersede emphasis on service quality. The tendency on the part of executives to focus on other objectives is illustrated in the following statement by Arnoldo Hax and Nicolas Majluf, authors in the field of strategic management: "Most U.S. firms suffer significantly from the use of short-term accounting-driven measures of performance to establish the reward mechanisms for high-level managers, who are mainly responsible for implementing strategic actions."[1]

Louis Gerstner, former president of American Express, suggests another powerful explanation for lack of management commitment

Factor and Definition	Specific Illustrative Issues
Management Commitment to Service Quality: Extent to which management views service quality as a key strategic goal.	• Are resources committed to departments to improve service quality? • Do internal programs exist for improving the quality of service to customers? • Are managers who improve the quality of service to customers more likely to be rewarded than other managers? • Does the company emphasize its sales goals as much as or more than it emphasizes serving customers? • Are upper and middle managers committed to providing quality service to their customers?
Perception of Feasibility: Extent to which managers believe that customer expectations can be met.	• Does the company have the necessary capabilities to meet customer requirements for service? • Can customer expectations be met without hindering financial performance? • Do existing operations systems enable customer expectations to be met? • Are resources and personnel available to deliver the level of service that customers demand? • Does management change existing policies and procedures to meet the needs of customers?
Task Standardization: Extent to which hard and soft technology are used to standardize service tasks.	• Is automation used to achieve consistency in serving customers? • Are programs in place to improve operating procedures so that consistent service is provided?
Goal-Setting: Extent to which service quality goals are based on customer standards and expectations rather than company standards.	• Is there a formal process for setting quality of service goals for employees? • Does the company have clear goals about what it wants to accomplish? • Does the company measure its performance in meeting its service quality goals? • Are service quality goals based on customer-oriented standards rather than company-oriented standards?

Exhibit 5–2 Conceptual Factors Pertaining to Gap 2

to service quality. "Because of the structure of most companies, the guy who puts in the service operation and bears the expense doesn't get the benefit. It'll show up in marketing, even in new product development. But the benefit never shows up in his own P&L statement."[2]

Many companies believe they are committed to service quality but their commitment is to quality from the company's own internal, technical perspective. Service quality in many firms means meeting the company's self-defined productivity or efficiency standards, many of which customers do not notice or desire. In other firms, quality is defined in terms of advanced technology—meeting standards required to keep pace with competitors on things which customers will not pay for and do not want. In our view, being committed to service quality means more than meeting company- or competitor-defined standards. Management commitment to service quality means providing service that the *customer perceives as high in quality*, as expressed by James Robinson of American Express: "Overriding all other values is our dedication to quality. We are a market-driven institution, committed to our customers in everything we do. We constantly seek improvement and we encourage the unusual, even the iconoclastic."[3]

When managers are not committed to service quality *from the customer's point of view*, they target resources only to other organizational goals such as sales, profits, or market share. They do not establish internal service-quality initiatives, and they do not see that attempts to improve service quality lead to better company performance.

CLOSING GAP 2: COMMITTING TO QUALITY

Delivering quality service requires leadership and commitment from top management, a point we stressed in chapter 1. Without this commitment—this willingness to temporarily accept the difficulties involved in change—quality service simply does not happen. Contact employees and middle management do not and cannot improve quality without strong leadership from management. Strong management commitment and leadership is illustrated by a poster prominently displayed at L. L. Bean, the successful direct-mail marketer.

> What Is a Customer? A Customer is the most important person even in this office . . . in person or by mail. A Customer is not dependent on us . . . we are dependent on him. A Customer is not an interruption of our work . . . he is the purpose of it. We are not doing a favor by serving him . . . he is doing us a favor by giving

us the opportunity to do so. A Customer is not someone to argue or match wits with. Nobody ever won an argument with a Customer. A Customer is a person who brings us his wants. It is our job to handle them profitably to him and to ourselves.[4]

Among companies that sell to other businesses, rather than to end customers, stand those whose customer-oriented philosophies lead them to be the best in their fields. DuPont, the top-rated firm among chemical companies, captures the reason for its success simply: "Our marketing effort starts with the customer."[5]

Top managers committed to quality must constantly and visibly express their commitment to the troops. Stew Leonard, of the highly respected dairy store of the same name, demonstrates his commitment to his customers with a three-ton granite block at the store's entrance reading:

Rule 1: The customer is always right.

Rule 2: If the customer is ever wrong, reread rule 1.[6]

Bill Marriott, Jr., continues his father's legendary commitment to customers and visibly expresses it by traveling the country to personally oversee operations. He claims: "It's a commitment. I'm the first in and the last out. If you are a leader, you better lead—and you lead by example. You have to motivate people, let them know you want to see what they can do."[7]

CLOSING GAP 2: GAINING COMMITMENT OF MIDDLE MANAGEMENT

If top-management commitment is the key to setting service standards to deliver quality, middle-management commitment is the key to making those standards work. Lack of support from middle management can derail the service-quality journey. Middle management often feels worn down by the "program of the month" treadmill and has inadequate time and support to keep up. If middle management perceives that service quality is just another program of the month, resistance rather than support will ensue. If middle management doesn't pass along top management's commitment to quality by communicating service standards, by setting service standards for their work units, and by reinforcing the standards with motivation and support, quality service simply does not happen.

Middle management must see that their efforts toward service quality are being noticed and appreciated. Incentives for managerial participation and improvements must be provided. Financial incentives linked to behavior that fosters high service quality, in addition to more typical performance goals such as sales, make service quality real for them. In one of the service organizations that sponsored our research, top management instituted a new 60-40 bonus plan to support the company's quest for quality. Instead of managerial bonuses based 100 percent on sales, the company rewarded managers on both sales (60 percent) and service quality (40 percent).

Training in the skills needed to lead service workers to deliver quality is often necessary. In its effort to enlist middle management's support and involvement in service quality, British Airways developed a five-day management training course called Managing People First. The course's objectives were to "make managers more decisive and creative, more responsive to the needs and concerns of their staff and colleagues, and more effective in motivating their subordinates to use their own judgment and initiative."[8] The airline also linked direct financial incentives to managers' behaviors in achieving these objectives through a strategy they call the three-legged stool:

> The seat of the stool represents the British Airways way of managing. The first leg is the "Managing People First" training program; the second leg is an evaluation program designed to measure not only what managers achieve, but how; and the third leg is a compensation program, whereby managers receive lump-sum bonus payments up to 20% of base salary, determined by what the manager achieves and how.[9]

GAP 2 PROBLEM: PERCEPTION OF INFEASIBILITY

Our research revealed that the size of Gap 2 is strongly affected by the extent to which managers perceive that meeting customers' expectations is feasible. As we saw in chapter 3, executives in the repair service firm participating in our exploratory study were fully aware that customers view quick response to appliance breakdowns as a vital aspect of high-quality service. However, they believed that establishing specifications to deliver a quick response consistently was not feasible for two reasons: (1) the time required to provide a specific repair service was difficult to forecast; and (2) skilled service technicians were less available in the peak summer season than at any other time. In this and many other situations, knowledge of customers' expectations exists but the perceived means to deliver to expectations apparently do not.

Perception of infeasibility is a managerial mind-set that may or may not be related to actual constraints on the organization. It may be true that technology available to improve a service delivery system does not exist, that financial constraints preclude the manager from aligning the firm to serve all the needs of customers, and that some customers' expectations and demands are simply too rigid and unrealistic. In these cases, managers may have no choice but to decide that meeting customers' expectations is infeasible. In our research, however, we found that the perception of infeasibility is often the result of short-term, narrow thinking on the part of managers—an unwillingness to think creatively and optimistically about customers' needs, and an excuse for maintaining the status quo.

CLOSING GAP 2: CREATING POSSIBILITIES

Being open to innovation, being receptive to different and possibly better ways of doing business—thinking big—is the key to perceiving feasibility. Managers in truly successful service companies have the perception that almost anything the customer wants is feasible. These managers are willing to change the way they do business, if necessary, and to invest money, time, and effort to fully satisfy their customers.

When hotel customers repeatedly complained that they didn't like to wait in lines to check out, most hotels threw up their hands and said that the problem couldn't be helped. Bill Marriott, Jr., however, thought it important enough to devise an alternative way to handle this recurring and pivotal customer request: the company invented Express Checkout. Customers, especially those in a hurry, could simply drop their keys at the counter if their bills, which had been slipped under their doors during the night, were accurate. Companies such as Marriott constantly pioneer customer-service advancements because they view customers' demands as challenges and puzzles rather than as problems.

American Express Company's Travel-Related Services (TRS) division found customers' expectations about credit-card services increased tremendously as competition in the industry intensified. Rather than accept performance that departed more and more from expectations as the competitive pressure built, the company decided that computer improvements were the answer to meeting customers' expectations. Through the computer improvements TRS developed, many important customer requests were met. The division reduced personal card processing from an average of 35 days to 15 days, replaced cards in an average of 2 days rather than 15 days, dropped response time to cardholder inquiries from 16 to 10 days, answered merchant inquiries in 4 days rather than 14, and reduced emergency service for card replacement to within 24 hours worldwide.[10]

American Airlines is another successful service company known for its innovative solutions to difficult service challenges. Over the years the airline has developed major service innovations that include in-flight entertainment, one-stop check-in, advance boarding passes, and automated reservations.[11] With the confusion and complexity that accompanied deregulation, American made the decision that the only way travel agents could cope was with computers. It responded by developing Sabre, a $200 million automated reservation system that revolutionized the industry. As an American executive explains:

> Most people think of Sabre as a computerized reservations system, and it is, but it also is much more than that. Sabre is a powerful, integrated data processing and communications system. It contains schedules for nearly 600 airlines. It has information on rental cars, hotels, broadway plays and foreign currency exchange rates. It lets travel agents sell their clients such things as flowers by wire, insurance and telex message capability.[12]

Another perplexing service problem involves the impact of weather on overnight mail delivery. Firms such as Airborne Express, Federal Express Corporation, and United Parcel Service set service standards and typically meet them as long as the weather is good. But customers want reliable, on-time, overnight delivery service even when weather makes delivery difficult or impossible. Most delivery companies settled for doing their best to adapt to weather, but Federal Express created possibilities by designing "nowcasting," a weather assessment and forecasting tool. Nowcasting assists its employees in achieving on-time performance no matter what the weather and provides "the most up-do-date, specific weather data to enable Federal Express to make contingency plans for its chief function: safe delivery of packages."[13]

Companies that create possibilities actively look for ways to provide better service to customers. Knowing that the detail involved in ordering supplies for hospitals can be overwhelming to customers, American Hospital Supply Corporation sought to turn this customer problem into a competitive advantage. The company developed an easier, customer-oriented ordering process by providing computer terminals to customers from which they could order all medical supplies quickly and conveniently. Customers were satisfied and the system made switching to a rival difficult; once customers were familiar with the computer system, the effort and learning cost of changing suppliers was high.[14]

Computer information systems are often the basis for setting standards to improve customer service. L. L. Bean, the direct marketer, earned its reputation for outstanding customer service using a computer data base that supplies moment-to-moment information about models, colors, and sizes of products in stock. With this system, the company can set and achieve high standards of customer service. The data base enables them to fill an incredible 99.8 percent of orders accurately.[15]

Marshall Field & Company uses a computer information system to deal with the difficult problem of scheduling employees. Having enough employees on the floor to serve customers well while not wasting resources is an ongoing challenge for large retail stores. Marshall Field developed a computer-based employee scheduling system to "maximize sales potential at point-of-sale, increase managerial effectiveness, and improve expense and productivity controls," all while setting high standards for service provided to customers. Using a personal computer, the company developed a program using as data daily sales plans by department, customer traffic patterns, store hours, company meal and break policies, and employee schedule availability. The computer generated weekly employee schedules with the right number of salespeople on duty at peak selling periods, even if that meant bringing extra help in to meet the levels of service the company wanted to provide its customers.[16]

All of these examples illustrate different approaches to creating possibilities, ways to provide the quality service customers expect.

GAP 2 PROBLEM: INADEQUATE STANDARDIZATION OF TASKS

The translation of managerial perceptions into specific service-quality standards depends on the degree to which tasks to be performed can be standardized or routinized. Some executives and managers believe that services cannot be standardized—that customization is essential for providing high-quality service. Somehow, standardizing tasks is perceived as being impersonal, inadequate, and not in the customer's best interests. Further, they feel that services are too intangible to be measured. This view leads to vague and loose standard setting with little or no measurement or feedback.

In reality, many service tasks are routine (such as those needed for opening checking accounts or spraying lawns for insects), and for these, specific rules and standards can be fairly easily established and effectively executed. If services are customized for individual customers (e.g., investment portfolio management or estate planning), specific standards (such as those relating to time spent with the customer) seem more difficult to establish. Even in highly customized services, however, some aspects of service provision can be routinized. Physicians and dentists, for example, can and do standardize recurring and nontechnical aspects of the service such as checking patients in, collecting payments, weighing patients, and taking temperatures. In delegating these routine tasks to assistants, physicians and dentists can spend more of their time on the more expert services of diagnosis or patient care.

CLOSING GAP 2: STANDARDIZING TASKS

According to Harvard's Ted Levitt, a long-time observer of service industries, standardization of service can take three forms: (1) substitution of hard technology for personal contact and human effort; (2) improvement in work methods or soft technology; and (3) combinations of these two methods.[17] Examples of hard technology include automatic teller machines, automatic car washes, and airport X-ray machines, all of which allow standardization of service provision by substituting machines for human effort. Soft technology is illustrated by restaurant salad bars and routinized tax and accounting services developed by firms such as H & R Block, Inc., and Comprehensive Accounting Corporation.

Hard and soft technologies facilitate the standardization of service necessary to provide consistent delivery to customers. By breaking tasks down and providing them efficiently, hard technology allows the firm to calibrate service standards such as the length of time a transaction takes, the accuracy with which operations are performed, and the number of problems that occur. In developing soft technology, the firm comes to understand completely the process by which the service is delivered; with this understanding, the firm more easily sets service standards.

Closing Gap 2 with Hard Technology

Hard technology can simplify and improve customer service, particularly when it frees company personnel by handling routine, repetitious tasks and transactions. Customer-service employees can then spend more time on the personal and possibly more essential portions of the job. American Airlines, whose standardized and automated baggage handling process is legendary, learned long ago that the standardization of its baggage system with hard technology could free the company to provide highly personalized service.

> A phone call to the lost-baggage number from any location at any hour is answered by a live sales rep at a center manned around the clock. The live voice didn't know any more than the tape message did but the reality was the sympathetic response the living person provided—a degree of comfort no tape machine could match.[18]

Some hard technology, in particular computer data bases that contain information on individual needs and interests of customers, allows the company to standardize the essential elements of service delivery. Basic delivery standards can then be established and measured. Some types of hard technology useful in standard setting include information data bases, automated transactions, and scheduling and delivery systems. Effective use of these types of technology is illustrated in the following company examples:

Information Data Bases. Campbell Soup Company receives regular requests for information about product ingredients, nutritional value, and flavors. Because many of these requests are repetitive, the company created a large computer data base to respond to these special requests. The data base allows Campbell to define service protocols, standard ways to respond quickly to customer requests, appearing to give individualized attention and answers to all questions. The data base frees up employees, as the only questions that must be handled personally by staff members are those that do not fall into the categories covered by the data base.[19]

Automating Tasks. Marshall Field eliminated "task-interfering duties" for salespeople. The retail store automated check approval, implemented in-store telephone directors to allow employees to contact other departments and other stores quickly, reorganized wrapping stations, and simplified order forms, all of which resulted in faster checkout and more attention to customers.[20] Each of these tasks had previously required varying amounts of time and blocked employees from responding quickly to customers' requests. With the new system, standards for service could be established and employees could quickly handle these simple tasks.

Scheduling and Delivery Systems. Pizza Hut centralized and computerized its home-delivery operations. Rather than having the separate tasks of order taking, baking, and delivery all in the same location, the company developed a system that works more effectively for both the company and its customers. Operators in a customer-service center (not a bakery) take requests for pizza. Working from a data base that shows past orders, trained operators take an average of 17 seconds to verify directions to a caller's home and enter his or her request. Operators then route the orders to the closest bake shops, which are strategically located throughout cities to ensure fast deliveries. Cooks in the satellite bakeshops prepare pizzas on instructions sent to bakeshop printers from order-takers' computers. Drivers aim to complete their deliveries within a half-hour of a customer's call and usually succeed.[21]

CLOSING GAP 2 WITH SOFT TECHNOLOGY: CHANGING THE WORK PROCESS

Standardizing some aspects of the service process is often desirable in providing consistent service quality. Mini-Maids Services, a firm that franchises home and office janitorial services, has successfully built a business by developing a repertoire of 22 standard daily cleaning chores. The company sends out crews of four who perform these 22 tasks in an average time of 55 minutes for a fee of $39.50 to $49.50.[22]

How does a company change the way work is done to gain these types of internal efficiencies without sacrificing perceived service quality? American Express's service-quality approach is an ideal illustration of the process. It "had all the earmarks of a classic industrial engineering study. It broke operations into discrete elements, measured how long each one took, set performance standards, and devised ways of meeting them."[23] First, the company defined four customer categories: traveler's-check purchasers, check sellers (banks), merchants who accept checks, and refund agents who reimburse the merchants. More than 100 managers from these areas joined with quality staffers to specify 50 separate services provided to these customers. Next, they determined how long these tasks were taking at the time and the ideal amount of time from their customers' perspectives. When these two measurements (present amount of time and ideal amount of time) differed, smaller groups of employees devised methods to improve them. As an example, by designing 13 new form letters and batching similar correspondence to help the word processing center better organize its workload,[24] response time to cardholders' written inquiries was cut to from 16 to 10 days.

When service to customers involves several different departments or areas in the firm, the company must link them together in meaningful ways from its customers' point of view. Merrill Lynch & Company designed a system called the Critical Path to track work as it passed through the company:

> Getting new products launched successfully requires many areas of the firm to work together. So we are standardizing the product introduction process . . . a checklist was designed so everyone knows what's needed and has adequate lead time to do their job. This checklist was administered by the New Product Committee . . . a Marketing Calendar was created and is being published monthly in an internal, management newsletter.[25]

Another important advantage to standardizing routine transactions is that the firm can free resources to personalize and improve service to its best customers. For this approach to work, the company must first define those best customers through criteria that make them easy to access. As an example, the Marriott Corporation defined as an Honored Guest those customers who spend at least 15 nights at a Marriott hotel or resort over a 12-month period. Guests who meet these qualifications receive service enhancements, amenities, and other benefits. The best Honored Guests, those who spend at least 75 nights over a 12-month period at a Marriott hotel or resort, receive the top treatment: an upgrade to a suite or concierge-level guestroom, direct billing, a room-service gift and a welcome note from the general manager. These special guests do not feel they are receiving treatment that is standardized, yet it is: Honored Guests get standard special treatment.[26]

Standardization, whether accomplished by hard or soft technology, reduces Gap 2. Both technology and improved work processes structure important elements of service provision. The process of standardization facilitates goal setting, which we discuss in the next section.

GAP 2 PROBLEM: ABSENCE OF GOAL SETTING

Companies that have been successful in delivering consistently high service quality are noted for establishing goals or standards to guide their employees in providing service quality. Of critical importance is the fact that the goals set by these companies are *based on customers' requirements and expectations* rather than internal company standards. While some similarity may exist between customers' requirements and company standards, we find many instances where service companies are measuring and monitoring internal standards for features that customers do not care about while ignoring other features that customers do care about.

CLOSING GAP 2: SETTING SERVICE-QUALITY GOALS

Effective service-quality goals have several common characteristics. Most important, they are based on customers' requirements. They are also specific. They are accepted by employees and cover important job dimensions. They are measured and reviewed with appropriate feedback. Finally, effective goals are challenging but realistic.[27]

1. *Designed to Meet Customers' Expectations.* American Express, after analyzing customers' complaints, surveys, and other customer data, found that timeliness, accuracy, and responsiveness were the important dimensions of quality to its customers. Management then identified 180 goals for different aspects of these customer-oriented dimensions rather than company-oriented dimensions of service quality.[28] Next, the company determined which performance levels the customers expected (rather than what the company wanted to establish) on each of the contacts customers had with the company.

2. *Specific.* Effective service goals are defined in *specific* ways that enable providers to understand what they are being asked to deliver. At best, these goals are set and measured in specific responses to human or machine performance. Goals should not be vague, as in "answer phones quickly" or "get the customer through the line as fast as possible." Instead, goals should be clear and specific as illustrated by the following quote from an American Airlines executive:

> We have goals and standards for almost every area of the operation, and we check them on a regular basis. We are constantly measuring how long it takes us to answer a reservations call, or process a customer in a ticket line, or get a plane-load of passengers on board the aircraft, or open the door of the airplane once it reaches its destination, or get food on, or get trash off.[29]

The specific measures of these activities form the baseline for performance at American Airlines and the standard on which all ensuing transactions are measured.

3. *Accepted by Employees.* Employees perform to standards consistently only if they understand and accept the goals. Imposing standards on unwilling employees often leads to resistance, resentment, absenteeism, or even turnover. Many companies establish standards for the amount of time it should take (rather than what it does take) for each service job and gradually cut back on the time to reduce labor costs. This practice inevitably leads to increasing tensions among employees. In these situations, managers, financial personnel, and union employees can work together to

determine new standards for the tasks. Through this participation, commitment of the line organization can be obtained and standards are accepted and more accurate.

4. *Important Job Dimensions.* As we saw in chapter 2, perceived service quality is a function of different dimensions. Most service workers cannot deliver to all of these dimensions at the same time. It is absolutely essential that management set priorities for these service workers, giving them clear messages about which aspects of the service job are most critical. One effective way to assure that the important tasks are accomplished by employees is to emphasize these important tasks in the goal-setting process. Most service customers in our research wanted reliability above all else. In the companies we studied, setting standards to do the job right the first time (reliability) would be emphasized above all else.

5. *Measured and Reviewed with Appropriate Feedback* To be effective, goals must be measured and reviewed regularly. Without measurement and feedback, corrections to quality problems will probably not occur. James Robinson of American Express puts it this way: "Employees do what management *inspects*, not what management *expects*."[30]

American Airlines' service goal approach illustrates the effective use of measurement and feedback:

> Reservation phones must be answered within 20 seconds, 85% of flights must take off within five minutes of departure time and land within 15 minutes of arrival time. Cabins must have their proper supply of magazines. Performance summaries drawn up every month tell management how the airline is doing and where the problems lie. The late arrivals may have been caused by disgruntled air controllers which can't be helped. But an outbreak of dirty ashtrays may be traced to a particular clean-up crew. The manager responsible for the crew will hear about it. His pay and promotion depend on meeting standards.[31]

American Express has an elaborate monitoring and tracking system for service quality. The system reflects the impact of any employee or department that interacts with customers. Called the Service Tracking Report, the system measures performance to the goals, such as the time it takes to process new applications, replace lost or stolen cards, or solve merchant problems. Quality assurance personnel regularly take samples of work and measure performance against these standards. The managers meet regularly to review recordings of telephone conversations and discuss ways to improve the handling of calls.[32]

6. *Challenging but Realistic.* A large number of studies on goal setting show that highest performance levels are obtained when goals are challenging but realistic. If goals are not challenging, employees get little reinforcement for mastering them. On the other hand, unrealistically high goals leave an employee feeling dissatisfied with performance and frustrated by not being able to attain the goal.

EMPIRICAL FINDINGS ABOUT GAP 2

We investigated the size of Gap 2 and the impact of the four factors described in this chapter in five major U.S. service companies. As described in chapter 4, we surveyed managers and contact personnel in these service companies, measuring their perceptions of the extent of Gap 2 and the factors likely to influence it. The results of this research are shown in exhibit 5–3 by company (numbered 1–5). On the left side of the charts, bar 1 shows the size of Gap 2 as perceived by managers and bar 2 by contact personnel. The solid sections of these bars indicate the current status of the gap in each of the companies (the higher the number, the smaller the gap). The patterned sections of these bars indicate opportunities for gap closure. For example, managers in company 1 perceive a bigger Gap 2 than those in company 3. The bars to the right show the levels of perceptions of individual factors (management's commitment to service quality, goal setting, task standardization, and perception of feasibility) responsible for Gap 2. As with Gap 2 bars on the left, the solid part of each bar on the right shows the current status on the factor as perceived by managers and the patterned section shows the opportunity for improvement in the factor. In company 1, for example, the smallest gap is in goal setting; it appears that the company has a goal-setting process in place. On the other hand, company 1 has a long way to go in management's commitment to service quality. If the company is serious about quality, management must become more committed, communicate that commitment to employees, and actually set goals focused on service quality.

An interesting pattern of results across companies is that contact personnel's perceptions of the size of Gap 2 are consistently higher (except in one case in which they are the same) than managers' perceptions of Gap 2 in the five companies. Contact personnel appear to have a more optimistic view of the size of the Gap 2 than does management.

The data shown in these charts reveal that different factors are likely to be responsible for Gap 2 in different companies. The size of the gaps

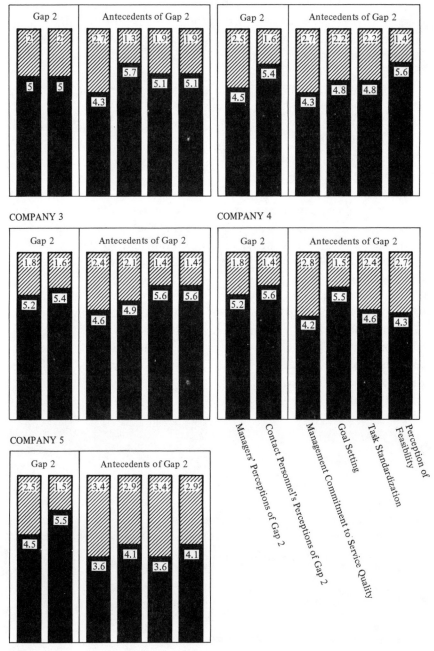

Exhibit 5-3 Gap 2 and Its Antecedents

in the individual factors are different across sample firms, suggesting that Gap 2 may have different drivers in different companies. For this reason, companies need to monitor all factors and determine through this type of analysis which factors are critical in their particular organizations. The factors identified as most critical would be targets for immediate attention for closing Gap 2.

Appendix B contains instructions and questionnaires for performing the type of gap analysis shown in exhibit 5–3.

SUMMARY

This chapter discussed Gap 2, the difference between management's perceptions of customers' expectations and the standards they set to fulfill these expectations. Our research indicates that the major reasons for Gap 2 include (1) inadequate management commitment to service quality; (2) lack of perception of feasibility; (3) inadequate task standardization; and (4) absence of goal setting.

Each of these reasons is discussed and detailed in this chapter, along with strategies to close the gap. To deliver high service quality, managers need the vision and commitment to change the systems of service delivery to meet customers' perceptions. This change often requires new equipment, technology, processes, and integration of executives from many different parts of the firm.

6

◇ ◇ ◇

GAP 3: THE SERVICE PERFORMANCE GAP

W E DEALT IN CHAPTER 4 with management's understanding of customers' expectations and in chapter 5 with the specifications management establishes to deliver to those expectations. In some cases management does understand customers' expectations and does set appropriate specifications (either informally or formally), and still the service delivered by the organization falls short of what customers expect. The difference between service specifications and the actual service delivery is the *service-performance gap*: when employees are unable and/or unwilling to perform the service at the desired level. Unfortunately, this service-performance gap is common in service businesses.

Organizations offering services that are highly interactive, labor intensive, and performed in multiple locations are especially vulnerable to Gap 3. Opportunities for mistakes and misunderstandings exist when service providers and customers interact: both customers and providers experience and respond to each other's mannerisms, attitudes, competencies, moods, and language. Greater variability is also more likely in labor-intensive services than when machines dominate service delivery. Bank customers who use human tellers experience far more service variability than those using automatic teller machines. Finally, when service is produced in a chain of outlets, quality control is complicated because the organizational layers between senior management and frontline service providers hinder two way communication and make it more difficult to assess individual employees' performance.

Service quality suffers when employees are unwilling or unable to perform a service at the level required. Willingness to perform may be described as discretionary effort, the difference "between the maximum amount of effort and care that an individual could bring to his or her job,

89

and the minimum amount of effort required to avoid being fired or penalized."[1] Employees who begin a new job giving 100 percent discretionary effort may be giving far less within weeks or months. This can happen because they have had to deal with too many long lines, too many unreasonable customers, too many rules and regulations, and too few pats on the back. It can also happen when they observe that few of their associates are giving their jobs their all.

In other cases, service providers may simply not have the ability to perform at specified levels. An organization may offer wage rates insufficient to attract skilled workers, or it may fail to train personnel adequately, or both. In addition, as a result of high turnover, workers may be moved into higher-level positions before they are ready. These factors are typical of many service industries, and all can lead to poor service quality.

Maintaining service quality, then, depends not only on recognizing customers' desires and establishing appropriate standards but also on maintaining a work force of people both willing and able to perform at specified levels.

Our extensive research focusing on the provider's side of our gaps model indicates that seven key conceptual factors contribute to Gap 3, the service-performance gap. These factors, illustrated in exhibit 6–1, include: (1) *role ambiguity*; (2) *role conflict*; (3) *poor employee-job fit*; (4) *poor technology-job fit*; (5) *inappropriate supervisory control systems* leading to an inappropriate evaluation/compensation system; (6) *lack of perceived control* on the part of employees; and (7) *lack of teamwork*. Exhibit 6–2 defines these factors and presents several specific issues about them. In this chapter, we describe the problems stemming from these factors and offer suggestions for dealing with them to close Gap 3. We then discuss empirical findings from our research pertaining to Gap 3 and the organizational factors contributing to it.

GAP 3 PROBLEM: EMPLOYEE ROLE AMBIGUITY

The role attached to any position in an organization represents the set of behaviors and activities to be performed by the person occupying that position.[2] The role is defined through the expectations, demands, and pressures communicated to employees by individuals (e.g., top managers, immediate supervisors, customers) who have a vested interest in how employees perform their jobs. When employees do not possess the information or training necessary to perform their jobs adequately, they

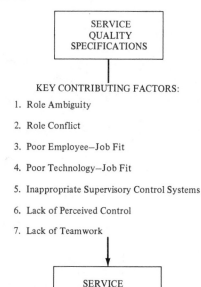

KEY CONTRIBUTING FACTORS:

1. Role Ambiguity

2. Role Conflict

3. Poor Employee–Job Fit

4. Poor Technology–Job Fit

5. Inappropriate Supervisory Control Systems

6. Lack of Perceived Control

7. Lack of Teamwork

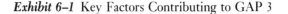

Exhibit 6–1 Key Factors Contributing to GAP 3

experience *role ambiguity*. They are uncertain about what managers or supervisors expect from them and how to satisfy those expectations. They do not have the training or the skills to provide the service necessary to satisfy customers. Further, they do not know how their performance will be evaluated and rewarded.

The status of training in many firms is bleak—too little too late. A customer-service representative in one of our studies commented: "It's really embarrassing—customers know about new products before we do. We're the company. We should know things before the customer does. But the training classes may be scheduled after the product comes out." During a focus group interview in banking, a lending officer expressed a similar complaint: "The bank will put out a product we don't understand— especially loans—and not tell us enough about it, not train us enough to sell it. With XYZ for example, I still have to get out the book [to look up how the loan works] and it takes me a good ten minutes." At this point, another participant in the group chimed in, "I just found out two weeks ago that we had the book." Then another said, "I just found out that we had XYZ!"

Training is essential in eliminating role ambiguity but employees sometimes lack role clarity in firms with good training. Unless training is supported by clear messages about what managers expect, unless em-

Factor and Definition	Specific Illustrative Issues
Role Ambiguity: Extent to which employees are uncertain about what managers or supervisors expect from them and how to satisfy those expectations.	• Does management provide accurate information to employees concerning job instruction, company policy and procedures, and performance assessment? • Do employees understand the products and services offered by the company? • Are employees able to keep up with changes that affect their jobs? • Are employees trained to interact effectively with customers? • How often does management communicate company goals and expectations to employees? • Do employees understand what managers expect from them and how to satisfy those expectations?
Role Conflict: Extent to which employees perceive that they cannot satisfy all the demands of all the individuals (internal and external customers) they must serve.	• Do customers and managers have the same expectations of employees? • How often do customer-contact employees have to depend on other support services employees to provide quality service to customers? • Do employees have more work to do than they have time to do it? • Does the number of demands in employees' jobs make it difficult to effectively serve customers? • Do too many customers want service at the same time? • Do employees cross-sell services to customers in situations where it is inappropriate?
Employee-Job Fit: The match between the skill of employees and their jobs.	• Do employees believe that they are able to perform their jobs well? • Does the company hire people who are qualified to do their jobs? • Does management devote sufficient time and resources to the hiring and selection of employees?
Technology-Job Fit: The appropriateness of the tools and technology that employees use to perform their jobs.	• Are employees given the tools and equipment needed to perform their jobs well? • How often does equipment fail to operate?

Exhibit 6-2 Conceptual Factors Pertaining to GAP 3

Factor and Definition	Specific Illustrative Issues
Supervisory Control Systems: The appropriateness of the evaluation and reward systems in the company.	• Do employees know what aspects of their jobs will be stressed most in performance evaluations? • Are employees evaluated on how well they interact with customers? • Are employees who do the best job serving customers more likely to be rewarded than other employees? • Do employees who make a special effort to serve customers receive increased financial rewards, career advancement, and/or recognition? • Do employees feel appreciated for their contributions?
Perceived Control: Extent to which employees perceive that they can act flexibly rather than by rote in problem situations encountered in providing services.	• Do employees spend time in their jobs trying to resolve problems over which they have little control? • Are employees given the freedom to make individual decisions to satisfy customers' needs? • Are employees encouraged to learn new ways to better serve their customers? • Are employees required to get approval from another department before delivering service to customers?
Teamwork: Extent to which employees and managers pull together for a common goal.	• Do employees and managers contribute to a team effort in servicing customers? • Do support services employees provide good service to customer-contact personnel? • Are employees personally involved and committed to the company? • Do customer-contact employees cooperate more than they compete with other employees in the company? • Are employees encouraged to work together to provide quality service to customers?

Exhibit 6–2 Continued

ployees know which of their behaviors are appropriate and inappropriate, unless feedback on performance is provided often enough to correct problems, Gap 3 can remain wide.

CLOSING GAP 3: PROVIDING ROLE CLARITY

Management can use four key tools to provide role clarity to employees: communication, feedback, confidence, and competence.[3] First, employees need accurate information about their roles in the organization. They need specific and frequent communication from supervisors and managers about what they are expected to do. They also need to know the goals, strategies, objectives, and philosophy of the company and of their own departments. They need current and complete information about the products and services the company offers. And they need to know the company's customers—who they are, what they expect, and which types of problems they encounter in using the service.

Next, employees need to know how well they are performing compared to the standards and expectations that management sets for them. Feedback provides reinforcement when employees perform well and offers the opportunity for correction when they perform poorly. This feedback need not always come directly from management; self-tracking of performance to key standards (such as the percentage of customer complaints handled within the expected time or the percentage of on-time deliveries) can provide the feedback necessary for employees to clearly understand their performance and roles.

Finally, employees need to feel confident and competent in their jobs. Companies can engender confidence in employees by training them in the skills needed to satisfy customers. Training that relates to the specific services offered by the firm help the contact person be and feel capable when dealing with customers. Training in communication skills, especially in listening to customers and understanding what customers expect, gives employees a sense of mastery over the inevitable problems that arise in service encounters. Training programs should be designed to increase employees' level of confidence and competence, which results in greater role clarity and helps close Gap 3.

Technical Training. It seems obvious that employees need training in the technical aspects of the services they provide. Yet many companies fall short of providing the technical knowledge and training necessary. One source of this problem is the proliferation of services in the service line—too many new services, too much added complexity, too short a lead time in introducing the services. Almost all the companies we studied were characterized by extensive additions to their service lines. In the case of the financial service firms, a clear impetus was deregulation. In the case of a repair firm, the impetus was electronics technology and its new product offspring: camcorders, videocassette recorders; home computers; and touch-sensitive, electronically timed washing machines.

To cope with new services, sophisticated customers, and technical complexity, firms need to develop strong training programs for employees. Merck & Company, the top-rated pharmaceutical firm in serving pharmacists and doctors, recognizes the necessity of training salespeople for the technical aspects of their jobs. The company's 11-month extensive program provides training in basic medical subjects (such as anatomy, physiology, and disease), Merck's products, presentation skills, and current topics in medicine. The program includes more than 13 weeks in a classroom, on-the-job training in the field, and medical classes conducted at universities known for the quality of their medical programs.[4]

Goodyear Tire & Rubber Company trains its entire service force to answer any and all questions customers may ask. To equip them for this challenge, the company designed a comprehensive training program that included specifics about the services and functions of the various departments as well as general training in consumer education and customer service. Similarly, Du Pont requires anyone who sells for its chemicals and pigments division to have worked in some other capacity at Du Pont for two years and also to have completed a year's training in business analysis and distribution.[5]

Training in Interpersonal Skills. Dealing with customers can be hard work, particularly when customers are demanding, hurried, dissatisfied, or angry. Unfortunately, demand fluctuations and other uncontrollable factors mean that all service workers at some point encounter disgruntled customers. Firms can and do develop employees to deal with these problems by training in interpersonal skills:

- British Airways is known for its training sessions in coping with the stress of customer contact that comes with intensive customer-service activities. The company put its entire 37,000-person customer-service staff through a training program called Putting People First which helps employees learn how to communicate effectively under pressure.[6] In one workshop exercise, half the participants were blindfolded and taken care of through a dinner meal by the other half. The purpose of this exercise and the training program as a whole was "to help people to ask for the kind of help they need on the one side, and on the other side to experience what it is like to give help that is required rather than the help you want to give."[7]

- At Stew Leonard's dairy store, over half of the 450 employees have gone through the Dale Carnegie program.[8]
- At Einstein Medical Center in Philadelphia, employees attend seminars where they take turns playing patient and learn a set of house rules for patient contact that include: "Make eye contact. Introduce yourself. Call people by name. Explain what you're doing." Einstein also has an ongoing campaign called HOSPITAL-ity to motivate everyone from janitors to doctors to be more courteous. Although doctors resisted initially, they "gradually discovered that they could act a great deal nicer and that patients noticed the difference." The service-quality excellence ratings of the center rose from 43 to 85 percent in three years.[9]
- Schaeffer & Sons Jewelers developed a training program to show employees how to transform complaints into sales. The four basic steps in the complaint handling process the company used were: open lines of communication; ask specific questions to get to the root of the problem; work within company policy to solve the problem; and reaffirm the customer's faith in the company's reputation.[10]

Teaching Employees about Customers. Although conventional wisdom holds that contact employees know customers well, perhaps even better than management knows them, we believe it essential to provide training about customers. One of our research studies (see exhibit 4–4) reveals that in the companies we studied, management perceives customers' expectations more accurately than contact employees perceive them. We speculate that managers in our study had access to research information about customers' needs and wants that they did not share with the contact employees. The more contact personnel know about customers' expectations, perceptions, and problems, the better they can serve them. Training contact personnel about their customers is emphasized in companies known for their service excellence. Milliken, the textiles company lauded for its customer service, includes an internship in manufacturing for all salespeople, and a stand-in-the-customer's-shoes training program. To provide quality service to their customers, salespeople must understand manufacturing operations because so many of Milliken's service products are used in manufacturing.[11]

GAP 3 PROBLEM: ROLE CONFLICT

Employees of service firms often experience *role conflict*, the perception that they cannot satisfy all the demands of all the individuals they must serve.[12] Many times this occurs because too many customers need or want service at the same time. Conflict between the expectations of the company and the expectations of customers also is not unusual in service firms. For example, conflict occurs when an income tax firm expects staff members to process as many customers as possible in a short time (i.e., limits the time with customers) and customers want personal attention from the staff (e.g., to discuss tax avoidance strategies for the future). Role conflict involves a poor fit among different elements of a service provider's job and creates feelings of tension, anxiety, and dissatisfaction.[13]

Role conflict often results when management emphasizes selling over service and expects employees to sell while they serve. Employees frequently feel they are expected to push these services on customers and many are torn between the company's expectations and their desire to serve customers. Employees in one of the banks we studied provide a clear example of role conflict. The bank had decided to introduce more aggressive personal selling at the branch level by emphasizing the sales component of branch employees' responsibilities. Many service providers view the sales and service elements of their jobs as conflicting. A teller observed: "If I am trying to cross-sell when there's a long line, the customers waiting in line give me that look: 'When is that girl going to shut up?' " One customer-service representative said: "You are torn sometimes between giving the customer what he or she wants and bringing money into the bank."

When faced with this conflict, does the employee take the time to cross-sell services to the customer or simply open the requested account and move on to the waiting customer? Complicating the issue is the reality that they may be measured—and rewarded—on the basis of cross-selling achievements.

Cross-selling is not always in conflict with service. When the employees and the customer have adequate time and the customer has interest, providing information about other company offerings may actually be part of quality service delivery. But when managers ask employees to sell in an aggressive manner or in a role (such as a teller) where selling is inappropriate, role conflict is the result.

The service-versus-sales dichotomy is not the only conflict employees experience. There are often simply too many demands on the employee's attention. The following comment is typical: "You are supposed to give your customer undivided attention, but you have already been interrupted seven times by telephone calls. You can't put the telephone caller on hold or send him elsewhere, because once I did that and the caller was a 'shopper' and my [performance] score was lowered."

The managers of service organizations can also inadvertently create role conflict for employees through excessive paperwork or unnecessary internal roadblocks. For example, customer-service personnel are often required to complete forms for the services they sell or the problems they handle. These employees may experience role conflict if other customers are waiting in a line or on the telephone to be served. Which master should be served, the waiting customer or the growing pile of paperwork?

A final source of role conflict is *role overload* which results from excessive contact with too many customers. Employees in service businesses experience a type of emotional overwork that author Arlie Russell Hochschild calls *contact overload* which leads to flat, frozen emotions.[14]

CLOSING GAP 3: ELIMINATING ROLE CONFLICT

Besides having a negative effect on employees' satisfaction and performance in the organization, role conflict can increase absenteeism and turnover.[15] A service organization that recognizes inherent conflicts in the service provider's job goes far in eliminating the distress of role conflict and its resulting distress on the organization.

If the company defines service roles and standards in terms of customers' expectations, role conflict is minimized. Many companies involve employees in the standard-setting process, believing that they are more knowledgeable than anyone else about their jobs. The advantage in this approach is that employees feel responsible for the service-quality changes they help develop, have a clear idea of what is expected of them, and accept change because they see why the new process is better.

Role conflict can be minimized by reinforcing change with other human resource systems. Use of performance measurement systems that focus on the customer in addition to (or rather than) internal efficiency goals is one way to clearly support the service-quality priority. Another is to train employees in priority setting and time management. Still another is compensation tied to delivery of service quality (by measures of customers' satisfaction, loyalty, perceived service quality) instead of, or as well as, other factors.

For employees suffering from role overload, frequent breaks and varied work tasks have been successful in managing the overload. Employees need time to relax mentally to avoid the burnout of contact overload.

GAP 3 PROBLEM: POOR EMPLOYEE-JOB FIT

Our research indicates that service-quality problems often occur because personnel are not well suited to their positions. Because customer-contact jobs tend to be situated at the lower levels of company organization charts (e.g., car rental agents, telephone operators, and repair technicians), personnel holding these jobs are frequently among the least-educated and lowest-paid employees in their companies. As a result, they may lack language, interpersonal, or other skills to serve customers effectively. Many service companies have high turnover among contact employees and are inclined to fill openings quickly, even if they must hire persons having background or skill deficiencies. Managers commonly do not give enough attention or devote sufficient resources to hiring and selection processes.

The overriding sentiment among disgruntled employees in one of our studies was that you get what you pay for, and the firm wasn't paying for much. One manager said, "We draw from the bottom of the barrel because that's the way we compensate." When management does not match employees to jobs through selection processes that identify those with ability or skill to perform the job well, Gap 3 widens.

GAP 3 PROBLEM: POOR TECHNOLOGY-JOB FIT

Provision of high service quality also depends on the appropriateness of the tools or technology employees use to perform the job. Technology and equipment, such as computers and diagnostic equipment, can enhance the service employee's performance. Appropriate and reliable technology must be provided for high-quality service delivery. Equipment inadequacies and failures can seriously interfere with adequate employee performance.

Our exploratory study revealed several instances in which service-quality shortfalls resulted from a lack of technology-job fit and/or employee-job fit. For example, a product-repair executive, in bemoaning the proliferation of new high-technology appliances, indicated problems stemming from a lack of both types of fit: "We may not have all the [technical] specifications needed to train technicians before a new product is marketed [technology-job fit]. Some technicians may never be capable of being trained to service these new 'high-tech' products [employee-job fit]. These products are coming too fast."

CLOSING GAP 3: IMPROVING
EMPLOYEE-TECHNOLOGY-JOB FIT

Competing effectively for first-rate service providers makes it easier to compete for customers. Successful service companies rely on careful selection of employees and technology and the fit among the employee, technology, and the job. Federal Express's company philosophy clearly illustrates the importance of human resources: "Hire the best people, give them the best training and compensation you can, and they'll deliver the high-level efficiency and service that translates into profit. People, service, profit—in that order."[16]

Because competing for talent promises to become more intense in the future—an issue we explore in depth in chapter 9—innovative recruitment and retention methods need to be developed.[17]

A number of major service companies are searching for and finding new ways to recruit and retain lower-level service employees. Service-Master Company, the successful franchised janitorial service, hires many people who are functionally illiterate. The company's CEO, recognizing the importance of these employees to the business, has adopted an approach that respects them and gains their loyalty. He believes that, "before asking someone to do something you have to help them to be something."[18] The company provides self-development programs to help the employees improve their lives. Another ServiceMaster Company slogan is "to help people grow." When a hospital served by the company decided to hire a deaf person as one of its contacts, ServiceMaster's local manager didn't object. Instead he authorized three of his supervisors to take a course in sign language.[19]

Wegman's, a large, successful grocery chain in Rochester, New York, suffered from the same problems as all employers who pay minimum wage. The company hired what it called the rawest of recruits and was plagued by high turnover among them. The company now has a program that develops these recruits personally and encourages them to stay with the firm. For those who work at Wegman's for at least a year, perform well in their jobs, and seem likely to do well in college or graduate school, the company offers scholarships for half their tuition. "Almost 1,000 of

Wegman's 11,000 full- and part-time employees have made the grade, stayed in school, and at Wegman's."[20]

Compensating employees at a higher-than-market level can also engender loyalty. Somerville Lumber & Supply, the Massachusetts company that retails lumber and other construction materials, pays employees more than other firms in its industry, starting them at an annual salary of about $20,000. The company pays an additional 15 percent of salary into a profit-sharing fund. Employees are entitled to a portion of that money if they stay for more than three years, and get the entire portion if they stay ten years. Many ten-year employees have accrued $100,000 and some longer-term employees are millionaires. Moreover, the profit-sharing plan is supplemented by a pension plan, under which another 10 percent of salary is set aside.[21]

Embassy Suites, Inc., a division of Holiday Corporation, believes that employees who have a chance to grow in their jobs are more likely to be satisfied and loyal to the company. To build growth into low-level positions such as housekeeping, the company offers an opportunity for all employees to cross-train for other positions in the company. Housekeeping personnel can learn how to work the front desk; food service personnel can learn housekeeping. For each new position employees learn, they receive a boost in their hourly pay. As employees develop personally and financially, the company creates a ready source of trained and flexible personnel for peak periods or understaffed times.[22]

Competing effectively for first-rate service providers is essential to success in a service business. Companies that excel in service select and develop employees carefully, choose appropriate technology, and concentrate on the fit among employees, technology, and jobs.

GAP 3 PROBLEM: INAPPROPRIATE
SUPERVISORY CONTROL SYSTEMS

In many service organizations, the performance of contact employees is measured by their output (e.g., the number of units produced per hour, the number or amount of sales per week). In these *output control systems*, the performance of individuals is monitored and rewarded not for service-quality delivery but for other company-defined goals.[23] These output measures alone are usually inappropriate or insufficient for measuring employees' performance relating to the provision of quality service. For example, most bank customers want bank tellers to be accurate, fast, and friendly. Banks that measure tellers' performance strictly on output measures, such as end-of-the day balancing of transactions, overlook key aspects of job performance that customers factor into quality-of-service perceptions.

CLOSING GAP 3: MEASURING AND REWARDING SERVICE PERFORMANCE

In service situations where the manner in which service is provided is essential to customers' satisfaction, performance also can be monitored through what are termed *behavioral control systems*. Behavioral control systems consist largely of observations or other reports on the way the employee works or behaves.[24] The use of behavioral control systems is illustrated by an ongoing "tone-of-service" survey with customers who have recently opened accounts at The Friendly National Bank of Oklahoma City.[25] Customers answer questions about the way they are treated by the customer-service representatives opening their accounts. Friendly also monitors customer-service representatives' performance through ongoing shopper research (researchers pretending to be customers) and a cross-sales index. Each month, customer-service representatives receive tone-of-service and shopper scores (behavioral measures) and a cross-sales score (output measure). The use of these behavioral measures encourages employees' performance to be consistent with customers' expectations of quality service.

A vital ingredient for excellent service-quality delivery is recognition of employees' performance. Employees' performance must be continually monitored, compared with service standards, and rewarded when outstanding. A performance-measurement system sensitive to high performance and tied to appropriate rewards can be very motivating, especially when workers know that others will learn how well they are performing. This system also helps management determine the specific effects of policy and personnel changes on operating performance and to weed out individuals who deliver substandard performance.

Performance measurement should extend beyond image tracking, isolated shopping visits, customer-complaint analyses, and other traditional approaches. Although a service performance-measurement system gets employees' attention, only a well-executed reward system keeps it. Workers realize that management is serious about quality when management is willing to pay for it. A good reward system, like a good measurement system, is one that is meaningful, timely, simple, accurate, and fair.

We recommend using a reward system under which employees are expected to meet service-quality standards and are rewarded for out-standing performance. Rewards can take many forms: direct financial rewards (merit salary increases and bonuses), career advancement, and recognition. The most effective system is one that incorporates all three approaches for both individuals and work groups. Singling out high-performing work units can energize peer pressure and lead to better performance.

Compensation and Direct Financial Incentives. The most convincing way to encourage active support for first-line service employees and middle managers is to tie compensation into performance and behaviors that lead to high service quality. At British Airways, middle managers are evaluated by bosses according to a list of 60 statements of behavior that had been identified as the key behavior characteristics necessary in providing quality customer service. Managers receive lump-sum bonuses worth up to 20 percent of their base salary, half determined by what they achieve and half by the behaviors by which they achieve it.[26]

Commitment to quality on the part of employees is also encouraged by profit-sharing programs. For example, at Publix Fruit & Produce, the food retailer, employees own 62 percent of the company's stock and get back 20 percent of the profits, "right down to the bagboys. . . . The result is workers who hustle. Energetic store clerks seem to be every-where. Happy employees, in turn, lead to happy customers."[27]

Recognition Programs that Work. Not all employee recognition programs have what it takes to be successful: challenging standards, acceptance by employees, neither too few nor too many rewards, and longevity. Federal Express has a tiered recognition program that works. At the first level, the Bravo Zulu award (meaning "well done" in military terms) of up to $100 can be given by anyone in management to any employee providing excellent customer service. A special flag stamp is affixed to the letter accompanying the award.[28] At the next higher level, Federal Express honors a handful of nonmanagement individuals with its Golden Falcon award each month, recognizing efforts that are "above and beyond their customary line of duty." This award includes a gold pin with the gold falcon emblem and ten shares of Federal Express stock.[29]

John Creedon, president and CEO of Metropolitan Life Insurance Company, instituted a highly creative and powerful recognition program in which 1,000 of the company's 36,000 plus service employees are eligible to win quality awards at $1,000 each. As in the previous Federal Express example, the awards were designed to recognize employees who performed uniquely to provide excellent service quality. Employees nominate themselves or are nominated by others by documenting in writing a single-page description of efforts resulting in a high level of customer satisfaction that also enhances Metropolitan Life's reputation for service quality. Creedon personally selects the final awardees after reviewing all the documented entries. The awards program is a strong signal of the value top management places on customer satisfaction and employee creativity in delivering it.[30]

Financial Rewards for Teams. Companies can use team rewards as an incentive. Domino's Pizza uses what it calls its TIPO (Team/Individual/Performance/Objectives) system to relate the monthly bonus to individual and team performance for a given period. The process begins by developing key satisfaction indicators for each unit and each specific job in quantifiable terms. Next, weights are assigned to the key indicators to emphasize the priority each key indicator has for customers. The expected level of performance is set, and then measured using phone surveys of customers. If the expected level is obtained, the team wins a monthly bonus.[31]

GAP 3 PROBLEM: LACK OF PERCEIVED CONTROL

Employees' reactions to stressful situations depend on whether they feel they can control those situations.[32] *Perceived control* involves the ability to make responses that influence threatening situations and the ability to choose outcomes or goals.[33] We believe that when service employees perceive themselves to be in control of situations they encounter in their jobs, they experience less stress. Lower levels of stress, in turn, lead to higher performance. When employees perceive that they can act flexibly rather than by rote in problem situations encountered in providing services, control increases and performance improves.

When employees do not feel a sense of personal control over the quality of service rendered, they feel helpless and discouraged about their jobs. In one of our studies in banks, for example, branch lenders used to process and approve loans. Then loan processing and credit decisions were transferred to remote operations centers. As a result, loan decisions move more slowly through the system and branch employees are not able to give customers timely information on the status of their applications. One branch lender said, "My number-one priority is working with other units over which I have no control." A branch manager put it this way: "We're offering terrible service now. We used to have control and now we don't. We used to know where everything is and now we don't."

Perceived control can be low when organizational rules, procedures, and culture limit the contact employees' flexibility in serving customers. It can also be low when the authority to achieve specific outcomes with customers lies elsewhere in the organization. Service companies commonly are organized internally in a way that makes providing fast service to customers difficult for service employees. When a contact person must get the approval of other departments in the organization before delivering a service, service quality is jeopardized. Though the contact person may be totally committed to serving the customer, he or she cannot perform well because control over the service is in the hands of an employee in another place in the organization. Finally, perceived control can be a function of the unpredictability of demand, a major problem in many service businesses.

CLOSING GAP 3: EMPOWERING SERVICE EMPLOYEES

Empowering service employees to satisfy customers helps them develop in the job and the company. Larry Wilson of Pecos Training puts it this way: "Help people find their power and use it in important ways. Give them a chance to find their courage . . . leadership is waking people up."[34] Empowered employees are committed employees, ones who serve the company and its customers well. Jim Kuhn, McDonald's corporate vice-president for individuality, says the key to motivating employees is to "Get out of their way. Believe in your folks and most will live up to your expectations."[35]

Empowerment means pushing decision-making power down to the lowest levels of the company. It means granting contact personnel the authority to make important decisions about serving customers. Empowerment also means replacing heavily standardized and mechanistic approaches for dealing with customers with looser structures that allow employees to individualize their skills and methods. Empowerment can create quick problem solutions for customers because permission to execute a transaction to satisfy customers need not be obtained from multiple employees.

Some service firms are legendary for their empowerment of contact people who go out of their way for their customers. A favorite legend at United Parcel Service is the regional manager who took it on himself to untangle a misdirected shipment of Christmas presents by hiring an entire train and diverting two UPS-owned 727s from their flight plans. When top management learned of his actions, it praised and rewarded him.[36]

Part of Federal Express's legendary company culture is its collection of stories of employee empowerment and dedication to customers. From a deliveryman hefting a 300-pound Fedex deposit box on a truck because he didn't have the key to open it, to a tracing agent who put in place the systems to rescue Baby Jessica from the well she had fallen into, Federal Express employees will do most anything the company allows them to do—and it allows, even encourages, them to do a lot. One legend describes a courier who spent Labor Day saving an ill child:

> A Federal Express courier responded to a Labor Day call from the Memphis trace department regarding a supply of matched blood needed by a child scheduled for surgery at Boston's Children's Hospital the next day. The Boston station's beeper was not functioning; the courier who then arrived at the station in person had to scale a barbed wire fence because his key would not open a new lock on the gate, explain the unusual circumstances to the security guard, find and deliver the package.[37]

One of the things that makes empowerment easier is an internal management information system that can provide unusually helpful information. At Walt Disney World, the story is told about a family who visited Epcot Center and neglected to make note of their parking area. Because Disney maintains daily computerized data that tells which parking lots are filled at what time in the day, employees were able to help the family find their car. With this data system, Disney employees located the car in less than 20 minutes using the family's time of arrival at the center. The guests were driven to the designated parking lot and up and down each row until their car was found.[38]

Empowerment is also effective at managerial levels of a company where department or field managers are given the power to make important company decisions to serve customers. At Byerly's, the grocery chain in Minnesota, deli managers are given complete control in their departments to create new products and expand the deli's selling potential.[39] Each Byerly's store is managed semi-independently by a single executive, who tailors the merchandising to neighborhood needs with little overseeing from top management.[40] The result? Satisfied customers who cannot get enough of the company and its products.

Executives often ask how it is possible to standardize service across departments and outlets and yet still provide sufficient perceived control to bring out the best in employees. Reconciling these two conflicting forces is admittedly difficult. One successful way to balance these forces is to require that managers or departments achieve certain essential goals and standards, allowing them to reach the goals in ways they choose. An example of attempting this balance is illustrated by Au Bon Pain, a chain of bakery and deli shops.

> Store managers are hired on the basis of wanting to solve their own problems. The company, in effect, leases the stores to its managers, gives them goals for labor and food costs, but agrees to split the controllable profits on a 50-50 basis. Like company owners, they have to solve their own problems, hire and fire their own people, set their own wage scale, cut their own deals. What they can't do is to compromise on food quality and customer service, which the company regularly monitors through in-store audits and visits by unidentified "mystery" shoppers. Aside from that, they're on their own. The stores have never run better or with less support from headquarters.[41]

GAP 3 PROBLEM: LACK OF TEAMWORK

The value of teamwork—employees and managers pulling together for a common goal—is a recurring theme in all our studies of service quality. The following statements from one of our studies illustrate a situation where bank employees did not feel they were working together well.

LENDING OFFICER: "I worked in the bank 13 years. There is a big difference in when I started and now in terms of how the employees feel about the bank. There used to be so much camaraderie. Now, it's like pulling teeth to get associates to help you."

CUSTOMER-SERVICE REPRESENTATIVE: "We're *not* working as a family and as a group. We may all come together again but it hasn't happened yet."

CUSTOMER-SERVICE REPRESENTATIVE: "Our cashier sits there and smokes cigarettes and drinks coffee. She doesn't help with any of our work. She says it isn't in her job description. She's a deadbeat."

One aspect of teamwork is the extent to which employees view other employees as customers. In many companies, support employees must provide good service to contact people to enable them to serve customers. Some businesses underestimate the importance to service quality of support services. While customer-contact personnel are obvious targets for quality-improvement efforts, the providers of internal support services are also critical. Poor service to customer-contact personnel results in poor service by those personnel.

Another aspect of teamwork involves the extent to which employees feel personally involved and committed to the firm. Strong belief in an organization and in the importance of one's contribution to it can inspire strong discretionary effort by workers; weak belief can have the opposite effect. To some extent, this employee commitment comes from the sense that management cares about them. In many companies, service people feel that individual performance goes unnoticed and unrewarded. One employee commented: "You feel like management doesn't know what you are doing. We need more support and recognition." Another said, "They should give recognition to people who are really performing. So many times you are judged by your immediate supervisor. That person may not like you. I wish other managers, higher up, would know how people are performing."

CLOSING GAP 3: BUILDING TEAMWORK

In organizations where teamwork exists, employees accomplish their goals by allowing group members to participate in decisions and to share in the group's success. Teamwork is the heart of service-quality initiatives—employees need to work together to have service come together for customers. Merrill Lynch has involved more than twenty-five hundred operations personnel in quality teams of 8 to 15 employees plus a supervisor; each team works to improve customer-service.[42] One group in the cashier's department saved Merrill $40,000 per year with a single idea: By daily updating of securities eligibility data from the Depository Trust Company, they could significantly reduce Merrill's reject ratio, saving money and improving customer service.[43]

Employees at all levels at American Express are required to learn the way that all departments work so that each understands the impact of his or her function on customers' perception of service.

> We concluded that the customer-service department is only the catcher's mitt. The real problems arise in other departments: data processing, mail room, new accounts, accounts receivable, etc. The fact that customer service has processed a customer order in two days is not helpful if the order stays in the mail room for four days, and another four days in data processing. Similarly, accounts receivable is just concerned about receiving funds. Well, that's fine if cus-

tomers really owe money. But we had better make sure before they start sending dunning letters.[44]

And at Shell Oil Company, more than 10,000 employees have participated in a quality-improvement training program focusing on working together in customer-supplier relationships. Vic Gigurelli, manager of quality improvement, comments: "Shell's emphasis on the internal customer is paying off. It has already provided a common language that engineers, craftsmen, clerical staff and business managers can all share to get work done."[45]

CLOSING GAP 3: MANAGING EXTERNAL CUSTOMERS

In many service businesses, part of the reason employees have difficulty delivering good service is that customers themselves are not fulfilling their roles in service delivery. When customers of an income tax preparation service do not save the necessary receipts, when customers in a bar become unruly, when customers at McDonald's do not clear their own tables—these and other examples of poor customer performance interfere with employees' abilities to deliver to standards set by management. What can a company do to encourage customers to accept their roles in service provision? David Bowen, an authority on the management of service employees, suggests that companies treat customers as "partial employees" and manage them by adapting many of the techniques discussed in this chapter for managing employees.[46] Answering the following questions may help to improve customers' service delivery.

Role clarity: Do customers understand how they are expected to perform their part of the transaction? Do employees provide clear instructions and feedback?

Ability: Are customers able to perform as expected? Are the right segments of customers being chosen?

Compensation: Are valuable rewards offered to customers for performing as expected? Is the price differential between full- and self-service adequate to induce customers to perform?

According to Bowen, management practices that can improve situations where customers are coproducers include providing customers with realistic service previews, training customers how to perform, providing visible rewards (airline personnel selecting passengers with first-class seats for early boarding over those with coach seats), selecting the participating

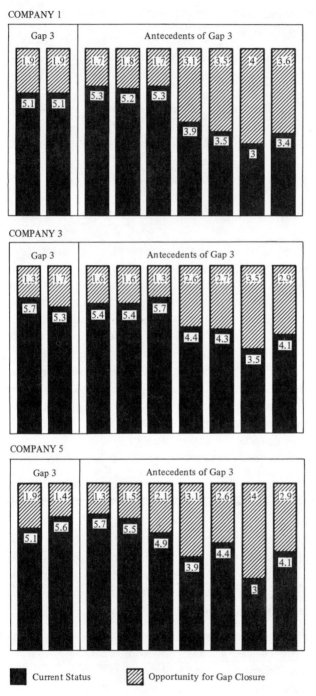

Exhibit 6–3 Gap 3 and Its Antecedents

COMPANY 2

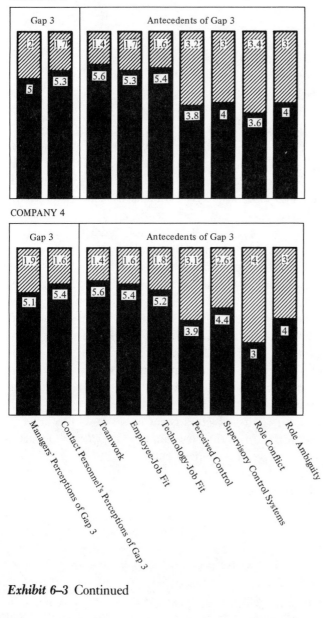

COMPANY 4

Exhibit 6–3 Continued

customer (e.g., those willing to use an automatic teller machine or pump their own gas), and providing customer scripts so that they know what is expected of them.

EMPIRICAL FINDINGS ABOUT GAP 3

We investigated the size of Gap 3 and the impact of the factors described in this chapter in five major U.S. service companies. As described in chapter 4, we measured managers' and contact personnel's perceptions of the extent of Gap 3 and the factors likely to influence it. The results of this research are shown in exhibit 6–3 by company (numbered 1–5). On the left side of the charts, bar 1 shows the size of Gap 3 as perceived by managers and bar 2 by contact personnel. The solid sections of these bars indicate the current status of the gap in each of the companies (the higher the number, the smaller the gap). The patterned sections of these bars indicate the opportunity for gap closure. For example, managers in company 3 perceive a smaller gap than those in any of the other companies. The bars to the right show the levels of individual factors (teamwork, employee-job fit, technology-job fit, perceived control, supervisory control systems, role conflict, and role ambiguity). As with the Gap 3 bars to the left, the solid part of the bar shows the current status on the factor and the patterned section shows the opportunity for improvement along the factor. (Both role conflict and role ambiguity have been reverse scored so that the interpretation of these factors is the same as with other factors.) A striking result is that in all five companies, *role conflict* is the factor with the biggest gap. It appears that in all our sample firms, employees feel that expectations of them are inconsistent or too demanding. Our sample companies have further to go in improving role conflict than in any other factor in Gap 3.

SUMMARY

We dealt in this chapter with the service-performance gap: when employees are unable and/or unwilling to perform the service at the level desired by management. Unwillingness to perform involves reduction in employees' discretionary effort, a result stemming from too many long lines, too many unreasonable customers, too many rules and regulations, and too few pats on the back.

Factors that contribute to the service-performance gap discussed in this chapter include: (1) role ambiguity; (2) role conflict; (3) poor employee-job fit; (4) poor technology-job fit; (5) inappropriate supervisory control systems leading to an inappropriate evaluation/reward system; (6) lack of perceived control on the part of employees; and (7) lack of teamwork. We described the problems stemming from these factors and offered suggestions for dealing with them to close Gap 3. Finally, we discussed empirical findings from our research pertaining to Gap 3 and its antecedents and explored the implications of those findings.

7

◇ ◇ ◇

GAP 4: WHEN PROMISES DO NOT MATCH DELIVERY

W E PROPOSE that the fourth major cause of low service-quality perceptions is the gap between what a firm promises about a service and what it actually delivers. Accurate and appropriate company communication—advertising, personal selling, and public relations that do not overpromise or misrepresent—is essential to delivering services that customers perceive as high in quality. Because company communications about services promise what people do, and because people cannot be controlled the way machines that produce physical goods can be controlled, the potential for overpromising is high.

Appropriate and accurate communication about services is the responsibility of both marketing and operations: marketing must accurately (if compellingly) reflect what happens in actual service encounters; operations, in turn, must deliver what is promised in communications. If advertising, personal selling, or any other external communication sets up unrealistic expectations for customers, actual encounters disappoint them.

As described in chapter 3, our research suggests that Gap 4 can also occur when companies neglect to inform customers of special quality assurance efforts that are not visible to customers. Customers are not always aware of everything done behind the scenes to serve them well. For instance, most hair styling firms have guarantees that ensure customer satisfaction with haircuts, permanents, and color treatments. However, only a few of them actively communicate these guarantees in advertising because they assume customers know about them. The firm that explicitly communicates the guarantee may be selected over others

115

by a customer who is uncertain about the quality of the service. Even though many competitors provide the same guarantees, the firm that communicates it to customers is the one chosen on that attribute. Making customers aware of standards or efforts to improve service when these efforts are not readily apparent to customers can improve service-quality perceptions. Customers who are aware that a firm is taking concrete steps to serve their best interests are likely to perceive a delivered service in a more favorable way.

Discrepancies between service delivery and external communications, in the form of exaggerated promises and/or the absence of information about service delivery aspects intended to serve customers well, can powerfully affect consumers' perceptions of service quality. Our extensive research focusing on the provider's side of our gaps model indicates that two key conceptual factors contribute to Gap 4. These factors, illustrated in exhibit 7–1, are: (1) *inadequate horizontal communication*, particularly among operations, marketing, and human resources, as well as across

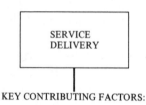

KEY CONTRIBUTING FACTORS:

1. Inadequate Horizontal Communication

    – Inadequate communication between
      advertising and operations

    – Inadequate communication between
      salespeople and operations

    – Inadequate communication between
      human resources, marketing, and
      operations

    – Differences in policies and procedures
      across branches or departments

2. Propensity to Overpromise

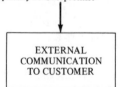

Exhibit 7–1 Key Factors Contributing to Gap 4

branches; and (2) *propensity to overpromise* in communications. Exhibit 7–2 defines these factors and presents several specific issues pertaining to them. In this chapter, we describe the problems stemming from these factors and offer suggestions for dealing with them to close Gap 4. We then discuss empirical findings from our research about Gap 4 and the organizational factors contributing to it.

GAP 4 PROBLEM: INADEQUATE HORIZONTAL COMMUNICATIONS

Communications between different functional areas in the firm, such as marketing and operations, are necessary to achieve the common goals of the organization. In situations where communication across functions, or *horizontal communication* channels are not open, perceived service quality is in jeopardy. If, for example, company advertising is developed independent of input from operations, contact personnel may not be able to deliver service that matches the image portrayed in advertising. This lack of communication is illustrated by Holiday Inns, Inc.'s unsuccessful No Surprises advertising campaign. Holiday Inns' advertising agency

Factor and Definition	Specific Illustrative Issues
Horizontal Communication: Extent to which communication occurs both within and between different departments of a company.	• Do customer contact personnel have input in advertising planning and execution? • Are customer contact personnel aware of external communications to customers before they occur? • Does the salesforce interact with customer contact personnel to discuss the level of service that can be delivered to customers? • Are the policies and procedures for serving customers consistent across departments and branches?
Propensity to Overpromise: Extent to which a company's external communications do not accurately reflect what customers receive in the service encounter.	• Is there increasing pressure inside the company to generate new business? • Do competitors overpromise to gain new customers?

Exhibit 7–2 Conceptual Factors Pertaining to Gap 4

found through consumer research that hotel customers wanted greater reliability in lodging and created a television campaign promising no surprises to customers. Top managers accepted the campaign in spite of the skepticism of operations executives who believed that this would be a difficult-to-live-up-to claim. The campaign raised consumers' expectations, gave dissatisfied customers additional reasons to be angry, and had to be discontinued.[1]

Not all organizations advertise, but all need coordination or integration across departments to be able to delivery quality service. All service organizations, for example, need horizontal communication between the sales force and service providers. If customers' expectations are unrealistically raised by salespeople, and if operations personnel cannot deliver on these promises, the size of Gap 4 widens.

Salespeople and operations employees in many companies are often in conflict, each function believing that the other makes work difficult. Operations employees feel that salespeople constantly promise more than they can deliver—usually more quickly than they can deliver—to get or maintain the business. Salespeople, on the other hand, believe that operations employees are unwilling to push hard enough to deliver to customers' expectations. A spirit of misunderstanding and mistrust can develop, enlarging Gap 4. When customers' expectations are raised by salespeople and then not met by service providers, quality perceptions are sacrificed.

Horizontal communication also must occur between the human resources and marketing departments. To deliver excellent customer service, firms must treat their employees as customers.[2] The extent to which the human resource function serves employees through training, motivation, compensation, and recognition has a powerful impact on the quality of service that employees deliver. Breaking down the walls between functions is difficult and time consuming, but high-quality service cannot be delivered without this communication.

CLOSING GAP 4: OPENING CHANNELS OF COMMUNICATION BETWEEN ADVERTISING AND OPERATIONS

When a company creates advertising that depicts the service encounter, it is essential that the advertising accurately reflect what customers experience in actual service encounters. Puffery or exaggeration puts service-quality perceptions at risk, especially when the firm is consistently unable to deliver to the level of service portrayed in advertising. Coordination and communication between advertising and service providers are pivotal in closing Gap 4.

Featuring actual employees doing their jobs or explaining their service in advertising is one way to coordinate advertising portrayals and the reality of the service encounter. Advertising that features actual employees doing their jobs can be very effective in communicating excellence, and the effect is present in both the primary audience (customers) and the secondary audience (employees).[3] An additional benefit is that featured employees become standards for other employees by modeling performance.

In featuring employees, the advertising department must interact directly with service providers. Therefore, the communication and coordination needed to create the advertising helps close the gap between external communications and delivery. Similar benefits can be achieved using other forms of advertising if employees are involved in the advertising process in other ways.

A common complaint of service employees in our studies is that companies run advertisements promising customers certain services or benefits before employees are told about the advertisements and *often before they are told about the services!* Customers come to them asking for the services and they feel uninformed, left out, and helpless.[4] This problem can be avoided by requesting input or opinions from operations employees during the advertising process or by monitoring actual service encounters.

Prior to running advertisements, it is desirable that service providers preview advertising campaigns to prepare them for the service customers will expect them to perform. After that point, the providers must be motivated to carry out the themes of courtesy, responsiveness, and reliability that are presented in advertising. High interdependence exist between advertising and operations, making cooperation and communication between these two functions critical if the promises-delivery gap is to be closed.

When advertising and operations personnel talk to each other, especially when contact personnel provide input to the advertising department about the feasibility of what is being promised in advertising, customers are led to expect what contact personnel can deliver, and Gap 4 can be narrowed.

CLOSING GAP 4: OPENING CHANNELS OF
COMMUNICATIONS BETWEEN SALES AND OPERATIONS

Mechanisms for opening channels of communications between sales and operations employees can take many forms, both formal and informal. Annual planning meetings, retreats, team meetings, or workshops where the departments interact can clarify the issues and allow each department to understand the goals, capabilities, and constraints of the other. A computer company we have worked with planned a "gap workshop" where employees from all functions of a service division met for two days to outline the four gaps in the division and to jointly make plans to close them.

Involving the operations staff in face-to-face meetings with external customers is a strategy that allows operations to more readily understand the salesperson's role and the needs and desires of customers. Rather than filtering customers' needs through the sales force, operations employees can witness firsthand the pressures and demands of customers. A frequent and desirable result is better service to the internal customer (the salesperson) from the operations staff as they become aware of their own roles in satisfying both external and internal customers.

CLOSING GAP 4: OPENING CHANNELS OF
COMMUNICATION BETWEEN HUMAN RESOURCES,
MARKETING, AND OPERATIONS

Because employees are internal customers of the human resource department, the service they receive strongly affects the way they serve external customers. Incentives, training, motivation, and selection must be aligned with service-quality objectives in the company if these internal customers are to deliver high-quality service to external customers.

One effective strategy for opening these channels is a staff position that formally links human resources and operations. The individual who fills this job, often called a service excellence manager, is responsible for developing programs and processes to motivate and facilitate the quality spirit in employees through techniques that include employee recognition and service goals of the company. Karen Caswell, service excellence manager at Citicorp/Citibank, has the full-time job of infusing the service-quality spirit in employees through techniques that include employee recognition and appreciation programs, acknowledgment of new service ideas, and employee newsletters. She views employees as her internal customers and bridges the human resources-marketing gap by educating, motivating, and advertising to employees in the same way that the marketing department communicates with external customers.

GAP 4 PROBLEM: DIFFERENCES IN POLICIES AND PROCEDURES ACROSS BRANCHES OR DEPARTMENTS

Another form of coordination central to providing service quality is consistency in policies and procedures across departments and branches. If a service organization operates many outlets under the same name, whether franchised or company-owned, customers expect similar performance across those outlets. If managers of individual branches or outlets have significant autonomy in procedures and policies, customers may not receive the same level of service quality across the branches. In this case, what they expect and receive from one branch may be different from what is delivered in other branches. Under these circumstances, the size of Gap 4 can be large.

A question frequently asked by companies is, "How much standardization can we achieve across branches without taking away the autonomy and perceived control of managers?" At issue is the need to assure consistency across outlets (so that expectations set by one outlet do not interfere with perceptions of service at another outlet) while allowing the managers autonomy to serve customers in their own ways. If one Command Performance hair styling salon provides hors d'oeuvres and wine for its customers—a touch that can make customers feel special—will customers expect hors d'oeuvres and wine at every Command Performance location and be disappointed if they do not receive the special service? If one McDonald's offers a contest or sweepstakes, won't customers expect it at every McDonald's?

Lack of consistency across outlets explains a large part of the financial and operational difficulties experienced by Jiffy Lube International, Inc., the Baltimore-based franchisor of quick-lube auto centers. Despite the tremendous demand for this new service, the brilliance of the service idea (a quick, efficient, and inexpensive lube job for which customers do not need an appointment), and herculean efforts to ensure similarity of the physical aspects of the service, service-quality perceptions of the firm are low. To respond to heavy demand and to penetrate the market quickly, the company grew from 400 outlets in 1987 to over 1,000 in 1989. Practices to deliver similar service were encouraged—but not required—by the franchisor and the unfortunate result was noticeably uneven service. In the geographic area of one of the authors, for example, three Jiffy Lube franchises produce very diverse service. One site offers outstanding personal service: the service manager consults with the customers several times during service, shows the customer samples of the fluids to be used, asks about problems, and answers questions directly and politely. At the second outlet, the service manager speaks to customers only on arrival and when they settle their bills. In this outlet, each customer must wait in the shop until service is provided because the.manager does not want cars that have already been serviced in the parking lot. In contrast, customers in the third outlet may leave their cars for at least an hour, allowing them to run errands or attend to other business in the nearby shopping center. This inconsistency of service, even within the same geographic region, has led to poor word of mouth and customer disappointment with Jiffy Lube and resulted in complaints and class-action suits that severely damage the firm's image.[5]

CLOSING GAP 4: PROVIDING CONSISTENT SERVICE ACROSS BRANCHES OR OUTLETS

If customers are to receive consistent service across branches or field units of a firm, a company must develop a mechanism for ensuring uniformity. In some successful companies, such as the Marriott Corporation, that mechanism is a set of standardized procedures fundamental to the business. Every functional area in Marriott hotels operates under standard operating procedure manuals where all processes and services are carefully documented. Housekeepers, for example, must perform 64 required steps in cleaning a room. These specific guidelines result in uniformly clean rooms anywhere in the Marriott chain. Marriott also allows flexibility and individuality in providing service: Employees are trained to follow these procedures *except when better service can be delivered by the employee* doing something above and beyond the standard to satisfy customers. Because Marriott wants to guarantee this consistently high service, the firm does not franchise its hotel operations but syndicates them instead to investor groups with Marriott retaining 70-year management contracts.

Andersen Consulting, a division of Arthur Andersen & Company and the largest consulting firm in the world, uses a corporate philosophy called the one-firm concept and a strong training program to develop consistency across its multiple locations. The one-firm concept means that all the separate offices operate as a whole—every employee works for Andersen Consulting first and their own office second. Among the ways that the one-firm concept is executed is through central training in suburban Chicago. Every professional employee from all over the world is trained in the same way at the same center. Cross-training of personnel, company communications, and the centralized training lead to such similarity of performance that some employees jokingly call themselves "Arthur Androids." Whatever difficulties experienced by employees using this philosophy, Andersen Consulting enjoys the best reputation for consistent service among the big-eight firms.

A firm may also choose other ways to obtain consistency, perhaps by setting standards or goals for service-quality outcomes that are visible to customers, but allowing the outlets to use their own process to achieve these goals.

GAP 4 PROBLEM: PROPENSITY TO OVERPROMISE

Because of increasing deregulation and intensifying competition in the services sector, many service firms feel more pressure than ever before to acquire new business and to meet or beat competition. To accomplish these ends, service firms often overpromise in selling, advertising, and other company communications. The greater the extent to which a service firm feels pressured to generate new customers, and perceives that the industry norm is to overpromise ("everyone else in our industry overpromises"), the greater is the firm's propensity to overpromise.

If advertising shows a smiling young lady at the counter in a McDonald's commercial, customers expect that—at least most of the time—there will be a smiling young lady in the local McDonald's. If advertising claims that a customer's wake-up call will *always* be on time at a Ramada Inn, customers expect no mistakes. Raising expectations to unrealistic levels may lead to more initial business, but invariably fosters customers' disappointment and discourages repeat business.[6] The propensity to overpromise generates external company communications that do not accurately reflect what customers receive in actual service encounters.

CLOSING GAP 4: DEVELOPING APPROPRIATE
AND EFFECTIVE COMMUNICATIONS
ABOUT SERVICE QUALITY

To be appropriate and effective, communications about service quality must (1) deal with the quality dimensions and features that are most important to customers; (2) accurately reflect what customers actually receive in the service encounter; and (3) help customers understand their roles in performing the service.

EMPHASIZE PRIMARY QUALITY DETERMINANTS

Communicating service quality begins with an understanding of the aspects of service quality that are most important to customers. Isolating quality dimensions most important to customers provides a focus for advertising efforts. Emphasizing the most important dimension or dimensions of service quality results in more effective communications than those focusing on other dimensions.

As we discussed in chapter 2, our research with SERVQUAL has provided surprisingly consistent rankings of the dimensions across service industries.[7] In virtually all the empirical work accomplished thus far, *reliability* stands above all others in importance, regardless of the specific service or industry studied. Customers' expectations of service providers are highest for reliability, and customers rank reliability as the most important of the five dimensions.

If reliability is central to service customers, why don't all companies focus on reliability in advertising? Who do many companies focus instead on other service dimensions such as empathy and tangibles? Our discussions with executives on this subject provides an explanation: On learning that bank customers ranked reliability as the pivotal quality dimension, a banking executive commented: "We're reliable, our competitors are reliable—why focus on something that everyone has?" What this executive perceived about bank reliability may be accurate in an objective sense, but our findings strongly indicate that customers' perceptions do not match managers' perceptions of reliability. In an era of bank closings, failed savings and loan institutions, and increasingly complicated computer technology, many customers doubt the reliability of banks. Executives often *misperceive* that customers of banks—and many other services as well—believe that reliability in their services exists. Customers clearly told us otherwise.

We believe it is essential to obtain perceptions of reliability from the customer before choosing dimensions that are less important than reliability for company advertising. SERVQUAL and related questions described in the appendixes provide a means to investigate these perceptions in individual firms and industries.

MANAGING CUSTOMERS' EXPECTATIONS

A major premise of our research has been that consumers' perceptions of service quality can be influenced either by raising consumers' perceptions or by lowering expectations. Managing customers' expectations, especially those created by the company itself through external communications and price, is an essential part of a strategy to attain perceived quality service.

The expectations customers bring to the service affect their evaluations of its quality: the higher the expectation, the higher the delivered service must be to be perceived as high quality. Therefore, *promising reliability in advertising is only appropriate when reliability is actually delivered.* Promising no surprises at a hotel, as Holiday Inns did, is disastrous if many surprises actually happen in the delivery process. As discussed earlier in this chapter, it is absolutely essential for the marketing or sales department to understand the actual levels of service delivery (e.g., percentage of times the service is provided correctly, percentage and number of problems that arise) before making promises about reliability.

Expectations are the standards or reference points against which a firm's performance is judged. We believe that Gap 4 can be closed by managing customers' expectations—letting customers know what is and is not possible and the reasons why. To manage these expectations, companies must first understand the factors that influence expectations.

"Uncontrollable" Sources of Expectations. As we discussed in chapter 2, our research suggests that word-of-mouth communication, customers' experience with the service, and customers' needs are key factors influencing consumers' expectations. These factors are rarely controllable by the firm; however, an in-depth understanding of these sources and their effects on expectations may lead to strategies that improve perceptions of service.

We are currently investigating the sources of expectations that customers have about service to understand more fully the role that experience plays in the formation of expectations. From our previous work, we have reason to believe that experience with a particular service provider, experience with competitive service providers, and experience with providers of other types of services all influence consumers' expectations. While the first two experiences are readily understood, the third is not so clear. We have found some evidence, for example, that customers' experience with telephone service affects expectations of service from all cable-television companies. Cable-television companies frequently provide service that is perceived by customers to be low in quality, largely because they were comparing the service to that of other service organizations—particularly telephone companies—that are considerably more reliable. This cross-service comparison is intriguing and may account for the unrealistic expectations customers bring with them into many new service encounters.

Firms wanting to investigate these issues may be able to examine research that currently exists in the company about customers' expectations. If research on expectations has yet to be conducted, an approach similar to the one we are using in our own expectations research may be useful. In each of the industries sponsoring our study, we are conducting focus-group interviews with current customers of the type of service the firm provides. An equal number of focus-group interviews involve experienced and inexperienced users of the service because we expect that the sources and levels of expectations will vary in important ways in these two groups. Each focus-group interview covers such topics as sources of customers' expectations of the service, the impact of uncontrollable variables such as word-of-mouth communication and competitors' offerings, as well as company-controlled factors such as those we discuss in the following section.

Controllable Sources of Customers' Expectations. Controllable factors such as company advertising, price, personal selling, and the tangibles associated with the service are likely to be critical in determining the expectations that customers hold for a service.

One of the most frequent questions we are asked on this topic is: "How can we lower expectations without losing business to a competitor who is inflating promises?" This question is particularly difficult when the industry as a whole is suffering from a poor image. Airlines were faced with difficult service delivery problems when the industry was deregulated: overcrowded airports, intense price and route competition, and scheduling problems led to poor service and declining customer perceptions. Airlines knew that reliability—getting to the destination on time safely— was the most important dimension of airline service, but also realized that this was never more difficult to deliver than during the intensely confusing and competitive postderegulation era. Developing an advertising campaign that did not overpromise but engendered awareness and positive perceptions toward a firm was a major challenge. American Airlines ran an advertisement with the headline "Why Does It Seem Like Every Airline Flight Is Late?" that identified with customers' frustrations and explained the key uncontrollable industry reasons for the problems. At the same time, the airline described efforts it was taking to improve the situation. American was comfortable with such claims because it had already documented that its on-time service was better than any of its competitors. Because American's reliability was the highest in the industry, the advertisement was believable and did not stimulate unrealistic expectations. Soon after, American was awarded top billing in service performance by a frequent flyer survey in North America. Later advertisements in the campaign made explicit reliability claims about American's service.

Another way to manage expectations is to describe the service delivery process and provide the customer a choice of quicker, lower-quality provision versus slower, higher-quality provision. In advertising or consulting, for example, speed is often essential but interferes with performance. If customers understand this tradeoff, and are asked to make a choice, they may be more satisfied with their choice because service expectations for each option are realistic.

In both these strategies, marketing reflects a full and accurate understanding of the operations function—how long it takes to accomplish a project, how successfully the company delivers, how often mistakes occur. This communication bridge between marketing and operations, as emphasized earlier in this chapter, is essential in managing expectations.

Price as an Indicator of Service Quality. We believe that price sets expectations for the quality of service, particularly when other cues to quality are not available. When customers lack information about the quality of a service (i.e., when service outcomes are difficult to judge in advance of purchase), they often use price as a surrogate for quality.[8] Because customers depend on price as a cue to quality and because price sets expectations of quality, service prices should be determined carefully. In addition to covering costs or matching competitors, prices must be chosen accurately to convey the appropriate quality signals. Pricing too low can lead to inaccurate inferences about the quality of the service. Pricing too high can set expectations that may be difficult to match in service delivery.

THE CUSTOMER'S ROLE IN SERVICE DELIVERY

Sometimes service problems and failures are caused by customers. Business customers of the postal service frequently put wrong or outdated addresses and zip codes on envelopes. Patients neglect to tell their doctors about unhealthy habits that lead to their medical problems. Restaurant customers are rowdy and interfere with the experience of other diners, and airline customers are irritable and let off steam by yelling at flight attendants. When customers do not accept their responsibilities and roles in service transactions, problems can occur. In many of these situations, communications can be used to encourage customers to be better customers.

New York State Electric and Gas Corporation (NYSEG) has developed many novel ways to help customers be better customers. The company created the *Senior Sun*, a large-type newspaper for senior citizens, to help them make wise and cost-efficient energy decisions. Representatives of the company speak regularly to senior groups about electric and gas safety and efficient energy use.[9] NYSEG also established an education advisory panel through which it offers aids and classroom materials for teachers to increase their understanding of energy issues and their ability to communicate these issues to students.[10]

EMPIRICAL FINDINGS ABOUT GAP 4

We investigated the size of Gap 4 and the impact of the two factors described in this chapter in five major U.S. service companies. As described in chapter 4, we measured managers' and contact personnel's perceptions of the extent of Gap 4 and the factors likely to influence it in service companies. The results of this research are shown in exhibit 7–3 by company (numbered 1–5). On the left side of the charts, bar 1 shows the size of the gap as perceived by managers and bar 2 by contact personnel. The solid sections of these bars indicate the current status of the gap in each of the companies. An interesting pattern that emerges in these charts is that contact personnel tended to perceive the current status of Gap 4 in their companies to be higher than managers' perceptions. In all but company 1, where manager and contact personnel scores are equal, contact people scored higher on the current status of the gap. This indicates that contact personnel in four of the companies have a more optimistic view of the size of the gap than do managers. The patterned sections of these bars indicate the opportunity for Gap 4 closure in each of the companies. Consistent with the observation just discussed, managers perceive that their companies have further to go in closing Gap 4 than contact personnel believe they do.

The bars to the right of the chart show the levels of individual factors of horizontal communication and propensity to overpromise in the five companies. The solid portion of the bar shows the current status on each factor and the patterned section shows the opportunity for gap closure. In company 1, the scores on both factors show large opportunities for gap closure, indicating that the company needs horizontal communication

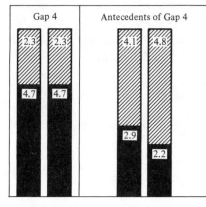

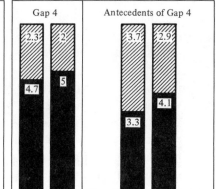

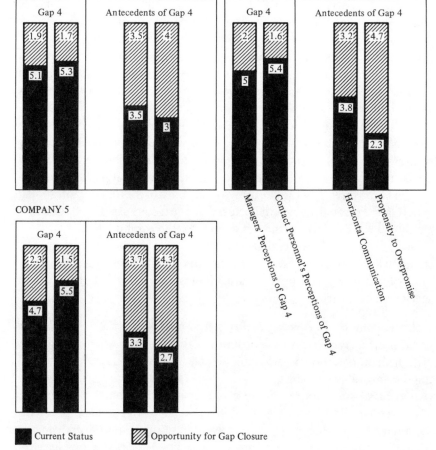

Exhibit 7–3 Gap 4 and Its Antecedents

and that the propensity to overpromise is high. With the exception of company 2, the scores on propensity to overpromise show wide opportunities for gap closure, indicating that overpromising is very high in the industries in which they compete. This pressure to overpromise is likely to inflate customers' expectations and consequently lead to diminished service-quality perceptions. These companies would be well advised to manage customers' expectations in ways suggested in this chapter to close Gap 4.

PUTTING IT ALL TOGETHER:
THE EXTENDED GAPS MODEL

The factors we describe in chapters 4 through 7 are germane to an understanding of service-quality shortfalls (i.e., Gaps 1 through 4) and in taking corrective action to ensure the delivery of high-quality service. Exhibit 7–4 is an extended model of service quality, showing the various organizational factors and their relationships to the service-quality gaps. As described in chapter 3, we tested this model by collecting data on the factors and the gaps in five major U.S. service companies. The empirical findings discussed throughout chapters 4–7 came from that extensive field study.

In this extended model, as in the basic gaps model, the gap between customers' expectations and perceptions of service quality (Gap 5) results from the four gaps on the organization's side of the model. As shown on the far right side of exhibit 7–4, customers have expectations and perceptions of Gap 5 on each of the five dimensions. Each of the four organizational gaps (Gaps 1 through 4) in turn is caused by the factors associated with that gap; these are itemized in the left column of the exhibit.

We developed the extended gaps model as a framework for understanding and researching service quality in organizations. The use of this model for research can help a company answer critical questions about service quality such as the following:

1. *Which of the four service-quality gaps is (are) most critical in explaining service-quality variation?* Is one or more of the four managerial gaps more critical than the others in affecting perceived service quality? Can creating one favorable gap (e.g., making Gap 4 favorable by employing effective external communications to create realistic consumer expectations and to enhance consumers' perceptions) offset service-quality problems stemming from other gaps? To answer these questions, firms can use SERVQUAL to capture customers' perceptions and the measures of

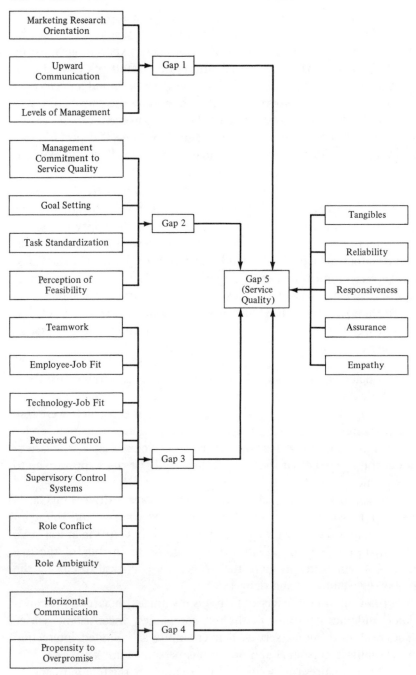

Exhibit 7-4 The Extended Gaps Model of Service Quality

Gaps 1 through 4 (described in chapter 3 and the appendixes) for employees' and managers' perceptions. Intuitively, it would seem that the first three gaps must be closed in order: customers' expectations must be understood before managers can set appropriate standards (Gap 2) and employees must be trained, motivated, compensated, and informed to close Gap 3. A logical progression, then, in closing the gaps is to try to close Gaps 1 through 3 sequentially. Gap 4, however, can be closed before working on the others by managing customers' expectations—bringing expectations in line with actual delivery by lowering expectations rather than improving service delivery.

2. *What are the main organizational factors responsible for the size of each of the four service-quality gaps?* A key managerial question involves the relative importance of the specific factors in delivering high-quality service to customers. If a company can implement only a few of the many organizational factors, which ones should be undertaken? To answer this question, we created measures of the organizational factors (e.g., amount of marketing research orientation, extent of teamwork, etc.) and related them to the measures of the four gaps. The results are shown in exhibit 7–5. The charts in this exhibit show Xs on the factors that were statistically significant in each of the five companies.

One conclusion that emerged from our empirical research is that there are multiple drivers of Gap 2. In the five firms, different combinations of factors emerged as significant. Especially important constructs were task standardization, goal setting, and management's commitment to service quality. This result indicates that companies can close Gap 2 in a variety of ways and suggests that there are no hard and fast rules appropriate to all companies.

As shown in the Gap 3 chart, the most important drivers of Gap 3 included teamwork, employee-job fit, perceived control, and role conflict. These four factors were significantly related to Gap 3 in at least two of the five sample firms. Teamwork is significant in four of the five companies, suggesting strongly that teamwork is critical in closing the gap between standards and delivery.

The most important driver of Gap 4 is insufficient horizontal communication, significant in four of the five companies. Inconsistent service policies among different service delivery units and limited interaction between contact personnel and operations personnel are key.

The questionnaires that we developed to measure the four gaps and 16 factors are in the appendixes along with instructions on methodology for implementing gap research in your company.

Gap 2

Factors	Company 1	Company 2	Company 3	Company 4	Company 5
Management Commitment	X				X
Goal Setting			X	X	
Task Standardization	X	X			
Perception of Feasibility			X		

Gap 3

Factors	Company 1	Company 2	Company 3.	Company 4	Company 5
Teamwork	X	X		X	X
Employee-Job Fit	X		X	X	
Technology-Job Fit		X			
Perceived Control			X		X
Supervisory Control Systems					
Role Conflict		X		X	
Role Ambiguity	X				

Gap 4

Factors	Company 1	Company 2	Company 3	Company 4	Company 5
Horizontal Communication	X	X	X	X	
Propensity to Overpromise				X	

Exhibit 7-5 Key Drivers of the Gaps: Factors that Are Statistically Significant

SUMMARY

Discrepancies between service delivery and external communications have a strong impact on customers' perceptions of service quality. In this chapter, we discussed the factors affecting the size of Gap 4, the gap between promises and delivery. These factors, illustrated in exhibit 7–1, included: (1) inadequate horizontal communication among operations, marketing, and human resources, as well as across branches; and (2) propensity to overpromise in communications. We defined these factors, described the problems they create in organizations, and offered suggestions for dealing with them to close Gap 4. Finally, we presented empirical findings from our research about Gap 4 and introduced the extended gaps model that integrates all of our research on service quality.

8

◇ ◇ ◇

GETTING STARTED ON THE SERVICE-QUALITY JOURNEY

IN A *WALL STREET JOURNAL* ARTICLE, "Service with a Smile? Not by a Mile," Jim Mitchell wrote: "The message of the commercials is 'We want you!' The message of the service is 'We want you unless we have to be creative or courteous or better than barely adequate. In that case, get lost.' " Mitchell's article appeared in 1984. Unfortunately, in the early 1990's, Mitchell's comment is still pertinent.

Clearly, many companies are still struggling to get out of first gear on the service-quality journey. The case for improving service is strong, yet outstanding service quality is more the exception than the rule.

The central question in many organizations is: How do we get started on service improvement? How do we move beyond the sterile hype, the start-stop program mentality, the organizational naysayers and doubters, and the constant pressure for short-term earnings growth? In this chapter we address the question of getting started in service improvement, of actually reshaping an organization's culture and competence. Our focus in the last four chapters has been on the ongoing efforts necessary to close service-quality gaps. In this chapter we shift our attention to *starting* the gap management process, to turning on the engine, backing out of the driveway, pointing the car in the right direction and embarking on the journey. We turn first to an analysis of why getting started is so problematic, and then suggest a series of guidelines for moving forward.

THE SERVICE STRUGGLE

The reason so many organizations are struggling with the challenge of improving service is insufficient leadership. It is a simple but important point. The root cause of deficient service quality is not inadequate structures, systems, or research. The root cause of deficient service is people in organizations with leadership responsibilities who, for whatever reason, do not put these necessaries in place.

Organizations are thwarted in improving service because senior managers, middle managers, and first-line service providers lack the will, knowledge, and/or skills to do their parts to move the organization forward. In service organizations everyone is responsible for quality. Some employees provide internal services in that their customers are inside the organization. Others primarily serve customers outside the organization. Still others serve both internal and external customers.

Each of these employees fits into one of the four "willingness/ability-to-serve" cells at any point in time, as shown in exhibit 8–1. A given employee may be both willing and able to perform excellent service (cell one), willing but unable (cell two), unwilling but able (cell three), or unwilling and unable (cell four). For an organization to "get off the dime" in service and make meaningful strides, it must find ways to move more people into cell one. Occupancy of the other cells at any level—senior or middle management or first-line workers—can foul up the machinery for moving forward. To get started in the gap management process we must think of moving three levels of employees from various states of deficiency to a state of effectiveness, so that they can start to close the gaps that they helped to create.

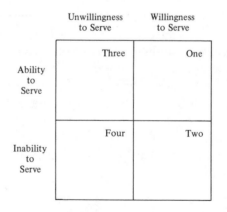

Exhibit 8–1 Willingness/Ability to Serve Matrix

TOP MANAGEMENT

It is unusual to think of senior executives as service providers, except in those instances in which they have contact with external customers. As we stressed in earlier chapters, however, senior management must perform a crucial internal service role, the role of service leadership. Only senior management has the position and clout to build an organization's value system on the pillars of satisfying customers, freedom of action, creative problem solving, and respect for employees—essential components of a service-minded culture.[1] Only senior management can build the cultural foundation for quality service in the organization.

To the extent that top management does not conceive and communicate a strong service vision for the firm, does not insist on high standards of internal and external service, does not deal effectively with the naysayers and political game players, does not give service workers the tools they need to do their jobs well, does not recognize and reward exemplary service performers—to the extent that top management does not do these things, they inadequately serve the rest of the organization. It is a simple but powerful truism: top management must provide a strong internal service to unleash a company's true capacity for service excellence.

So what is the problem? Why aren't more top executives like the service leaders we described in chapter 1? For many, the answer is poor understanding and/or skills germane to service leadership, that is, an ability-to-serve problem. It is our experience that some senior executives do not understand the dynamics of service quality well enough to know what to do. This leads to efforts destined for failure, for example, initiating quick-fix programs such as a one-day "smile" training course, delegating primary responsibility for quality improvement to a staff department, or focusing attention strictly on contact personnel and ignoring the critical relationship between internal and external service providers.

Other top executives may know what to do but still may not be able to do it. They may lack the self-confidence to truly lead other people, they may be poor communicators, unable to express a service vision, or they may not have the sensitivity to really understand what others in the organization are saying and feeling.

And for still other senior executives, the key deficiency is one of will, that is, a willingness-to-serve problem. They lack the obsession, the spirit, the commitment to lead the development of a service culture. Service quality is simply not a priority.

- "Average service is good enough."
- "Financial deals drive profits; service issues are just so much mush."
- "Customers won't pay for service, so go for price."
- "American workers are lazy, the work ethic is dead, and mediocre service is inevitable."

These are just a few of the sentiments we hear from top managers—either literally or when we "listen" with our eyes. Consider the sobering words of marketing researcher Mimi Lieber:

> underneath all of the lists, rules, manuals and consumer insight is a core problem we need to address: that our spirit at the top has to change and our attitude toward front-line service be improved. Service is a spiritual and cultural issue. . . . Few on top have been frontline. American managers are still short-term, bottom-line focused. They got where they are generally without concern for spiritual values. They want competitive volume levels *today*, are often more motivated by how to look to the next job in the next company than what *this* company will be in ten years' time. Devoting energy and heart to internal morale, creating the esprit de corps, listening to each other is still considered a job for "personnel."[2]

The task of significantly improving service in large, complex organizations with hundreds or thousands of employees can appear awesome and overwhelming. In addition, improving service generally involves spending money before making money. Without a strong will at the top of the organization, without what Mimi Lieber calls "heart," the service-quality journey will be problematic at best, fruitless at worst.

MIDDLE MANAGERS

One critical group that is often overlooked or given short shrift in the service-quality journey is middle managers—that eclectic body of department heads, supervisors, and others who often serve external customers but who provide internal service as well. The best way to recognize middle-managers' importance in any quest to improve service is simply to reflect on the fact that everyone in the organization works for middle managers, except top managers.

Middle managers are appropriately labeled in one sense, inappropriately labeled in the other. The term *middle* is certainly appropriate. Middle managers are right smack in the middle—of everything. Top management works through middle managers; first-line service providers work for middle managers. Middle managers represent the linkage between the top and bottom of the organizational structure. They can be a conduit for progress or a black hole into which promising ideas mysteriously disappear, for suffocation and burial.

The term *manager*, on the other hand, is less satisfactory. For an organization to truly pursue service excellence, it needs people in the middle who go beyond managing and lead; it needs people in the middle who reinforce the service vision, build a culture of achievement and teamwork in the immediate work unit, and act as role models that show the way and remove service obstacles from the path of subordinates.

Excellent service is not only a function of inspired leadership at the top of organizations; it is also a function of inspired leadership in the middle of organizations. Without question, the quality of leadership service provided by people in the middle of the organization influences directly the quality of service provided by people lower in the organization.

Where the rub comes in is that middle managers in many firms are often ill equipped to be effective service leaders. They may have been promoted to management positions because of their success in technical or sales roles; their leadership qualities and service philosophy may not have been considered at all. And once in these management positions, they may not be held accountable for their willingness or ability to coach, communicate, or model a service ethic.

In many organizations managing is defined as "getting things done through people"; how managers accomplish this task is of little concern. But as our research summarized in this book so clearly shows, the how of management is crucial to improving service; how superiors relate to subordinates can be the difference between awful service and excellent service.

Just how important are middle managers in the service-quality journey? Here is what one prominent bank marketing executive has to say:

> The weakest link in banks, which is an undermining factor of service quality, is middle management. That's where it falls apart.
> This comes from high turnover at this level, lack of commitment, lack of understanding "the big picture," lack of motivation, and lack of senior management communications. If service quality is ultimately provided by lower levels—tellers, proof operators, transit clerks, loan processors, and the like—then managers of these people are the enforcing link, as well as the promoting link.[3]

And just how tough can it be to transform middle managers from service stranglers to service champions? Here is what Corning Glass Works CEO James Houghton had to say when an interviewer asked him about the resistance he experienced while starting a total quality process at Corning:

> The hardest people to reach are middle managers, and specifically first-line supervisors, because it means a very significant change. Instead of saying, "Do this, do that," first-line supervisors are now being asked to be coaches, to be part of a team, and to listen to their employees on how things could be done better. That takes away some of their management prerogative, which is very hard to deal with. It's very hard for someone who's been doing things the same way for 30 years to be told, "You're still the boss, but you're a different boss."[4]

Middle managers are clearly more central to the twin questions of what causes service-quality problems and what can be done to improve quality than is commonly suggested on the lecture circuit or in the literature. The tendency is for speakers and writers to focus on top managers (who have the clout to lead cultural shifts) and first-line employees (who directly perform services for customers). But, as we have shown, middle managers are in the center of everything and can either put fuel or sand in the gas tank. This is why one of the most critical internal services top management performs in the organization is promoting the right people into middle management, to be in charge of other people.

First-Line Service Providers

When service providers do not provide the quality of service that management asks them to provide—Gap 3 in the service-quality model —it is because they are unwilling and/or unable to do so. Like management personnel, all first-line service providers fit somewhere in the willingness/ability to serve matrix. Unlike management personnel, however, these employees do not by and large perform an internal leadership service; instead, they are the receivers of this service, for better or for worse.

To fully understand how the willingness factor operates in service performances, one needs to recall from chapter 6 the concept of discretionary effort—the difference between the maximum amount of energy and care an individual can bring to his or her work, and the minimum amount required to avoid penalty or termination.[5] Most service jobs are high in discretionary effort content, meaning that it is up to the individual employee whether to give a 100 percent service effort or to give something substantially less.

What happens often in service organizations is that poor teamwork, role conflict, and other organizational failings discussed in chapter 6 diminish discretionary effort. It is not that American service providers are slovenly or lazy. We have found absolutely no evidence in our research of a poor work ethic in America. Rather, what happens is that new, high-energy service employees do not receive the organizational support and inspiration they need to sustain them through the inevitable travail of service work. And without the support of good leaders, good teammates, clear direction, consistent signals, and most everything else we've discussed in this book, many of these service providers lose energy and effectiveness over time even as they increase in competence. They lose the will to serve.

In organizations that benefit from strong service leadership, the difference in discretionary effort between new and experienced employees is likely to be minimal. In organizations that are poorly led, the difference is likely to be striking. Exhibit 8–2 illustrates these patterns.

Constructs discussed in chapter 6 can also have an adverse effect on employees' ability to perform the service. We have found evidence in our research of companies "force-fitting" people into jobs for which they were ill-suited because the firms were unwilling to pay more to attract qualified candidates, because many openings existed and this ruled out other considerations in filling them, or because a good understanding of the required skill set did not exist which meant that almost anyone was

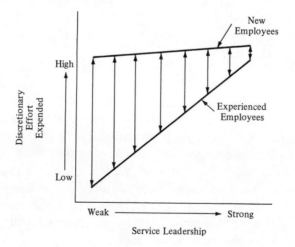

Exhibit 8–2 Difference in Discretionary Effort Expended by New and Experienced Employees

qualified. Hiring the wrong people for service jobs manifests itself in poor employee-job fit.

Moreover, service providers may not be able to properly serve their customers simply because they lack full control over the service's delivery, depending instead on other organizational units to come through for them and their customers. Perceived control is a key construct in closing Gap 3, as we have discussed.

First-line service providers—telephone installers, television repair technicians, beauticians, truck drivers, medical laboratory analysts, loan processors, accounting personnel, tax preparers, dental hygienists, secretaries, and many, many others—are often considered the root cause of America's service malaise. We disagree.

Yes, many service workers are unwilling and/or unable to meet the service expectations of their customers. But this need not be the case. If people in service roles lack the direction or the training or the support tools or the control over the service to be successful, whose fault is it? If they are hired into service roles for which they lack the basic intelligence, whose fault is it? If they are given no sense of how their role fits into the overall scheme of things, of what their customers expect, or why their work is important, whose fault is it?

The success or failure of first-line service providers is influenced greatly by the quality of service leadership they receive. When managers lead, service excellence is within reach. When managers do not, excellent service is a pipe dream. This is why we make such a fuss about leadership in this book. And this is why in the next section we focus on what management needs to do.

GUIDELINES FOR GETTING STARTED

Changing the mind-sets, habits, skills, and knowledge of human beings—which is what most organizations must do to materially improve service—is no small challenge. It involves undoing what exists—clearing out impediments to change—not only creating what does not exist. No magic formulas, simple solutions, or quick-fixes exist to get started and make headway. Overnight service-quality miracles are more a figment of lecture-circuit rhetoric than organizational reality. The truth is that it usually takes longer to materially improve service than the sponsors of this change anticipate, and then it takes longer still for the customers to notice. Quality service is a "fix" but it is almost always a "slow fix."

So in this part of the chapter we lay no claims to breakthrough thinking that will quickly raise an organization's SERVQUAL scores. Instead, we discuss some practical necessities for giving an organization a decent chance to move forward on quality. What follows are guidelines to build a *foundation for change*.

GET READY TO WORK HARD

Redirecting an organization's paths of habit and convenience is very hard work. If senior managers are to assume the mantle of service leadership, they best be prepared to work at it. Senior managers cannot delegate responsibility for service-quality improvement; they themselves must lead the charge or nothing will happen.

As Corning CEO Houghton puts it: "You almost have to have a messianic view of this. You must be willing to travel, to go and see people and talk. You can't communicate or show your commitment on a videotape or in written form all the time. You have got to believe."[6]

Consider the case of a CEO with whom we work. He runs an automobile services company, the biggest in its field, and the largest subsidiary of its parent firm. The CEO has been on the job about a year and is anxious to improve service quality to better differentiate his firm from competitors, and to command premium prices in an increasingly cut-throat pricing environment. He thinks improved service is absolutely essential and yet he faces a very complex service process (with many functions touching the service before it gets to the customer), employee morale problems traceable in part to a poorly handled reduction in force several years prior, and tremendous needs for upgraded technology. All the while, he confronts hungry, price-cutting competitors on the one hand, and a corporate parent with high profit expectations on the other hand.

Our CEO friend is very determined on the service-quality issue, having moved aggressively to open lines of communication with employees, commission research, and fund a series of specific quality-improvement projects. Progress is slow and the pressures just outlined are ever present. Does our CEO friend have a hard road to travel? You bet he does! And this is why the willingness-to-lead factor discussed earlier is so critical. Without this CEO's personal resolve, the entire service-improvement effort in his company would have crashed by now.

One of the leading academics in the service-quality field, Professor Ben Schneider of the University of Maryland, makes the hard work point well:

Service is not as mushy and touchy-feely as it has been made out to be; the delivery of consistently excellent service . . . requires the kind of hard work any business requires—hard work in mapping out responsibilities, hard work in mapping out people needs for training and superior leadership and management, hard work in designing the kinds of equipment and software service deliverers require, and hard work in identifying, continuously, customer requirements and wants. The biggest challenge is a change in mindset from easy countables . . . to measuring what is important.[7]

The superb service companies we have studied over the years all have two things in common: a good service idea and a willingness to work incredibly hard to make the idea work. Highly successful service companies do something that is important to customers, and they do it better than their competitors. As consultant G. Lynn Shostack likes to say, delivering truly superb service, day after day after day, is a bitch.

It is claimed that the average life span of a piece of trash on the grounds of Disney World is four seconds. We do not know if this statistic is absolutely true. So we shall be conservative and say that the figure is less than 30 seconds. The point is, what this company has done over the years in transforming customers into "guests in a fantasyland" is the result of obsessive dedication and commitment to the founder's dream. It was not magic that built the Magic Kingdom, it was the grind of hard work.

BASE DECISIONS ON DATA

We can offer no better advice on getting started in service improvement than to start with data. The potential effectiveness of a service-quality journey critically hinges on accurately answering the questions posed in the process model for quality improvement we presented in exhibit 3–7. So much depends on decision makers knowing what customers expect from the service, what customers perceive the service to be, and what is getting in the way of the organization meeting customers' expectations.

Without empirically based answers to these questions, the likelihood of wrong decisions and wasted resources is very great. Individual biases, assumptions, and games playing are likely to rule service-improvement planning in the absence of data. In matters of service quality, there is no substitute for knowing what is going on.

As suggested earlier, one of the biggest psychological hurdles for executives to clear in starting a service-improvement effort is the sheer magnitude of the challenge. So many customers to serve. So many transactions every day. So many employees to reach. So many different services to perform. So many "fail points" for each of the services. So many bad past decisions to overcome. So many contrary pressures to reconcile.

The best way to cope with the overwhelming part of getting started is to be selective in what is done rather than try to do everything all at once. And this requires information—information concerning (1) what target markets desire most from the service; (2) how well the firm serves these wants compared to competitors; and (3) the causes of service weaknesses that need to be corrected. This type of information gives executives a basis for prioritizing and sequencing service-improvement actions. And in doing so, the information contributes to executives' willingness and ability to provide service leadership.

Within the framework of service-quality research as we have discussed it in this book, there is another consideration in setting priorities for service interventions. This is the identification of what Berry, Bennett, and Brown call lighthouses for change—specific service initiatives that are most likely to have a positive, timely, and visible impact in focusing organizational attention on the potential for quality.[8] Some early successes in the service-improvement process, when the credibility of the effort is most at risk, can pay rich dividends in getting the attention of reluctant senior and middle managers. In general, funding decisions should favor the projects and people most likely to succeed—which requires sensitive antennae that come from information gathering.

Here are four guidelines to keep in mind in implementing a data-before-decision approach to improving service quality:

1. *Use a portfolio of research methods.* Every service research methodology has weaknesses and limitations; it is wise to use multiple methods to transcend the weaknesses of any one approach and to provide richer, more comprehensive insight. We recommend using both qualitative research (e.g., customer focus groups and managers regularly phoning customers for feedback) and more quantitative methods (e.g., expectation/perception research, "mystery" shopping of service providers, and surveying customers soon after they have received service).

2. *Do ongoing research.* Data start to get old as soon as they are collected. Any study of service gives a "snapshot" for a particular time period. It is only when these snapshots are taken regularly, when they can be lined up side-by-side, that they tell a story of patterns and trends. SERVQUAL and the other research approaches discussed in this book should be administered on a regular basis so that data patterns can be evaluated and emerging concerns spotted quickly. The right way to start a service-improvement initiative is to install an ongoing service research process, not just do a single study.

3. *Do employee research.* Often overlooked in service research is the importance of employee research. This is a serious oversight as employee research is just as critical as customer research because employees are customers, too. Who other than employees can assess the quality of internal services? Moreover, no one has a better vantage point for identifying obstacles to service than the very employees performing the service on a daily basis.

In our own research with employees, we have used with great success two key questions as part of a broader group of questions:

- What is the biggest problem you face day in and day out trying to deliver a high quality of service to your customers?
- If you were president of this company for one day, and could make only one decision to improve quality of service, what decision would you make?

We can suggest no questions that are more important to ask employees when starting a service-improvement effort than these two. These questions cut through the surface issues, exposing some of the most serious service impediments in the organization.

4. *Share research with employees.* Service research is not only valuable in guiding managerial decision making, it is also valuable in guiding first-line employee decision making. Our data show that managers had a better grasp of customers' service expectations and priorities than did first-line customer-contact employees. We do not know for sure why we found this, but one plausible explanation is that the companies we studied do considerable service-quality research which is shared with managers but not first-line employees. Because service employees are more likely to meet customers' service expectations if they first understand these expectations, we urge that service research be shared with employees. This could entail using videotaped customer focus-group sessions in employee training, issuing to employees periodic research summaries written in lay language, and even involving employees in data collection—for example, interviewing customers on the telephone.

We advise treating first-line service providers as though they were management when it comes to sharing service-quality research. It is better to be generous with information than stingy. Otherwise, employees may not know what they are supposed to do, or why they need to do it.

ORGANIZE FOR CHANGE

A readiness to work hard at quality improvement and data to guide the work are two critical pieces of the getting started puzzle. A structure that can harness energy and facilitate change is a critical third piece. Knowing what to do and being ready to do it are insufficient in and of themselves; organizing systems for replacing inertia with action must also be created. If well conceived, these organizing systems enhance both the willingness and the ability of managerial and first-line service employees to improve service.

Successful efforts in organizing for service improvement at companies such as American Express, Metropolitan Life, and National Westminster Bank USA, suggest the following principles:

1. *Create service improvement roles.* Casual, "let's-get-together-when-we-can-talk-about-service-quality" initiatives fail. Most people in organizations are already busy and preoccupied with their main responsibilities. And if this wasn't true a few years ago, it is true now given the belt-tightening, layoffs, and restructurings that many U.S. companies underwent in the late 1980's.

For service improvement to have a chance, it has to become part of people's main responsibilities and this means creating formal and informal organizational roles for people to perform. Formal roles might include membership in one type or another service-improvement group. A good example of formalizing service-improvement roles comes from Metropolitan Life's quality improvement process. In this process, Met Life's management asked each organizational unit to identify the principal services it delivered and the customers for these services. Once a unit's major services were identified, a quality-improvement team was established for each service with the mandate of assessing and improving it. Each team was headed by a member of middle management and made up of representatives from every organizational unit involved in creating the final service. Ultimately all the people in the company were formally involved in a quality-improvement team.[9]

Informal roles could involve being a service defender or service champion. *Service defenders*, typically respected senior line executives, protect the culture-change process from the naysayers, resistors, and budget cutters; the defenders give credibility, substance, and clout to the service-improvement effort. They make it clear that excellent service is "the way it's going to be." *Service champions* are those who actually plan, steer, coordinate, and nurse the change process; they are the heads of service-improvement units (from task forces or committees to actual departments) who provide the inspiration, energy, and cohesion required to transform talk into action. The service defender and service champion roles are both essential prerequisities to substantive cultural change. Sometimes the defender and champion roles are performed by the same person; more often, they are performed by different people.[10]

2. *Create an integrative mechanism.* One constant in virtually all successful service-improvement case studies we have examined is a high-level, interdepartmental steering group to energize, manage, and coordinate the service-improvement effort. Comprised mostly of line executives who retain their respective positions in the organization, these groups provide an ongoing mechanism for generating, evaluating, and recommending service-improvement ideas organizationwide, and for bringing cohesion to the service-improvement process. The interdepartmental makeup of these groups provides the opportunity for systemic solutions to service problems; their high-level members provide collective power to get things done (for example, getting proposals funded); their continuing presence provides an organizational rudder around which additional service-improvement entities can emerge.

It is crucial to drive service-improvement efforts from the line, not just the staff, for reasons of organizational credibility, clout, and ownership. Although a staff service-quality department may work in tandem with a service-quality steering group in implementing research, training, communications, and other initiatives, the staff function cannot replace the steering group. After all, if the staff "owns" the service-improvement process, why should line executives (or anyone else) be interested?

3. *Develop a statement of direction.* One of the principal functions of the service-quality steering group is to develop a strategic sense of what needs to be done in the company to improve service. This involves a realistic assessment of the present and a definition of what is needed in the future.

One large U.S. bank with which we are familiar has committed this appraisal to one sheet of paper, an adaptation of which is shown in exhibit 8–3. This document is helpful in capturing the direction the bank needs to take, and offering criteria by which service-improvement proposals can be evaluated.

To get started in service improvement, we recommend preparing a succinct, written statement of direction that can be a continuing guidepost for the service-related decisions that follow. The document need not be in the form or cover the particular categories of the exhibit. However, the document should be strategic rather than tactical, long term in focus rather than short term, and grounded in empirical assessment rather than based on a few people's assumptions or opinions. A good starting point for drafting a statement of direction is a research-based assessment of the various service-quality gaps present in the organization and the key causes underlying these gaps.

Exhibit 8–3 Sample Service-Quality Statement of Direction

Strategy	Achieve competitive advantage through superior customer service.	
	Now	**Needed**
Structure	Hierarchical/bureaucratic	Flat/decentralized
	Independent	Collaborative
	Market oriented	Market oriented
Style	Competition	Teamwork and
	Upward delegation	collaboration
	Variable, Random	Downward delegation
		Consistent, Reliable
Shared Values	One-way	Two-way
	communication	communication
	Confusion re: tradeoffs	Stakeholder balance
	"Life's too short"	Superior/excellent
	Risk-aversion	service
		Innovation/creativity
Staff	Weak, unseasoned	Strong managers and
	managers	leaders
	Survivor ethic	Professional ethic
Skills	Credit evaluation	Financial markets
	Product specialist	expertise
	Financial management	Relationship managers
		Sales/marketing
		management
Systems	Profit center emphasis	Customer
	Incongruent with	information/profits
	strategy	Congruent with
	Reinforce competition	strategy
	and lack of trust	Reinforce teamwork
	Control oriented	and trust
		Support oriented

4. *Involve many and emphasize teamwork.* The right way to approach the service-improvement challenge is to get as many people involved as possible and to get them involved in *teams.* Our research clearly shows the importance of teamwork in improving service, as we pointed out in chapter 6. For one thing, involvement in a team is renewing, stimulating, invigorating. The concept of a team raises the ante for individual performance. To let down the boss is bad, but to let down the team is often

worse. The aggressive use of service-improvement teams unleashes one of the most potent of all motivators—the recognition and respect of peers when one does well, and their disdain when one does poorly.

The concept of service teams is important in another respect and this is that people in organizations depend on one another to deliver an excellent service. The service process normally involves a chain of related services and servers; service quality is rarely the sole result of isolated, individual action. Feinberg and Levenstein make the point well:

> The weak links in an organization are usually at the point where departments are supposed to meet. It's at these joints that institutional arthritis attacks. When departments are separated like national frontiers, fully equipped with barbed-wire fences, bristling watchtowers, and buried mine fields, serious losses occur.[11]

In getting started on service improvement, organizations need to emphasize the development of *vertical teams* (people performing different services that contribute to the overall service) and *project or solution teams* (people who come together to solve specific problems) in addition to *horizontal teams* (people performing the same type of services).

Building a sense of service teamwork into a culture involves many of the concepts already touched on in this book. Teams have to be able to meet and exchange information on a regular basis, they need to celebrate their victories and learn from their defeats, they need recognition and reinforcement, and they need leadership from within and from above. Teamwork is a high-octane fuel for the service-quality journey; there is no better energy source than the team.

5. *Think evolution rather than revolution.* Organizational theorist Karl Weick observes that because we tend to define social problems in such grand terms (for example, the drug problem or the national debt) we paralyze our ability to act. The problem appears to be so big that we either freeze up at the enormity of the issue or we become apathetic.[12] Weick's observation is germane in the present context. As mentioned earlier in the chapter, the complexity and enormity of the service-quality challenge often inhibits management's willingness to act.

An antidote to this problem is to take the approach of steady improvement rather than breakthrough change. Improving service becomes a more inviting challenge, a more practical endeavor when one breaks big problems into little problems and seeks continuous improvement.

Developing a service-minded culture must be an evolutionary process. Revolution breeds fear and skepticism; evolution signals determination and commitment. A steady, unwavering, systematic, multifaceted approach to service improvement in which people can get their hands around definable issues and produce results is the best way to move from paralysis to action.

For the last several years, National Westminster Bank USA has had more than 100 quality-action teams, comprised of employees at all levels of the organization, working to improve quality for specific services and functions in the company. As a result, Nat West USA has reduced missorts in the mail room, reduced the error rate on applications of all types generated from the bank's 130 plus branches, improved the time-liness of operations for such services as letters of credit, reduced ATM downtime, eliminated unnecessary paperwork, improved response time to inquiries, improved fee capture, and reduced float losses.[13] Nat West executives Howard Deutsch and Neil Metviner write:

> People are getting involved, improving their own functions, cutting out the "hassles" that get in their way and looking at bettering each aspect of their jobs. Managers are finding more time to manage, motivate and develop the talents of their staffs by reducing the time spent on rework and "fire fighting." . . . People are seeing that they can make a difference, that their suggestions can become reality and that they will be rewarded and recognized for these achievements.[14]

LEVERAGE THE FREEDOM FACTOR

One of the most potent ways to get started on the service-quality journey is to "thin the rule book." Many service organizations operate with thick policy and procedure manuals that have the effect of strangling service initiative and judgment. These thick manuals benefit neither customer nor service provider, producing a regimented service when a flexible one is needed, a by-the-book service when a by-the-customer one is required.

Too many policies and procedures take the fun out of serving. For one thing, delivering inflexible service when the situation calls for flexible service angers customers and interacting with angry customers is no fun for employees. Also problematic is the frustration many employees feel when they know certain operating procedures keep them from doing good jobs in serving their customers. Which of you reading this book would relish not being able to do what you know is right for the customer and the business because to do it might result in a reprimand, penalty, or even the loss of your job?

Many service firms are unwittingly tying their employees up in knots, saying to them with the thick rule books that they are supposed to be robot servers rather than thinking servers. And in the process, these firms are reducing employees' perceived control and sapping their willingness and ability to serve customers effectively. Why on earth would a company's management choose to operate in such a dysfunctional way? Often, it is for the worst of reasons:

- because many managers do not trust employees' judgment, they make all kinds of rules that in effect represent management's judgment; and
- because thinking employees appear to threaten management prerogatives, control, and power.

To jump-start quality improvement, managers have to give back to service providers the freedom to serve that they have unnecessarily and unproductively taken away from them. Managers have to select their people well, provide them with a strong foundational culture in which to work, offer them strategic direction, and equip them with the company-specific skills and knowledge they need to perform their roles. And then the managers need to get out of the way, so the people can get the job done. Managers cannot make the transition to leadership as long as employees are so bundled in red tape that they cannot follow the lead.

We do recognize that some rules are necessary in organizational life and that certain policies need to be consistent across organizational units. Indeed, inconsistencies across service-delivery units in the same organization can create Gap 4 problems, as noted in chapter 7. We do believe service providers need boundaries and they certainly need direction. What we are advocating to help get the service improvement process started is empowerment, a concept we discussed at length in chapter 6 as it is crucial in ongoing gap management. It is also crucial for getting started.

Empowerment simply means removing the barriers that prevent workers from exercising judgment and creativity in performing their work.[15] We agree with Robert Waterman when he writes: "When managers guide instead of control, the sky's the limit on what people can accomplish."[16]

We recommend that organizations appoint one or more task forces to systematically review existing policies and procedures for the express purpose of revising or eliminating those that unnecessarily restrict service providers' freedom of action.

We recommend also that companies tackle head-on the issue of empowerment in the education and training of senior and middle managers. Managers need to learn about the dangers of overmanagement; they need to learn to ask their subordinates for ideas, widen the solution boundaries for their people, and walk away from decisions for which they are not needed.[17] Managers need to learn the freedom lesson of A. S. Neill who advises: "Think of your role as that of a release valve, not that of a restraining force. We need more green flags and less yellow; more rivers and less dams."[18]

SYMBOLIZE SERVICE QUALITY

Still another key to getting started on the service journey is the use of symbols—sayings, objects, behaviors, stories—that convey management's commitment to quality. Although symbols alone will not change a company's culture, they can reinforce shifts in organizational structure, operating policies, and performance measurement and reward systems, collectively signaling to employees that what is occurring is real.

Indeed, much of what we have covered already in this book (from the types of on-the-job behaviors that are measured to the tone and thickness of the rule book) are themselves highly symbolic, communicating to employees what is really important in the organization. Our intent in this section is to go beyond the symbolic importance of management actions that have been taken for other reasons and to discuss the importance of symbolization for its own sake.

Symbols in organizations communicate volumes to employees, including those symbols that are unintended by management and damaging. It is better to manage symbolization than not, better to think about and plan the organization's symbolic message system than leave it to chance and hope for the best.

The symbolization of quality can come in many forms, from polishing the lobby floor in The Friendly Bank daily to picking up the trash at Disney World instantly, from putting the store manager's office near the checkout area so that managers are close to the action, as is done at Randall's Food and Drugs, to featuring the most outstanding service employees in the company's annual report, as is done at Norwest Bank.

Examples of the proactive use of symbols to reinforce service-mindedness abound. Alliance Fund Services begins staff meetings with "story telling" in which participants discuss recent examples of excellent service from their respective units. National Westminster Bank USA has created a cartoon character named DIRF (an acronym for Do It Right First) who appears on employee posters, key rings, memo pads, and a variety of other internal media. A fable titled "The Legend of DIRF" was sent to the bank staff.[19]

We have found no company, however, that has been more proactive in service symbolization than Sewell Village Cadillac, a Dallas company that consistently ranks among the top U.S. Cadillac dealerships in customer satisfaction ratings and sales volume. Sewell Village displays a "leader board" that lists the top service technicians as judged by customer feedback, posts in the lunchroom service-quality scores for each technician, and awards technicians gold medallions for display at their work stations and badges for their uniform sleeves in recognition of error-free service. The floors in the repair and maintenance areas of the facilities are spotless, as clean and polished as in a well-run bank or department store. In most automobile dealerships, the sales manager makes far more money than the service manager, but at Sewell Village the service manager earns on the same level as the sales manager. In most automobile dealerships, the employees who park and retrieve cars brought in for servicing are called "lot lizards." At Sewell Village they are called customer-service representatives.

Using symbols to foster and reinforce a service ethic can encourage strong discretionary effort by adding meaning to people's work. From bank tellers to automobile mechanics, the prospect of being defeated by the rigors and grind of the service role with an accompanying loss of discretionary effort is ever present. Effective service symbols present an honest reflection of management's service commitment, appear in multiple internal media, and are ongoing, imaginative and fun. These service symbols can help recharge employees' batteries, challenge them to greater efforts, and serve as a constant reminder of the service priority.

PROMOTE THE RIGHT PEOPLE TO MANAGEMENT POSITIONS

Getting started on the service-quality journey—and then keeping going—is, in the final analysis, a result of leadership. Leadership is the only engine that can transform organizations from service mediocrity to service excellence—a point that we have not been shy about making. It follows that one of the surest ways to nurture service improvement in an organization is to identify those individuals with the strongest service leadership potential for promotion opportunities.

Earlier in the chapter we discussed the common tendency in organizations to overlook service leadership potential when promoting people into middle-management positions. This leads to the wrong people being put in charge right in the heart of the organization.

Distinguishing leaders from managers requires conscious effort. On the surface, they may look quite alike. Here are two tests to apply in identifying leaders:

1. *The footprints-in-the-sand test.* With people, the best predictor of the future is the past. The key is to study a person's past qualitatively, not just quantitatively, and to examine methods not just outcomes. Some of the key questions to ask and answer are:
   - What are the person's greatest career accomplishments—and why?
   - When in positions of authority, what innovations or new directions did this person sponsor?
   - What is this person's philosophy of service? What evidence exists that this individual can be a service champion or service defender? What evidence exists that this person is obsessive about service?
   - Do signs exist that this person inspires others and builds followership? Do others believe in this individual? Do they believe in his or her integrity?
   - Is there evidence of informal leadership in this person's background, that is, the ability to influence a group without the benefit of an official position or title?

2. *The stand-for-something test.* True leaders are determined pursuers of their vision for the future. They are clear about the direction they wish to go and why. They do not straddle the fence, are not wishy-washy, do not play it safe. As Peter Drucker has written, the leader's first task is to be the trumpet with a clear sound.[20] Thus, a crucial leadership test is the extent to which an individual's beliefs and priorities are on the table, visible for all to see.

When individuals with service leadership values and capability advance in the organization, three good things occur. First, these people have more of a chance to help the firm improve service by virtue of their greater responsibilities. Second, they get the chance to develop their leadership capabilities further. Third, as they progress in the organization, others see for themselves that service leadership is winning behavior.

One of the most important ways that top management can exercise service leadership is to replace incomplete, incorrect, or superficial criteria with leadership-based criteria and a willingness to do some digging when promoting people into middle-management positions. Otherwise, middle managers may be the black hole we wrote about earlier, thwarting the *initiatives* of senior management and the *initiative* of first-line employees.

SUMMARY

It is far easier to talk about improving service than to actually improve it. To improve service, three levels of employees—top managers, middle managers and first-line service providers—have to be willing and able to improve the services they provide.

Many firms are struggling to get started in service improvement because they lack a foundation for service-oriented cultural change and the old culture refuses to die. To build this foundation for change, top management must provide a strong internal leadership service. If top management is willing and able to do this, then the other pieces of the getting started puzzle start to fall into place; if top management is unwilling and/or unable to lead the charge, then it is unlikely that attitudes and behavior at the middle-management and first-line levels will change materially.

Chapters 4 through 7 suggest a critical role for top management in the ongoing process of service gap management; in this chapter we make the case for top management's active involvement in getting started in service improvement. Exhibit 8–4 summarizes the key steps.

These prescriptions apply to middle managers, too, and they certainly affect first-line service providers; but, in all cases, they require the support and involvement of senior management. It is up to management to get things started.

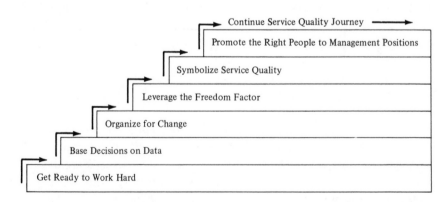

Exhibit 8–4 Steps Necessary for Getting Service-Quality Improvement off the Ground

9

◇ ◇ ◇

SERVICE-QUALITY CHALLENGES FOR THE 1990'S

W E HAVE WRITTEN this book to share the purposes, nature, and findings of our ongoing service-quality research sponsored by the Marketing Science Institute. In this volume we have discussed the critical importance of quality service, defined its salient dimensions, introduced the SERVQUAL methodology for measuring service quality, and used our gaps model to frame a discussion on service-quality problems and solutions. We have also presented our ideas about how firms can get started on the service-quality journey.

In this, our final chapter, we look ahead to the new decade and pose four challenges that are particularly important to closing service-quality gaps:

- designing quality into the service;
- making technology a servant;
- attacking the labor shortfall;
- raising our service aspirations.

DESIGNING QUALITY INTO THE SERVICE

One of the key service-quality challenges for the 1990's is service design. Service design is a form of architecture that involves processes rather than bricks and mortar.[1] The idea is to design high quality into the service system from the outset, to consider and respond to customers' expectations in designing each element of the service.

157

The quality of virtually any service depends on how well myriad elements function together in the same service process to meet customers' expectations. These elements include people who perform various services that relate to the overall service, equipment that supports these performances, and the physical environment in which the services are performed.

Design flaws in any part of a service system can and do play havoc with service quality. As college professors we can relate many stories of how elements in our educational service system have detracted from the quality of our teaching service. These include swivel classroom seats that squeak whenever students shift position (which is often) and classroom lighting systems designed to be turned totally on or off (with no dimming option for using visuals). Shostack writes:

> Every detail in the overall design is important and can affect the service encounter. I have seen corporate reputations undone by envelopes containing confidential customer data that popped open in transit due to inferior glue. I have seen computer programs changed to improve operations efficiency, with the result that statements became impossible for customers to understand.[2]

Designing quality into service requires melding the precision of the engineer, the holistic view of the architect, and the customer-mindedness of the marketer. We need to be more rigorous, more detail-oriented and more comprehensive in the design of services. Indeed, to truly design quality into a service, one needs not only to understand the customer, but one needs also to understand the service!

SERVICE BLUEPRINTING

The most promising tool for service design is "service blueprinting." Although Shostack wrote about service blueprinting as early as 1984, few organizations actually used this tool during the 1980's.[3] The real opportunity for blueprinting lies ahead.

A service blueprint is a visual definition of a service process. It displays each subprocess (or step) in the service system, linking the various steps in the sequence in which they appear. A service blueprint is essentially a detailed map or flow chart of the service process.

Two concepts used in service blueprints are especially helpful in improving quality; they are "lines of visibility" and "fail points." The line of visibility in a service blueprint separates those processes visible to the customer from those that are behind the scenes. What is important about this concept is the need to understand the interconnection between "below-the-line" and "above-the-line" service processes and to recognize that the latter processes that customers experience directly are dependent in part on the former processes that customers do not experience. Attention must be paid to designing quality into the service below the line of visibility even though customers are frequently unaware of these processes.[4] Shostack's example of a company purchasing inferior glue resulting in confidential correspondence coming open in transit illustrates the below-the-line, above-the-line connection.

Fail points are the processes in the service system where deficiencies are most likely to occur. Identifying fail points in a service blueprint focuses attention on the need for special training, additional inspection, building in corrective subprocesses, or even redesign of the original process. Reducing the vulnerability in a service system is one of the most important objectives of service design.

HARD BUT WORTHWHILE WORK

Service blueprinting is slow, laborious, painstaking work. And yet the benefits are well worth the effort. The very act of creating a service blueprint provides rich insight into the service and ways to improve it. By breaking down the service process into its key elements, blueprinting also facilitates the setting of appropriate service standards for the performance of each element.

What is ideal is to blueprint new service concepts as they are being developed. The best way to design quality into a service is to do it as the service is first taking shape.

Consider, for example, the mundane subject of hotel room bathrooms. The best time to think of all the design details that make the bathroom truly workable for hotel guests is before the hotel is built. This is the optimum time to design a clothing hook for the bathroom door, a hand towel rack close to the sink, a bath towel rack close to the shower, shower curtains that are wide and long enough to keep the floor from getting soaked, and a countertop near the sink that is big enough to accommodate a toiletry kit and hair dryer. To think of these details after the hotel opens means frustrating many guests and possibly having to invest in expensive retrofits.

Although blueprinting is most ideal for designing brand new services, it is also a valuable tool for redesigning quality into existing services. As long as the service is still being offered, it is not too late to map out the service, understand it better, and correct design flaws.

Consider, for example, traditional compensation systems that pay life insurance agents generous rewards for generating new business and skimpy rewards for servicing existing business. These systems, we believe, are seriously flawed, manufacturing for life insurance agents the sales-versus-service role conflict discussed in chapter 6. The agent that conscientiously serves existing clients with information updates, annual policy review sessions, and attention to special requests (such as beneficiary changes) may not make nearly the income of agents who spend the vast majority of their time seeking new clients. Of course, in the long run service-minded agents benefit from favorable word-of-mouth advertising if—and it is a big if—they can survive during the early years.

Life insurance companies need to redesign agent performance measurement and reward systems to encourage excellent service to existing clients, a step that some companies such as Metropolitan Life and Jefferson-Pilot Life Insurance Company are already taking. Changing such a culturally entrenched system is not easy, but to not change it commits the industry to a future of client dissatisfaction, unnecessarily high rates of dropped policies, credibility/image problems, and high agent turnover rates.

One of the challenges for the 1990's, then, is to consider service quality to be a design issue. With rigorous, detailed attention to customers' expectations for each step in a service process, it is possible to design quality into the service. It is possible to eliminate or compensate for service fail points, and more intelligently link up subprocesses by combining solid understanding of customers and service in the same design exercise. The most customer-minded executives need to come off the sidelines and become directly involved in the technical design of services. And in so doing, they need to adapt some of the methods of engineers and architects. In service quality, a picture can be worth a thousand words.

MAKING TECHNOLOGY A SERVANT

Another challenge for the 1990's is to more fully realize technology's potential as a powerful service ally. It is often tempting, and sometimes chic, to view technology as a service evil. Heartless computers spew out form letters, foul up billing statements, and even answer the telephone. And the so-called personal touch seems to get lost in the shuffle.

In truth, technology, wisely conceived and used, is a liberating force that makes possible better service. The right technology used in the right way is integral to delivering the dimensions of service that customers expect: tangibles, reliability, responsiveness, assurance, and empathy. Merrill Lynch's Cash Management Account with its automated funds-shifting capability and its integrated, all-on-one-page statement—one of the most successful financial service innovations ever—is a product of technology. So are the bar-code scanners that speed up checkout lines and reduce out-of-stock conditions in retail stores, the automatic teller machines that make it easier for users to access their deposit accounts, and the computerized reservation systems that allow travel agents to make an airline reservation, reserve a specific seat, order a special meal, make hotel and car rental reservations, and print tickets and confirmations *in a matter of minutes!*

Although great strides in the use of technology have been made during the 1980's, the primary impetus for much of this change were the objectives of lowering costs and increasing productivity. Improved service was a spin-off benefit in some cases and a casualty in other cases. A key for the 1990's is to view technology as *a primary means for improving service.* The possibilities for the 1990's are considerable if service improvement can become a true driving force for technological innovation. We believe technology is one of the principal means for upgrading service in the new decade and it is in this spirit that we offer the following guidelines:

1. *Combine high tech with high touch.* For most service firms, the best opportunities for improving service come from combining technology and personal service, rather than stressing one over the other. Technology-based processes can reduce to seconds service functions that would require hours or days if performed manually. Technology can also offer greater accuracy and precision than even the most conscientious and talented of human beings.

Technology alone, however, is not nearly the service weapon of technology and personal service combined. Whereas a bank can improve service delivery with a network of well-located automatic teller machines, it could improve service even more by coupling the ATM network with personal bankers in various branch locations who serve assigned customers for their nonroutine banking needs. Thus, bank customers can use automatic or human tellers for their routine banking needs and a personal banker for their nonroutine needs, such as loans and investments. The service system offers customers both high-tech and high-touch service capabilities which customers will use depending on their overall preferences and their needs of the moment; for example, for cash or for financial advice. The synergy between technology and personal service provides a multiplicative impact.

Valley National Bank of Arizona's 1989 introduction of a 15-minute loan illustrates the power of tech and touch. Valley Bank's capability to deliver in 15 minutes a service that had required several days to deliver is made possible by what the bank calls integrated platform automation. The entire lending process is automated with personal computers in the branches communicating directly to the bank's mainframe computer. Personal bankers put required information into their personal computers and the computer system takes over, retrieving data from the customer's files, conducting a credit bureau check, approving the loan, even printing the documentation for the client to sign and the check. If additional review or approval is necessary, the system allows the personal banker to immediately transmit the information to a loan center where a loan officer makes the lending decision and transmits it back to the personal banker.[5]

Technology and personal service can be mutually supportive, interconnected keys to excellent service. If technology and personal service are in conflict, it is because management has put them in conflict. Properly blending technology and personal service requires understanding the service well enough to know which elements can be automated, and understanding the customer's service expectations well enough to know which service elements require the personal touch.[6]

2. *Use technology to support the service strategy.* Technology is a tool to improve service. Its potential for doing so relates directly to the clarity of the service strategy. When the strategy is unclear, the sense of which technology is needed to support the strategy is unclear, too.

To ask the question, "What is the best technology?" is to ask the wrong question. The proper question is: "What is our service strategy and how can we best use technology to implement this strategy?" Service strategy decisions should always precede technology decisions.

Consider the case of Florida Power & Light Company (FPL) and its quest for improved service reliability. Its strategy involves reducing the duration and frequency of service interruptions, a major cause of customers' complaints. Serving a part of the country that annually averages 80 days of thunderstorms with associated lightning causing service interruptions, company engineers teamed with suppliers to develop advanced surge protectors that protect transformers from lightning damage. The company has developed a sophisticated, computer-based lightning tracking system to anticipate where weather-related problems might occur and strategically position crews at these locations to quicken recovery response time. These and other initiatives have enabled FPL to reduce service unavailabiliity (customer minutes interrupted divided by customers served) from 70 minutes at year-end 1987 to 48.37 minutes at year-end 1988. The company's target for 1991 is 36.41 minutes.[7]

3. *Focus technology on the customer.* All technologies have a customer. The customer may be inside the organization or outside, but in either case a technology's success hinges on whether it adds value for its user. A successful technology may help service employees work smarter or faster. Or it may free them up from tedious chores, unleashing them to perform more creative and fulfilling service. Technologies that aid service employees usually aid external customers as well in ways ranging from faster service (due to improved productivity) to more reliable service (due to automating labor-intensive functions). Recall from chapter 6 that technology-job fit (employees having the appropriate technology to perform the service) is an important factor in influencing Gap 3. Of course, technology also benefits external customers directly, as the universal product code, automatic teller machine, and other examples used in this section illustrate.

Taking a customer-oriented approach to technology means identifying the customers for each technological initiative, learning their service expectations and perceptions, and eliciting their feedback to new technology concepts and prototypes. A new technology should be viewed as a new product; and like any new product, technology should be market-based.

No service company illustrates better the potential for improving service and profits through market-driven technology than McKesson Corporation, a pharmaceutical distribution company. Investing millions of dollars to develop an electronic data interchange capability to improve its service to ten thousand plus independent pharmacists, McKesson grew its business from $1 billion at the start of the 1980's to $6 billion at the end of the decade.

What McKesson did was develop information systems to help independents compete with drug chains in inventory management, pricing, credit, and other ways. With *Economost* and *Econoscan*, independent retailers could use a hand-held computer and optical character scanner for electronic order entry, inventory control, and shelf management. In addition, the retailers could use *Econocharge*, a store credit-card system; *Econoclaim*, a system for processing prescription information and insurance claims; *Econosure*, a business insurance policy; and *Pharmaserve*, an in-store computer system. Clearly, it would not be an easy task for a McKesson competitor to dislodge customers who are linked up to these data interchange systems.[8]

Materially improving service through technology requires an eclectic, open view to blending technology and people; a clear strategy; and a customer focus. It also requires a willingness to experiment, modify, learn from mistakes, and experience pain before gain. And it requires patient money. Some of the service sector's biggest technology winners for the 1990's—from American Airlines' Sabre reservation system to Citibank's state-of-the-art ATM network—involved huge, up-front investments in the 1970's and 1980's. Turning technology into a servant requires that management take the long view.

ATTACKING THE LABOR SHORTFALL

One of the most vexing problems for the service sector in the 1990's concerns labor-force shortfalls. The problem is very serious and cuts to the heart of the service-improvement challenge that many companies face. Not enough young people are available to do the nation's entry-level service work, and, of those available, many lack the basic required skills.

At the low-wage end of America's restaurant industry, 200,000 jobs were unfilled in 1989. Compounding the problem is a 250 percent employee turnover rate.[9] Some of the nation's top hotel chains have actually closed down wings of certain properties because they cannot hire enough maids to clean the rooms. New York Telephone Company had to test 60,000 applicants in 1987 to hire 3,000 deemed qualified to assume entry-level positions.[10]

What is occurring is a rapid expansion of service-sector jobs and an elevation of the basic and technical skills needed for these jobs just as changing demographics are shrinking the labor pool of young people who in many instances are not receiving the education they need to be marketable. In essence, we have labor shortages and labor mismatches rolled into one big, alarming problem.

Because people born between 1946 and 1964—the so-called baby boomers—have been having only about half as many children as their parents did, about 2 million fewer 16- to 24-year-olds will enter the labor force in 1995 compared to 1987. During this same period, the Bureau of Labor Statistics (BLS) expects the number of jobs available to grow by 10 percent, the vast majority in the service sector.[11]

A Labor Mismatch

Taking a longer view, the BLS estimates that private sector service jobs will expand by about 16 million jobs between 1988 and the year 2000. This growth alone almost equals the total number of people employed in the manufacturing sector in 1988. Significantly, many of the new service-sector jobs will be in high-skill areas such as engineering, medical technology, and computer programming, and medium-skill areas such as retail sales and financial services.[12]

The Labor Department has developed a methodology for measuring on a one-to-six scale the levels of reading, writing, and vocabulary skills required to perform a wide range of jobs. The Hudson Institute evaluated the new jobs the economy will create between 1985 and the year 2000 against these scales. The Hudson Institute concludes that more than three-fourths of the country's new workers will be at levels 1 and 2 (limited verbal and writing skills) while more than 50 percent of the new jobs available will be at levels 3 and above. For example, retail sales employees will have to function at level 3, writing up orders and reading merchandise information. The Hudson Institute estimates that only 22 percent of the new employees will be able to operate at level 3 or better.[13]

One million American youth drop out of school each year; for many urban high schools, dropout rates exceed 50 percent. One of every eight 17-year-olds is functionally illiterate.[14] Writes Pat Choate in *The High-Flex Society:* "The top third of America's young people is the best educated in the world, but the middle third is slipping into mediocrity, and the bottom third is at Third World standards."[15]

The implications of quantity and quality labor shortfalls for the service sector are sobering. For one thing, there will be great pressure on service organizations to lower their service-quality standards—which is the exact opposite of what needs to be done as we discuss in the next section. Thus, we may see Gap 2 in the service-quality model affected adversely.

We may also see growing Gap 3 problems in many companies as critical service positions either remain unfilled or are filled by people ill-equipped to perform in them. As we write this book, our impression is that the staffs of major hotels in Stockholm, Sweden, speak better English than the staffs of major hotels in New York City. In fact, this may not be quite true but it is close enough to the truth to signal the depth of the labor-pool challenge facing service firms.

THE NEED FOR INNOVATIVE APPROACHES

America's best-managed service companies are starting to deal with the labor-pool problem in innovative ways. In so doing, they are setting examples for others to follow. McDonald's established its McMasters training program in 1986 to attract more older workers into employment. McDonald's and other fast-food chains are installing self-service drink-dispensing equipment. Customers get free refills but it alleviates the need for extra employees to pour drinks.

Walt Disney World trains existing employees to recruit new employees. Each division is responsible for its own recruiting on the basis that people actually performing a job know it better than anyone else and are more likely to hire good people.[16] Wal-Mart provides scholarship assistance to employees so that they can attend colleges or universities while continuing to work part time. Successful graduates are then promoted into management. Approximately 40 percent of Wal-Mart's managers started as hourly trainees.[17]

A growing number of service companies are tackling worker skill deficiencies head-on—teaching employees to read and write. By the late 1980's, American firms were investing $300 million a year to teach employees basic skills.[18] And more corporate executives are investing their personal time and their firms' resources to assist local schools in curriculum development, teaching, equipment acquisition, and funding.

The key to this complex labor-pool puzzle is new mind-sets at the highest corporate levels. Service companies need to compete as hard for talent as they compete for market share. They need to assume direct responsibility for developing talent, for not only recruiting the best available people but also encouraging and helping them to get better once they are employed. They need to work every angle to cope with the problem, from substituting new service designs and technology for people to taking a marketing approach to recruiting through aggressive advertising, career fairs, employee-get-an-employee campaigns and more. There is no law after all that forces service companies to restrict employee recruiting to small-type ads buried in the classified sections of newspapers!

Most of all, service companies have to work harder at improving the jobs they wish to fill. It is important to think of jobs as products that employees buy and to tailor these job-products to fulfill employees' wants and needs. This is what service companies must do most of all to attract and retain employees who are able and willing to provide excellent service. Companies must seek to attract and retain a larger market share of the most qualified employment candidates through superior job-products.

No company in America better illustrates the internal marketing approach we are proposing than Walt Disney World. Disney World is at the same time a no-nonsense employer with rigorous training regimens and strict personal grooming standards for all "cast members" and a generous employer that invests heavily to create good jobs. For example, Disney World operates a 75-acre recreation complex including a lake for the exclusive use of employees and their families. The company posts available positions every week through its "Casting Call," choosing to promote from within. It publishes a weekly employee newspaper, *Eyes and Ears;* sells Disney merchandise to employees at substantial discounts; and provides continuing education classes, stock purchase plans, a housing referral service, and many other services to employees.

Everyone employed by Disney World is on a first-name basis. If Walt Disney were alive today, all employees would refer to him as "Walt."

Disney World is indeed a special place to work: a culture that attracts good people and spurs their achievement, satisfaction, and enjoyment on the job. As Walt Disney once said himself, "You can dream, create, design and build the most wonderful place in the world . . . but it takes people to make the dream a reality."[19]

RAISING OUR SERVICE ASPIRATIONS

The most significant service challenge of them all for the 1990's is to raise our service aspirations. It is time for American executives to declare war on service mediocrity, to become indignant in the face of shoddy service, intolerant in the face of so-so service.

If the 1980's were a decade of growing service consciousness in America, the 1990's must be the decade in which we decide collectively, as executives and as consumers, to seek superior service, to settle for nothing less, to be more determined, more obsessive, more committed than ever before.

The stakes are very high. It is more than a matter of economics although the issue of economic superiority within industries and among countries is at stake. It is also a matter of national pride. The rising clamor for better service in America is reflected in developments ranging from cover stories in national magazines to legislation requiring airlines to publish their on-time performance records. This is really a clamor to return to the country's roots of craftsmanship, integrity, generosity, and civility. The service issue, so visible and so much a part of everyone's everyday, seems to have become a barometer of a declining culture.

Roger Hale, the chairman of Tennant Company, a manufacturer of industrial floor cleaning equipment, was recently named Minnesota's Executive of the Year in recognition of his company's commitment to quality. In explaining his obsession for quality, Hale exposes the cultural challenge we face as a country.

Tennant Company was known for producing top-quality floor maintenance equipment. But during my visits with our Japanese joint-

venture partner in the late 1970's, I had been hearing complaints—
sometimes bitter—about hydraulic leaks in our most successful
machines. Back home, I began asking questions: Why were the hydraulic leaks happening only in the machines we sent to Japan? . . .
As it turned out, the leaks weren't just happening in Japan. The
difference was that U.S. customers accepted the leaks. If a drop of
oil appeared on a freshly polished floor, they simply wiped it up.[20]

Role Models Exist

We do have examples of American companies unwilling to play second
fiddle on service quality to the Japanese or any other country. What we
need now is for many executives to become zealous about service, to
become as competitive concerning their quality standards as they are on
other matters, such as market share and stock price. Indeed, if they
become this committed to quality, market share and stock price will be
favorably affected, as we discussed at the beginning of the book.

We need more companies such as Smith & Hawken, Deluxe Corporation, and Dunkin' Donuts Incorporated. Gap 2 is not a problem in
these companies; if anything, the companies' service standards are higher
than the customers' expectations!

Smith & Hawken is a California-based firm that sells garden products
via catalog. Early on its management saw the need to overcompensate
through exemplary service for the customer's perceived loss of control in
purchasing by catalog. In the mid-1980's, the company codified its principles of service. The following partial list has brief explanatory notes in
parentheses:

- *Our goal as a company is to have customer service that is not just the best, but
  legendary.* (Legendary may seem grandiose but you need a goal that
  is ever expanding rather than merely attainable.)
- *You are the customer.* (When a customer is upset, service personnel
  need to be the customer and feel the customer's unhappiness. Service
  personnel have permission to do whatever it will take to make the
  customer feel good again about the company.)
- *You are the company.* (Each employee must carry the authority, dig-
  nity, and bearing of ownership.)
- *There is no such thing as taking too much time with a customer.* (Our
  business lives, breathes, and dies according to one simple activity:
  repeat business.)

- *The phone is mightier than the pen.* (When customers have questions or concerns, we call. Calling collapses the time between problem and solution, as well as eliminates paperwork.)
- *A job isn't done until it is checked.* (If we don't build in redundancies, the customers will do our error checking for us and they may not be forgiving.)
- *Do it once and do it yourself.* (Whenever possible, one employee should follow through on the entire customer service episode.)[21]

Deluxe Corporation (formerly Deluxe Check Printers) of St. Paul, Minnesota, is one of America's most profitable companies, a success that traces back to August 18, 1936, when company founder, W. R. Hotchkiss decreed, "Starting immediately, regardless of expense, energy and effort involved, every order will be shipped by the end of the day after it arrives." Deluxe still adheres to this standard of service today, reporting its service-quality statistics in the shareholders letter appearing in its annual report. In 1988 Deluxe shipped 94.4 percent of its orders by the day-after deadline and printed 98.7 percent of them without error. So obsessed is Deluxe with service quality that it pushed legislation through Congress to allow it to put U.S. Postal Service stations inside its plants to improve average delivery time.[22]

Deluxe Corporation's obsession with being the best in its field is matched by Dunkin' Donuts' obsession with serving the best coffee to be found anywhere. The company seems to be succeeding, selling 405 million cups of coffee in the United States in 1988.[23] Here is how Clifford and Cavanaugh describe Dunkin' Donuts' obsession with making excellent coffee in the book *The Winning Performance:*

> Dunkin' Donuts really cares about the quality of its coffee. Its goal is to serve the "best cup of coffee in the world." Dunkin' Donuts has a 23-page specification of what it requires in a coffee bean. But buying high-quality, specially blended coffee beans is just the beginning. Dunkin' Donuts franchisees have to make sure their coffee is fresh. Beans are to be used within ten days of their delivery; if they are not, they are returned on the next Dunkin' Donuts supply truck. Once the coffee is brewed, it can be served for only 18 minutes; after that it must be thrown out. And the coffee must be brewed between 196 and 198 degrees Fahrenheit exactly. Dunkin' is one of the few chains that still use real cream—*not* half and half, *not* milk, *not* the sugar-based powder.[24]

TENETS TO LIVE BY

From retailing garden tools to delivering checks to making coffee, superior service is within reach if we are willing to reach for it. Here are four tenets to follow in reaching for superior service:

1. *Seek constant improvement.* Service excellence is an attitude, a mind-set; it is also competence and design. The only option is to continually strive for a stronger service attitude, more competence and better design every day of every week of every month of every year.

Service quality is *not* a program; it does not have an end point. One commonality in the best-serving companies in America is a burning desire to improve, to be better next week and next year than this week and this year.

Senior managers cannot build a service-minded culture within their companies by investing in service when earnings are good and putting service issues on the back burner when earnings are poor. Executives cannot build a service-minded culture by turning the service issue on and off like a water faucet. Service excellence requires a full-court press—all of the time.[25]

2. *Forget about being a commodity business.* There is no such thing as a commodity business; rather, there are only businesses that we think of in this way. Commodity is a mind-set. Whereas some observers might consider bank checks or coffee to be commodities, executives at Deluxe Corporation and Dunkin' Donuts clearly do not and this is their competitive advantage. Executives in these companies see service excellence as the primary opportunity to differentiate their offering from competitors, as the primary means for competing on value rather than price. These executives view service quality as the one dimension of business performance that their competitors may be unable to match. They view service excellence as the opportunity to be a company in a commodity industry that does not offer a commodity.

3. *Do the service right the first time.* Our research has shown consistently that consumers consider reliability to be the single most important dimension in judging service. Consumers want service providers to look good, be responsive, be knowledgeable and nice, and be empathetic. But most of all, consumers expect service providers to perform the service they promised to perform accurately and dependably.

For most consumers, reliability is the core service. Service providers' apologies start to wear thin when a company is unreliable. When a company is careless in performing the service, when it makes frequent mistakes, when it is casual about keeping its service promises, customers lose confidence in the firm's reliability and little can be done to regain it.

Our data show our sample companies to be more deficient on the reliability dimension than on any other. These firms have the most negative SERVQUAL scores on the dimension of service quality that is most important to consumers.

American executives need to set their sights higher for service reliability. They need to place a higher premium on error-free service; they need to value zero defects and back up their conviction with resources. In service design; in the application of technology; in the goal-setting process; in the hiring, training, measuring, and rewarding of staff, executives need to keep pursuing better and better reliability. Reliability is the heart of excellent service.

4. *Do the service very right the second time.* It is sometimes suggested on the lecture circuit that it is okay for companies to be careless in the primary service as long as they are effective in solving the problems that carelessness creates. However, as our data from chapter 2 show, this notion is false. It is far better to be excellent in reliability and recovery than to be fair in reliability and excellent in recovery.

Excellent reliability and recovery represent a powerful one-two punch in service quality. Companies need to aspire to doing the service right the first time and, on those occasions when this does not occur, doing the service very right the second time.

How a company handles service problems tells consumers a great deal about the firm's service values and priorities. Customers are used to experiencing additional hassles and disappointments when attempting to resolve problems with service organizations. Thus, quick, competent, courteous problem resolution gives organizations an excellent opportunity to impress customers and recover much of—but probably not all of—the confidence lost via the original service encounter.

Being excellent in problem resolution service involves encouraging customers to communicate their problems to the company so the company has the chance to recover. It involves having enough staff, and the right kind of staff: personable, resilient, well-trained. It involves systems, structure, and authority that allow the staff to solve the problem on the first contact with the customer. It involves taking the long view toward creating true customers, rather than the short view of maximizing near-term profits.[26] Most of all, being excellent in problem resolution requires wanting to be excellent in problem resolution, viewing this as a genuine opportunity to build and improve the business rather than as a peripheral activity or necessary evil.

Seeking continuous improvement, seeking differentiation from competitors no matter which type of product is involved, combining ultrareliable service with excellent recovery—these four tenets convey collectively that even good service isn't good enough for the 1990's. It is time to raise our service standards in America and aspire to be the best servers in the world. This is the signal challenge for the new decade; the potential payoff—for companies and country—is rich indeed.

FINAL WORDS

In this chapter we have discussed four challenges for the 1990's that are especially important in closing the service-quality gaps in our model. Designing quality into the service, using technology to enhance service, attacking labor-pool shortfalls, and raising our service aspirations are all critical for the new decade.

We believe excellent service is a genuine key to a better future—for those who give service as well as for those who receive it, for companies that make things as well as for companies traditionally labeled service businesses, for our country's national pride, as well as its economic competitiveness.

This is the new age of the service economy in America and elsewhere. What kind of future is in store for our citizens, our communities, our industries, our economy, and our national self-respect if our service is slovenly, uncaring, incompetent?

The spirit of this book is that service quality need not be an amorphous or mystical idea. Through the framework of our research-based gaps model and our methodology anchored in SERVQUAL we have attempted in this volume to convey that service *is* definable, *is* measurable, *is* improvable. What is needed now in organizations is the internal service of service leadership.

Executives must assume the mantle of service leadership to inspire people to be the best they can be; give them the systems, tools, and technologies to facilitate their work; remove unnecessary obstacles and discouragements from their paths; allow them the freedom to truly serve their customers; and build internal cultures of teamwork, congruence, and achievement. Companies ranging from American Express to Federal Express, Deluxe Corporation to L. L. Bean, McKesson to Disney, are winning big with excellent service. And so can many more of our companies.

Our book's publication coincides with the onset of a brand new decade. This is perfect. The 1980's were the service-quality awareness decade in the United States. Let's make the 1990's the service-quality action decade.

APPENDIXES

IN THE FOLLOWING APPENDIXES, we discuss the approaches we have developed to quantify and analyze the five gaps in our conceptual model of service quality. Appendix A presents SERVQUAL, the instrument for measuring customer's perceptions of service quality (Gap 5), and discusses its applications. Appendix B presents approaches for quantifying Gaps 1 through 4 and the factors associated with them (i.e., their potential causes).

SERVQUAL AND ITS APPLICATIONS

S ERVQUAL IS a concise multiple-item scale with good reliability and validity that companies can use to better understand the service expectations and perceptions of their customers.[1] We have designed the instrument to be applicable across a broad spectrum of services. As such, it provides a basic skeleton through its expectations/perceptions format encompassing statements for each of the five service-quality dimensions (tangibles, reliability, responsiveness, assurance, and empathy). The skeleton, when necessary, can be adapted or supplemented to fit the characteristics or specific research needs of a company.

We should also mention that we have refined the original SERV-QUAL instrument based on our experience in using it in a number of studies. The instrument we present in this appendix is the latest version that has benefited from several refinements and improvements.

THE SERVQUAL INSTRUMENT

Exhibit A–1 on page 180 contains the SERVQUAL instrument. The questionnaire in exhibit A–1, in addition to containing an expectations section consisting of 22 statements and a perceptions section consisting of a matching set of company-specific statements, also contains a section to ascertain customers' assessment of the relative importance of the five dimensions. This section is placed between the expectations and perceptions sections.

In addition to including the sections in exhibit A–1, our customer questionnaire contained a section on customers' experience with, and overall impressions about, the service (e.g., had they encountered a problem with the service, would they recommend the service to a friend) and a section on demographics (e.g., age, sex, income, education). Depending on the specific information needs of a company, appropriate sections like these can be added to the basic instrument shown in exhibit A–1.

COMPUTING THE SERVQUAL GAP SCORES

The SERVQUAL statements (in both the expectations and perceptions sections) are grouped into the five dimensions as follows:

Dimension	Statements Pertaining to the Dimension
Tangibles	Statements 1–4
Reliability	Statements 5–9
Responsiveness	Statements 10–13
Assurance	Statements 14–17
Empathy	Statements 18–22

Assessing the quality of service using SERVQUAL involves computing the difference between the ratings customers assign to the paired expectation/perception statements. Specifically, a Gap 5 or SERVQUAL score for each statement pair, for each customer, is computed as follows:

SERVQUAL Score = Perception Score − Expectation Score

A company's quality of service along each of the five dimensions can then be assessed across all customers by averaging their SERVQUAL scores on statements making up the dimension. For instance, if N customers responded to a SERVQUAL survey, the average SERVQUAL score along each dimension is obtained through the following two steps:

1. For each customer, add the SERVQUAL scores on the statements pertaining to the dimension and divide the sum by the number of statements making up the dimension.
2. Add the quantity obtained in step 1 across all N customers and divide the total by N.

The SERVQUAL scores for the five dimensions obtained in the preceding fashion can themselves be averaged (i.e., summed and divided by five) to obtain an overall measure of service quality. This overall measure is an *unweighted* SERVQUAL score because it does not take into account the relative importance that customers attach to the various dimensions.

An overall *weighted* SERVQUAL score that takes into account the relative importance of the dimensions is obtained through the following four steps:

1. For each customer, compute the average SERVQUAL score for each of the five dimensions (this step is the same as the first step in the two-step procedure outlined earlier).

2. For each customer, multiply the SERVQUAL score for each dimension (obtained in step 1) by the importance weight assigned by the customer to that dimension (the importance weight is simply the points the customer allocated to the dimension divided by 100).

3. For each customer, add the weighted SERVQUAL scores (obtained in step 2) across all five dimensions to obtain a combined weighted SERVQUAL score.

4. Add the scores obtained in step 3 across all N customers and divide the total by N.

APPLICATIONS OF SERVQUAL

As described in the preceding section, data obtained through the SERVQUAL instrument can be used to compute service-quality gap scores at different levels of detail: for each statement pair, for each dimension, or combined across all dimensions. By examining these various gap scores a company can not only assess its overall quality of service as perceived by customers but also identify the key dimensions, and facets within those dimensions, on which it should focus its quality-improvement efforts. The SERVQUAL instrument and the data generated by it can also be used in a variety of other ways as discussed next.

COMPARING CUSTOMERS' EXPECTATIONS AND PERCEPTIONS OVER TIME

While examining SERVQUAL scores (which represent the gap between customers' expectations and perceptions) can be insightful, additional insight can be gained by tracking the levels of expectations and perceptions through repeated administration of SERVQUAL (e.g., once every six months or once a year). Such a comparison of expectations and perceptions over time reveals not only how the gap between the two is changing but also whether the changes are stemming from changing expectations, changing perceptions, or both. The illustrative chart in exhibit A–2 tracks customers' expectations and perceptions along the

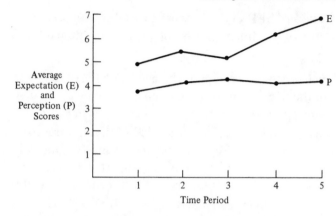

Exhibit A–2 Illustrative Tracking of Customers' Expectations and Perceptions along the Reliability Dimension

reliability dimension (similar charts can be constructed for the other dimensions). The chart shows that quality along the reliability dimension has deteriorated sharply in periods 4 and 5, apparently due to a significant increase in expectations without a corresponding improvement in perceptions.

COMPARING YOUR OWN SERVQUAL SCORES AGAINST COMPETITORS' SCORES

The two-section format of SERVQUAL, with separate expectation and perception sections, makes it convenient to measure the service quality of several competing companies simply by including a set of perception statements for each company. The expectations section need not be repeated for each company. A company can, therefore, easily adapt SERVQUAL and use it to track its quality of service against that of its leading competitors. Exhibit A–3 illustrates such competitive tracking along the reliability dimension. Similar charts constructed for the other dimensions, as well as for overall service quality, would provide valuable insights about the company's relative strengths and weaknesses and how they are changing over time.

EXAMINING CUSTOMER SEGMENTS WITH DIFFERING QUALITY PERCEPTIONS

One potential application of SERVQUAL is its use in categorizing a company's customers into several perceived-quality segments (e.g., high,

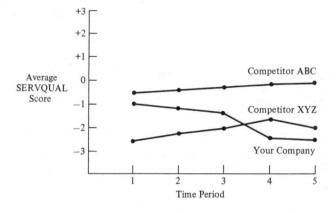

Exhibit A–3 Illustrative Tracking of SERVQUAL Scores along the Reliability Dimension

medium, and low) on the basis of their individual SERVQUAL scores. These segments then can be analyzed on the basis of (1) demographic, psychographic, and/or other profiles; (2) the relative importance of the five dimensions in influencing service-quality perceptions; and (3) the reasons behind the perceptions reported. For example, suppose a company found that a large number of SERVQUAL respondents falling in the medium perceived-quality group fit its prime target market based on demographic and psychographic criteria. Suppose further that reliability and assurance were found to be the most important quality dimensions and, based on perception-expectation gap scores for items concerning these dimensions, the items relating to record-keeping accuracy and behavior of contact personnel revealed the biggest gaps. With these data, the company's management would understand better what needs to be done to improve its image in the eyes of a very important group—customers within the company's prime target market who give the company medium service quality scores and who are in position to either respond to improved service from the company or defect to the competition.

A company might also benefit by examining the differences, if any, in the service-quality perceptions of customers segmented on the basis of demographic characteristics (e.g., sex, age, income), length of association with the company, willingness to recommend the company, and so forth. Overall SERVQUAL scores, as well as scores on individual dimensions, can be computed for each segment and compared across segments. A prerequisite for this application (and the preceding one) is inclusion in the

SERVQUAL questionnaire of questions pertaining to the relevant segmentation variables.

Assessing Quality Perceptions of Internal Customers

SERVQUAL, with appropriate adaptation, can be used by departments and divisions within a company to ascertain the quality of service they provide to employees in other departments and divisions. For instance, suppose the data processing department in XYZ Company wishes to use SERVQUAL to determine how its internal customers rate its quality of service. To do so, it can modify SERVQUAL by incorporating "excellent data processing departments" as the frame of reference throughout the expectations section and replacing "XYZ Co." with "XYZ's data processing department" in the perceptions section. The modified instrument can be administered to a sample of internal customers, or to all such customers if the data processing department's internal customer base is fairly small (e.g., 200 or less).

Exhibit A–1 SERVQUAL Questionnaire

Directions: Based on your experiences as a consumer of _____ services, please think about the kind of _____ company that would deliver excellent quality of service. Think about the kind of _____ company with which you would be pleased to do business. Please show the extent to which you think such a _____ company would possess the feature described by each statement. If you feel a feature is *not at all essential* for excellent _____ companies such as the one you have in mind, circle the number **1.** If you feel a feature is *absolutely essential* for excellent _____ companies, circle **7.** If your feelings are less strong, circle one of the numbers in the middle. There are no right or wrong answers—all we are interested in is a number that truly reflects your feelings regarding companies that would deliver excellent quality of service.

	Strongly Disagree						Strongly Agree
1. Excellent_____ companies will have modern-looking equipment.	1	2	3	4	5	6	7
2. The physical facilities at excellent _____ companies will be visually appealing.	1	2	3	4	5	6	7
3. Employees at excellent _____ companies will be neat-appearing.	1	2	3	4	5	6	7
4. Materials associated with the service (such as pamphlets or statements) will be visually appealing in an excellent _____ company.	1	2	3	4	5	6	7
5. When excellent _____ companies promise to do something by a certain time, they will do so.	1	2	3	4	5	6	7
6. When a customer has a problem, excellent _____ companies will show a sincere interest in solving it.	1	2	3	4	5	6	7
7. Excellent _____ companies will perform the service right the first time.	1	2	3	4	5	6	7
8. Excellent _____ companies will provide their services at the time they promise to do so.	1	2	3	4	5	6	7

(continued)

	Strongly Disagree						Strongly Agree
9. Excellent _____ companies will insist on error-free records.	1	2	3	4	5	6	7
10. Employees in excellent _____ companies will tell customers exactly when services will be performed.	1	2	3	4	5	6	7
11. Employees in excellent _____ companies will give prompt service to customers.	1	2	3	4	5	6	7
12. Employees in excellent _____ companies will always be willing to help customers.	1	2	3	4	5	6	7
13. Employees in excellent _____ companies will never be too busy to respond to customers' requests.	1	2	3	4	5	6	7
14. The behavior of employees in excellent _____ companies will instill confidence in customers.	1	2	3	4	5	6	7
15. Customers of excellent _____ companies will feel safe in their transactions.	1	2	3	4	5	6	7
16. Employees in excellent _____ companies will be consistently courteous with customers.	1	2	3	4	5	6	7

	Strongly Disagree						Strongly Agree
17. Employees in excellent _____ companies will have the knowledge to answer customers' questions.	1	2	3	4	5	6	7
18. Excellent _____ companies will give customers individual attention.	1	2	3	4	5	6	7
19. Excellent _____ companies will have operating hours convenient to all their customers.	1	2	3	4	5	6	7
20. Excellent _____ companies will have employees who give customers personal attention.	1	2	3	4	5	6	7
21. Excellent _____ companies will have the customer's best interests at heart.	1	2	3	4	5	6	7
22. The employees of excellent _____ companies will understand the specific needs of their customers.	1	2	3	4	5	6	7

Directions: Listed below are five features pertaining to _____ companies and the services they offer. We would like to know how important each of these features is to *you* when you evaluate a _____ company's quality of service. Please allocate a total of 100 points among the five features *according to how important each feature is to you*—the more important a feature is to you, the more points you should allocate to it. Please ensure that the points you allocate to the five features add up to 100.

1. The appearance of the
   _____ company's physical facilities,
   equipment, personnel, and
   communication materials. _____ points

2. The _____ company's ability to
   perform the promised service
   dependably and accurately. _____ points

3. The _____ company's willingness to
   help customers and provide prompt
   service. _____ points

4. The knowledge and courtesy of the
   _____ company's employees and their
   ability to convey trust and confidence. _____ points

5. The caring, individualized attention the
   _____ company provides its
   customers. _____ points

   TOTAL points allocated　　　　　　　　　　**100**　　**points**

   Which *one* feature among the above five
   is *most important* to you? (please enter
   the feature's number) _____

   Which feature is *second* most important
   to you? _____
   Which feature is *least important* to you? _____

Directions: The following set of statements relate to your feelings about XYZ Company. For each statement, please show the extent to which you believe XYZ Company has the feature described by the statement. Once again, circling a 1 means that you strongly disagree that XYZ Company has that feature, and circling a 7 means that you strongly agree. You may circle any of the numbers in the middle that show how strong your feelings are. There are no right or wrong answers—all we are interested in is a number that best shows your perceptions about XYZ Company.

	Strongly Disagree						Strongly Agree
1. XYZ Co. has modern-looking equipment.	1	2	3	4	5	6	7
2. XYZ Co.'s physical facilities are visually appealing.	1	2	3	4	5	6	7
3. XYZ Co.'s employees are neat-appearing.	1	2	3	4	5	6	7
4. Materials associated with the service (such as pamphlets or statements) are visually appealing at XYZ Co.	1	2	3	4	5	6	7
5. When XYZ Co. promises to do something by a certain time, it does so.	1	2	3	4	5	6	7
6. When you have a problem, XYZ Co. shows a sincere interest in solving it.	1	2	3	4	5	6	7
7. XYZ Co. performs the service right the first time.	1	2	3	4	5	6	7
8. XYZ Co. provides its services at the time it promises to do so.	1	2	3	4	5	6	7
9. XYZ Co. insists on error-free records.	1	2	3	4	5	6	7
10. Employees in XYZ Co. tell you exactly when services will be performed.	1	2	3	4	5	6	7
11. Employees in XYZ Co. give you prompt service.	1	2	3	4	5	6	7
12. Employees in XYZ Co. are always willing to help you.	1	2	3	4	5	6	7

(Continued)

		Strongly Disagree						Strongly Agree
13.	Employees in XYZ Co. are never too busy to respond to your requests.	1	2	3	4	5	6	7
14.	The behavior of employees in XYZ Co. instills confidence in you.	1	2	3	4	5	6	7
15.	You feel safe in your transactions with XYZ Co.	1	2	3	4	5	6	7
16.	Employees in XYZ Co. are consistently courteous with you.	1	2	3	4	5	6	7
17.	Employees in XYZ Co. have the knowledge to answer your questions.	1	2	3	4	5	6	7
18.	XYZ Co. gives you individual attention.	1	2	3	4	5	6	7
19.	XYZ Co. has operating hours convenient to all its customers.	1	2	3	4	5	6	7
20.	XYZ Co. has employees who give you personal attention.	1	2	3	4	5	6	7
21.	XYZ Co. has your best interests at heart.	1	2	3	4	5	6	7
22.	Employees of XYZ Co. understand your specific needs.	1	2	3	4	5	6	7

B

APPROACHES FOR MEASURING SERVICE-PROVIDER GAPS AND THEIR CAUSES

I<small>N THIS APPENDIX</small> we first describe the approach and questions we have used to quantify the extent of Gaps 1 through 4. We then present the items to measure the factors or antecedents (discussed in chapters 4–7) pertaining to each of the four gaps.

MEASURING GAPS 1 THROUGH 4

G<small>AP</small> 1

From a measurement standpoint, Gap 1 is different from the other three service-provider gaps because it crosses the boundary between the customer and provider sides of our conceptual model (please refer to exhibit 3–6). Specifically, its measurement requires a comparison of responses pertaining to expectations from two different samples— customers and managers. Therefore, in the latest empirical phase of our research we included the expectations section of SERVQUAL (with modified directions) along with the section for measuring the relative importance of the five dimensions, in the questionnaire we used to survey

187

managers. These are the first two sections of the instrument shown in exhibit B–1.

As the directions for the first two sections of exhibit B–1 imply, the data generated from those sections pertain to managers' perceptions of customers' expectations and the relative importance customers attach to the five quality dimensions. The extent of Gap 1 can, therefore, be measured by determining the discrepancy between the managers' ratings and the customers' ratings on the corresponding questions on the SERV-QUAL questionnaire (exhibit A–1). Specifically, a Gap 1 score along each of the five dimensions is computed as follows:

1. Determine the average expectation score along the dimension for the customer sample. (This can be done by using a procedure similar to the two-step procedure outlined in appendix A for determining the average SERVQUAL score along each dimension.)
2. Determine the average expectation score along the dimension as perceived by the manager sample, using the same procedure as under step 1 but on data from the manager sample.
3. Subtract the average score determined in step 1 from the average score determined in step 2. The resulting difference is the Gap 1 score along the dimension (the more negative the Gap 1 score, the worse the gap).

An *overall* Gap 1 score can also be computed by first averaging the scores across the five dimensions for each sample separately and then computing the difference between the two sample averages. To compute a *weighted* overall Gap 1 score, one needs to first compute a weighted expectation score for each sample separately (using a procedure similar to the four-step procedure outlined in appendix A for computing a weighted SERVQUAL score) and then compute the difference between the two weighted sample scores. The weighted overall Gap 1 score captures the discrepancies between customers and managers on both expectations along the five dimensions and the relative importance of the dimensions.

GAPS 2 THROUGH 4

We measured Gaps 2 through 4 by asking samples of employees in the companies participating in this phase of our research to directly indicate their perceptions of the extent of those gaps. Specifically, for each gap, employee respondents used a seven-point scale to indicate the extent of the gap along each of the five service quality dimensions. The last three sections of the instrument in exhibit B–1 contain, respectively, the rating scales we used to measure gaps 2, 3, and 4. On these scales, *higher* numbers imply *smaller* gaps. An *overall* measure of each gap is obtained by averaging the scores across the five rating scales pertaining to the gap.

APPROPRIATE RESPONDENTS FOR MEASURING GAPS 1 THROUGH 4

In our gap model (shown in exhibit 3–6), Gaps 1 and 2 are managerial gaps in that the key company employees to whom they pertain are *managers*—Gap 1 stems from managers' lack of understanding of customers' expectations and Gap 2 represents managers' failure to set appropriate service specifications. Gaps 3 and 4, in contrast, pertain more to *first-line service employees* because they are the ones whose service-delivery performance may fall short of service specifications (Gap 3) and/or promises made to customers through external communications (Gap 4). Therefore, on the basis of closeness to and knowledge about the various gaps, the most appropriate survey respondents are managers for measuring Gaps 1 and 2 and customer-contact personnel for measuring Gaps 3 and 4.

In addition to obtaining the most appropriate measures of the four gaps, we also wanted to ascertain the differences, if any, between managers' and contact personnel's perceptions of all four gaps. We therefore included measures of all four gaps in both the manager and contact personnel surveys. And, as described in chapters 4 through 7, our results showed that managers had a better understanding of customers' expectations than contact personnel had (i.e., managers had a smaller Gap 1 than contact personnel), but that contact personnel's perceptions of Gaps 2, 3, and 4 were generally more optimistic (i.e., implied smaller gaps).

MEASURING ANTECEDENTS OF GAPS 1 THROUGH 4

In chapters 4 through 7, we identified, defined, and discussed a number of key factors that are potential antecedents of Gaps 1 through 4. To measure the extent to which these factors were present in the companies participating in the empirical phase of our research, we developed specific statements pertaining to the factors. We developed these statements based on information obtained from our earlier qualitative research phases and on scales available in the literature to measure several of the factors (e.g., role conflict, role ambiguity). We attached seven-point scales (ranging from Strongly Disagree to Strongly Agree) to the statements to obtain the respondents' ratings.

Exhibit B–2 contains the set of statements in the questionnaire we used to survey managers. These statements pertain to potential antecedents of the two managerial gaps (i.e., Gaps 1 and 2). The specific antecedents and statements on the questionnaire pertaining to them follow:

Antecedents of Gap 1	Corresponding Statements
Marketing research orientation	Statements 1–4
Upward communication	Statements 5–8
Levels of management	Statement 9
Antecedents of Gap 2	Corresponding Statements
Management's commitment to service quality	Statements 10–13
Goal setting	Statements 14–15
Task standardization	Statements 16–17
Perception of feasibility	Statements 18–20

Exhibit B–3 contains the set of statements in the questionnaire that we used to survey contact personnel. These statements pertain to potential antecedents of the two gaps representing performance shortfalls on the part of contact personnel (i.e., Gaps 3 and 4). The specific antecedents and the questionnaire statements pertaining to them follow:

Antecedents of Gap 3	Corresponding Statements
Teamwork	Statements 1–5
Employee-job fit	Statements 6–7
Technology-job fit	Statement 8
Perceived control	Statements 9–12
Supervisory control systems	Statements 13–15
Role conflict	Statements 16–19
Role ambiguity	Statements 20–24
Antecedents of Gap 4	Corresponding Statements
Horizontal communication	Statements 25–28
Propensity to overpromise	Statements 29–30

DETERMINING SCORES FOR THE ANTECEDENTS OF GAPS 1 THROUGH 4

The average score for each antecedent (on a scale of 1 to 7 on which the higher the score the more favorable the current status of the antecedent) can be computed through the following three steps:

1. For negatively worded statements pertaining to the antecedent, reverse the ratings given by the respondents (i.e., score 7 as 1, 6 as 2, etc.).
2. For each respondent, add the scores on the statements comprising the antecedent and divide the total by the number of statements.
3. Add the scores obtained in step 2 across all respondents and divide the total by the number of respondents.

A final note on the instruments included in appendix B: Because we only recently developed these instruments and have used them in just the latest phase of our research, they have not been subjected to the same degree of testing and refining as our SERVQUAL instrument included in appendix A. We intend to further refine our instruments and procedures for measuring the internal gaps and their antecedents as we use them in future studies.

Exhibit B–1 Instrument to Measure Gaps 1 Through 4

PART I

Directions: This portion of the survey deals with how you think your customers feel about a _____ company that, in their view, delivers excellent quality of service. Please indicate the extent to which your customers feel that excellent _____ companies would possess the feature described by each statement. If your customers are likely to feel a feature is *not at all essential* for excellent _____ companies, circle the number **1**. If your customers are likely to feel a feature is *absolutely essential*, circle **7**. If your customers' feelings are likely to be less strong, circle one of the numbers in the middle. Remember, there are no right or wrong answers—we are interested in what you think your customers' feelings are regarding _____ companies that would deliver excellent quality of service.

	Our Customers Would Strongly Disagree					Our Customers Would Strongly Agree	
1. Excellent _____ companies will have modern-looking equipment.	1	2	3	4	5	6	7
2. The physical facilities at excellent _____ companies will be visually appealing.	1	2	3	4	5	6	7
3. Employees at excellent _____ companies will be neat-appearing.	1	2	3	4	5	6	7
4. Materials associated with the service (such as pamphlets or statements) will be visually appealing in an excellent _____ company.	1	2	3	4	5	6	7
5. When excellent _____ companies promise to do something by a certain time, they will do so.	1	2	3	4	5	6	7
6. When a customer has a problem, excellent _____ companies will show a sincere interest in solving it.	1	2	3	4	5	6	7
7. Excellent _____ companies will perform the service right the first time.	1	2	3	4	5	6	7
8. Excellent _____ companies will provide their services at the time they promise to do so.	1	2	3	4	5	6	7

	Our Customers Would Strongly Disagree					Our Customers Would Strongly Agree	
9. Excellent _____ companies will insist on error-free records.	1	2	3	4	5	6	7
10. Employees in excellent _____ companies will tell customers exactly when services will be performed.	1	2	3	4	5	6	7
11. Employees in excellent _____ companies will give prompt service to customers.	1	2	3	4	5	6	7
12. Employees in excellent _____ companies will always be willing to help customers.	1	2	3	4	5	6	7
13. Employees in excellent _____ companies will never be too busy to respond to customers' requests.	1	2	3	4	5	6	7
14. The behavior of employees in excellent _____ companies will instill confidence in customers.	1	2	3	4	5	6	7
15. Customers of excellent _____ companies will feel safe in their transactions.	1	2	3	4	5	6	7
16. Employees in excellent _____ companies will be consistently courteous with customers.	1	2	3	4	5	6	7

(Continued)

	Our Customers Would Strongly Disagree						Our Customers Would Strongly Agree
17. Employees in excellent _____ companies will have the knowledge to answer customers' questions.	1	2	3	4	5	6	7
18. Excellent _____ companies will give customerss individual attention.	1	2	3	4	5	6	7
19. Excellent _____ companies will have operating hours convenient to all their customers.	1	2	3	4	5	6	7
20. Excellent _____ companies will have employees who give customers personal attention.	1	2	3	4	5	6	7
21. Excellent _____ companies will have the customer's best interests at heart.	1	2	3	4	5	6	7
22. The employees of excellent _____ companies will understand the specific needs of their customers.	1	2	3	4	5	6	7

PART II

Directions: Listed below are five features pertaining to _____ companies and the services they offer. We would like to know how important each of these features is to *your customers* when they evaluate a _____ company's quality of service. Please allocate a total of 100 points among the five features *according to how important each feature is to your customers*—the more important a feature is likely to be to your customers, the more points you should allocate to it. Please ensure that the points you allocate to the five features add up to 100.

1. The appearance of the _____ company's physical facilities, equipment, personnel, and communication materials.   _____ points

2. The _____ company's ability to perform the promised service dependably and accurately.   _____ points

3. The _____ company's willingness to help customers and provide prompt service.   _____ points

4. The knowledge and courtesy of the company's employees and their ability to convey trust and confidence.   _____ points

5. The caring, individualized attention the _____ company provides its customers.   _____ points

TOTAL points allocated   **100**   **points**

Which *one* feature among the above five is likely to be *most important* to your customers? (please enter the feature's number)   _____

Which feature is likely to be *second* most important to your customers?   _____

Which feature is likely to be *least important* to your customers?   _____

Directions: Performance standards in companies can be **formal**—written, explicit, and communicated to employees. They can also be **informal**—verbal, implicit, and assumed to be understood by employees. For each of the following features, circle the number that best describes the extent to which performance standards are formalized in your company. If there are no standards in your company, check the appropriate box.

	Informal Standards						Formal Standards	No Standards Exist
1. The appearance of the company's physical facilities, equipment, personnel, and communication materials.	1	2	3	4	5	6	7	[ ]

(Continued)

	Informal Standards					Formal Standards		No Standards Exist
2. The ability of the company to perform the promised service dependably and accurately.	1	2	3	4	5	6	7	[ ]
3. The willingness of the company to help customers and provide prompt service.	1	2	3	4	5	6	7	[ ]
4. The knowledge and courtesy of the company's employees and their ability to convey trust and confidence.	1	2	3	4	5	6	7	[ ]
5. The caring, individualized attention the company provides its customers.	1	2	3	4	5	6	7	[ ]

Directions: Listed below are the same five features. Employees and units sometimes experience difficulty in achieving the standards established for them. For each feature below, circle the number that best represents the degree to which your company and its employees are able to meet the performance standards established. Remember, there are no right or wrong answers—we need your candid assessments for this question to be helpful.

	Unable to Meet Standards Consistently				Able to Meet Standards Consistently		No Standards Exist
1. The appearance of the company's physical facilities, equipment, personnel, and communication materials.	1	2	3	4	5	6	7	[ ]
2. The ability of the company to perform the promised service dependably and accurately.	1	2	3	4	5	6	7	[ ]
3. The willingness of the company to help customers and provide prompt service.	1	2	3	4	5	6	7	[ ]
4. The knowledge and courtesy of the company's employees and their ability to convey trust and confidence.	1	2	3	4	5	6	7	[ ]
5. The caring, individualized attention the company provides its customers.	1	2	3	4	5	6	7	[ ]

Directions: Salespeople, advertising, and other company communications often make promises about the level of service a company will deliver. In some organizations, it is not always possible to fulfill these promises. For each feature below, we want to know the extent to which you believe that your company and its employees deliver the level of service promised to customers. Circle the number that best describes your perception.

	Unable to Meet Promises Consistently					Able to Meet Promises Consistently	
1. The appearance of the company's physical facilities, equipment, personnel, and communication materials.	1	2	3	4	5	6	7
2. The ability of the company to perform the promised service dependably and accurately.	1	2	3	4	5	6	7
3. The willingness of the company to help customers and provide prompt service.	1	2	3	4	5	6	7
4. The knowledge and courtesy of the company's employees and their ability to convey trust and confidence.	1	2	3	4	5	6	7
5. The caring, individualized attention the company provides its customers.	1	2	3	4	5	6	7

Exhibit B–2 Statements to Measure Antecedents of Gaps 1 and 2*

Directions: Listed below are a number of statements intended to measure your perceptions about your company and its operations. Please indicate the extent to which you disagree or agree with each statement by circling one of the seven numbers next to each statement. If you strongly disagree circle **1.** If you strongly agree, circle **7.** If your feelings are not strong, circle one of the numbers in the middle. There are no right or wrong answers. Please tell us honestly how you feel.

	Strongly Disagree						Strongly Agree
1. We regularly collect information about the needs of our customers.	1	2	3	4	5	6	7
2. We rarely use marketing research information that is collected about our customers.($-$)	1	2	3	4	5	6	7
3. We regularly collect information about the service-quality expectations of our customers.	1	2	3	4	5	6	7
4. The managers in our company rarely interact with customers.($-$)	1	2	3	4	5	6	7
5. The customer-contact personnel in our company frequently communicate with management.	1	2	3	4	5	6	7
6. Managers in our company rarely seek suggestions about serving customers from customer-contact personnel.($-$)	1	2	3	4	5	6	7
7. The managers in our company frequently have face-to-face interactions with customer-contact personnel.	1	2	3	4	5	6	7

(Continued)

	Strongly Disagree						Strongly Agree
8. The primary means of communication in our company between contact personnel and upper-level managers is through memos.(–)	1	2	3	4	5	6	7
9. Our company has too many levels of management between contact personnel and top management.(–)	1	2	3	4	5	6	7
10. Our company does not commit the necessary resources for service quality.(–)	1	2	3	4	5	6	7
11. Our company has internal programs for improving the quality of service to customers.	1	2	3	4	5	6	7
12. In our company, managers who improve quality of service are more likely to be rewarded than other managers.	1	2	3	4	5	6	7
13. Our company emphasizes selling as much as or more than it emphasizes serving customers.(–)	1	2	3	4	5	6	7
14. Our company has a formal process for setting quality of service goals for employees.	1	2	3	4	5	6	7
15. In our company we try to set specific quality of service goals.	1	2	3	4	5	6	7

	Strongly Disagree						Strongly Agree
16. Our company effectively uses automation to achieve consistency in serving customers.	1	2	3	4	5	6	7
17. Programs are in place in our company to improve operating procedures so as to provide consistent service.	1	2	3	4	5	6	7
18. Our company has the necessary capabilities to meet customers' requirements for service.	1	2	3	4	5	6	7
19. If we gave our customers the level of service they really want, we would go broke.(−)	1	2	3	4	5	6	7
20. Our company has the operating systems to deliver the level of service customers demand.	1	2	3	4	5	6	7

* Statements with a (−) sign at the end are negatively worded and therefore should be reverse-scored (i.e., a rating of 7 should be scored as 1, 6 as 2, 5 as 3, and so on).

Exhibit B–3 Statements to Measure Antecedents of Gaps 3 and 4*

Directions: Listed below are a number of statements intended to measure your perceptions about your company and its operations. Please indicate the extent to which you disagree or agree with each statement by circling one of the seven numbers next to each statement. If you strongly disagree, circle 1. If you strongly agree, circle 7. If your feelings are not strong, circle one of the numbers in the middle. There are no right or wrong answers. Please tell us honestly how you feel.

		Strongly Disagree						Strongly Agree
1.	I feel that I am part of a team in my company.	1	2	3	4	5	6	7
2.	Everyone in my company contributes to a team effort in servicing customers.	1	2	3	4	5	6	7
3.	I feel a sense of responsibility to help my fellow employees do their jobs well.	1	2	3	4	5	6	7
4.	My fellow employees and I cooperate more often than we compete.	1	2	3	4	5	6	7
5.	I feel that I am an important member of this company.	1	2	3	4	5	6	7
6.	I feel comfortable in my job in the sense that I am able to perform the job well.	1	2	3	4	5	6	7
7.	My company hires people who are qualified to do their jobs.	1	2	3	4	5	6	7
8.	My company gives me the tools and equipment that I need to perform my job well.	1	2	3	4	5	6	7
9.	I spend a lot of time in my job trying to resolve problems over which I have little control.(−)	1	2	3	4	5	6	7
10.	I have the freedom in my job to truly satisfy my customers' needs.	1	2	3	4	5	6	7

	Strongly Disagree						Strongly Agree
11. I sometimes feel a lack of control over my job because too many customers demand service at the same time.(−)	1	2	3	4	5	6	7
12. One of my frustrations on the job is that I sometimes have to depend on other employees in serving my customers.(−)	1	2	3	4	5	6	7
13. My supervisor's appraisal of my job performance includes how well I interact with customers.	1	2	3	4	5	6	7
14. In our company, making a special effort to serve customers well does not result in more pay or recognition.(−)	1	2	3	4	5	6	7
15. In our company, employees who do the best job serving their customers are more likely to be rewarded than other employees.	1	2	3	4	5	6	7
16. The amount of paperwork in my job makes it hard for me to effectively serve my customers.(−)	1	2	3	4	5	6	7
17. The company places so much emphasis on selling to customers that it is difficult to serve customers properly.(−)	1	2	3	4	5	6	7

(Continued)

	Strongly Disagree						Strongly Agree
18. What my customers want me to do and what management wants me to do are usually the same thing.	1	2	3	4	5	6	7
19. My company and I have the same ideas about how my job should be performed.	1	2	3	4	5	6	7
20. I receive a sufficient amount of information from management concerning what I am supposed to do in my job.	1	2	3	4	5	6	7
21. I often feel that I do not understand the services offered by my company.(−)	1	2	3	4	5	6	7
22. I am able to keep up with changes in my company that affect my job.	1	2	3	4	5	6	7
23. I feel that I have not been well trained by my company in how to interact effectively with customers.(−)	1	2	3	4	5	6	7
24. I am not sure which aspects of my job my supervisor will stress most in evaluating my performance.(−)	1	2	3	4	5	6	7
25. The people who develop our advertising consult employees like me about the realism of promises made in the advertising.	1	2	3	4	5	6	7

	Strongly Disagree						Strongly Agree
26. I am often not aware in advance of the promises made in our company's advertising campaigns.(–)	1	2	3	4	5	6	7
27. Employees like me interact with operations people to discuss the level of service the company can deliver to customers.	1	2	3	4	5	6	7
28. Our company's policies on serving customers are consistent in the different offices that service customers.	1	2	3	4	5	6	7
29. Intense competition is creating more pressure inside this company to generate new business.(–)	1	2	3	4	5	6	7
30. Our key competitors make promises they cannot possibly keep in an effort to gain new customers.(–)	1	2	3	4	5	6	7

* Statements with a (–) sign at the end are negatively worded and therefore should be reverse-scored (i.e., a rating of 7 should be scored as 1, 6 as 2, 5 as 3, and so on).

NOTES AND REFERENCES

Chapter 1
SERVICE LEADERSHIP SPELLS PROFITS

1. David Birch, "The Atomization of America," *Inc.*, March 1987, pp. 21–22.
2. James Brian Quinn and Christopher E. Gagnon, "Will Services Follow Manufacturing into Decline?" *Harvard Business Review*, November–December 1986, p. 103.
3. Jay Rosenstein, "Top Consumer Complaint: Account Errors," *American Banker*, November 1, 1988, pp. 1, 14–15.
4. "How Readers Rate Service in U.S.: 'The Animals Are Running the Zoo,' " *Atlanta Journal*, March 1, 1987.
5. "Pul-eeze! Will Somebody Help Me?" *Time*, February 2, 1987, p. 49.
6. Alan L. Otten, "How Medical Advances Often Worsen Illnesses and Even Cause Death," *Wall Street Journal*, July 27, 1988, p. 1.
7. Based on an interview with Lowell Levin published in *Bottom Line*, June 30, 1988, p. 1.
8. Stanley Marcus, "Fire a Buyer and Hire a Seller," *International Trends in Retailing*, Fall 1985, p. 49.
9. James G. Carr, "We Flatties Don't Come Back!" *Pace*, November–December 1982, p. 17.
10. Warren Bennis and Burt Nanus, *Leaders: The Strategies for Taking Charge* (New York: Harper & Row, 1985), p. 92.
11. The inspiration for the phrase "providing a service good enough that people will pay a profit to have it" comes from an *Inc.* magazine interview with retailer Stanley Marcus who was quoting the Dayton family in Minneapolis, founders of the Dayton-Hudson Corporation.
12. As quoted in "Companies That Serve You Best," *Fortune*, December 7, 1987, p. 98.

13. Lecture delivered by Robert Onstead at Texas A&M University, College Station, Texas, October 29, 1985.

14. Speech by Joseph Ellis, Center for Retailing Studies Symposium, San Antonio, Texas, October 2, 1986.

15. Peter F. Drucker, "Leadership: More Doing than Dash," *Wall Street Journal*, January 6, 1988.

16. Leonard L. Berry, "Delivering Excellent Service in Retailing," *Arthur Andersen Retailing Issues Letter*, April 1988.

17. "The Quest for Quality," *The Royal Bank Letter*, November–December 1988.

18. Same as note 5, p. 52.

19. Robert D. Buzzell and Bradley T. Gale, *The PIMS Principles—Linking Strategy to Performance* (New York: Free Press, 1987), p. 7.

20. Stew Leonard, "Love Your Customer," *Newsweek*, June 27, 1988, special advertising supplement.

21. As quoted in "Do You Know Me?" *Business Week*, January 25, 1988, p. 79.

22. Valarie A. Zeithaml, "Consumer Perceptions of Price, Quality, and Value: A Means-End Model and Synthesis of Evidence," *Journal of Marketing*, July 1988, p. 14.

23. Same as note 22, p.11.

24. "Brokerage House Embarks on Journey to Quality Service," *Marketing News*, December 21, 1984, p. 9.

25. John A. Goodman, Ted Marra, and Liz Brigham, "Customer Service: Costly Nuisance or Low-Cost Profit Strategy?" *Journal of Retail Banking*, Fall 1986, p. 12.

26. Raymond J. Larkin, "The History of Quality at American Express," *FYI.*, American Express corporate affairs publication, October 9, 1987, p. 4.

Chapter 2
THE CUSTOMERS' VIEW OF SERVICE QUALITY

1. See, for example, Philip B. Crosby, *Quality Is Free: The Art of Making Quality Certain* (New York: New American Library, 1979); and David A. Garvin, "Quality on the Line," *Harvard Business Review*, September–October 1983, pp. 65–73.

2. Writings focusing on service quality include: Christian Gronroos, *Strategic Management and Marketing in the Service Sector* (Helsingfors: Swedish School of Economics and Business Administration, 1982); Uolevi Lehtinen and Jarmo R. Lehtinen, "Service Quality: A Study of Quality Dimensions," unpublished working paper, Service Management Group OY, Helsinki, Finland, 1982; Robert C. Lewis and Bernard H. Booms, "The Marketing Aspects of Quality," in *Emerging Perspectives on Service Marketing*, ed. L. Berry, L. Shostack, and G. Upah (Chicago: American Marketing Association, 1983), pp.

99–107; W. Earl Sasser, Jr., R. Paul Olsen, and D. Daryl Wychoff, *Management of Service Operations: Text and Cases* (Boston: Allyn and Bacon, 1978).

3. A comprehensive scheme for classifying services has been developed by Christopher H. Lovelock, "Classifying Services to Gain Strategic Marketing Insights," *Journal of Marketing*, Summer 1983, pp. 9–20.

4. Further details concerning the development and testing of the SERVQUAL instrument can be found in A. Parasuraman, Valarie A. Zeithaml, and Leonard L. Berry, "SERVQUAL: A Multiple-Item Scale for Measuring Consumer Perceptions of Service Quality," *Journal of Retailing*, Spring 1988, pp. 12–40.

5. Only unweighted mean SERVQUAL scores are shown in this exhibit. The weighted mean SERVQUAL scores, while more negative than the unweighted mean scores, display a similar pattern for each pair of subgroups shown in the exhibit.

6. Patricia Sellers, "How to Handle Customers' Gripes," *Fortune*, October 24, 1988, pp. 88–100.

7. Same reference as in note 6, p. 89.

8. William R. George and Leonard L. Berry, "Guidelines for Advertising Services," *Business Horizons*, July–August 1981, pp. 52–56; Valarie A. Zeithaml, A. Parasuraman, and Leonard L. Berry, "Problems and Strategies in Services Marketing," *Journal of Marketing*, Spring 1985, pp. 33–46.

Chapter 3

POTENTIAL CAUSES OF SERVICE-QUALITY SHORTFALLS

1. David A. Garvin, "Quality on the Line," *Harvard Business Review*, September–October 1983, p. 68.

2. Quoted in "Beyond Customer Satisfaction through Quality Improvement," *Fortune*, September 26, 1988, special advertising section.

Chapter 4

GAP 1: NOT KNOWING WHAT CUSTOMERS EXPECT

1. As discussed in C. Gronroos, *Strategic Management and Marketing in the Service Sector* (Helsingfors: Swedish School of Economics and Business Administration, 1982).

2. Christopher H. Lovelock, "Why Marketing Management Needs to Be Different for Services," *Marketing of Services* (Chicago: American Marketing Association, 1981), pp. 5–9.

3. Karl Albrecht and Ron Zemke, *Service America! Doing Business in the New Economy* (Homewood, Ill.: Dow Jones-Irwin, 1985), p. 6.

4. Thomas J. Peters and Nancy Austin, *A Passion for Excellence* (New York: Random House, 1985), p. 84.

5. Don Lee Bohl, ed., "Close to the Customer," *An American Management Association Research Report on Consumer Affairs* (New York: American Management Association, 1987).

6. Same as note 4, p. 94.

7. *CNN News*, May 25, 1987.

8. J. Carey, J. Buckley, and J. Smith, "Hospital Hospitality," *Newsweek*, February 11, 1985, p. 78.

9. As discussed in "Customer Perceptions of GE Aerospacce," *Customer Focus*, General Electric Company publication, December 1986.

10. Same as note 5.

11. Same as note 5.

12. Kate Bertrand, "In Service, Perception Counts," *Business Marketing*, April 1989, p. 46.

13. "How American Express Measures Quality of Its Customer Service," *AMA Forum*, March 1982, pp. 29–31.

14. Same as note 4.

15. Same as note 5.

16. Mary J. Rudie and H. B. Wansley, "The Merrill Lynch Quality Program," *Services Marketing in a Changing Environment* (Chicago: American Marketing Association, 1985), p. 9.

17. W. E. Crosby, "American Airlines—A Commitment to Excellence," *Services Marketing in a Changing Environment* (Chicago: American Marketing Association, 1985), p. 12.

18. Lisa McGurrin. "Hillbilly Music in the Frozen Peas at Stew Leonard's," *New England Business*, February 17, 1986, pp. 38–41.

19. Same as note 5.

20. J. Curry, "Service: Retail's No. 1 Problem," *Chain Store Age*, January 1987, p. 20.

21. Same as note 17.

22. David Goyne, "Customer Service in Retailing," presentation at Center for Retailing Studies Fall Conference, Houston, Texas, October 11, 1985.

23. "Weinstock's Tackles the Problem of Service," *Chain Store Age*, January 1987, p. 16.

24. Same as note 4, p. 16.

25. Stephen Koepp, "Make that Sale, Mr. Sam," *Time*, May 18, 1987, pp. 54–55.

26. Same as note 25.

27. As quoted in speech by Richard C. Whiteley, "Creating Customer Focus," The Forum Corporation, Philadelphia, Pennsylvania, June 15, 1988.

28. Same as note 3, p. 145.

29. Mike Sheridan, "J. W. Marriott, Jr., Chairman and President, Marriott Corporation," *Sky*, March 1987, p. 48.

30. Same as note 29.

31. Same as note 4.

32. "McDonald's Tries to Keep Personal Touch," *Bryan-College Station Eagle*, May 28, 1985, p. 7A.

Chapter 5

GAP 2: THE WRONG SERVICE-QUALITY STANDARDS

1. Arnoldo Hax and Nicolas S. Majluf, *Strategic Management: An Integrative Perspective* (Englewood Cliffs, N.J.: Prentice-Hall, 1984), p. 90.

2. "Making Service a Potent Marketing Tool," *Business Week*, June 11, 1984, p. 170.

3. "Boosting Productivity at American Express," October 5, 1981, pp. 62, 66.

4. Thomas J. Peters and Nancy Austin, *A Passion for Excellence* (New York: Random House, 1985), p. 95.

5. "At Du Pont, Everybody Sells," *Sales & Marketing Management*, December 3, 1984, p. 33.

6. Lisa McGurrin, "Hillbilly Music in the Frozen Peas at Stew Leonard's," *New England Business*, February 17, 1986, pp. 38–41.

7. Mike Sheridan, "J. W. Marriott, Jr., Chairman and President, Marriott Corporation," *Sky*, March 1987, p. 48.

8. Leigh Bruce, "British Airways Jolts Staff with a Cultural Revolution," *International Management*, March 1987, p. 36.

9. Same as note 8, p. 37.

10. Same as note 3.

11. W. E. Crosby, "American Airlines—A Commitment to Excellence," *Services Marketing in a Changing Environment* (Chicago: American Marketing Association, 1985), p. 11.

12. Same as note 11, p. 10.

13. J. Ott, "Federal Express Starts 24-hour Weather Forecasting System," *Aviation Week*, February 7, 1987, p. 38.

14. "Customers Come First," *The Economist*, December 6, 1986, p. 79.

15. George Russell, "Where the Customer Is Still King," *Time*, February 2, 1987.

16. As discussed in speech by Walter Brown, vice-president of productivity and staffing, Marshall Field's, "Field's Computes Enriched Customer Service," at 1987 National Retail Marketing Association meeting in New York.

17. Ted Levitt, "Industrialization of Service," *Harvard Business Review*, September–October 1976, pp. 63–74.

18. Same as note 4, p. 78.

19. Don Lee Bohl, ed., "Close to the Customer," *An American Management Association Research Report on Consumer Affairs* (New York: American Management Association, 1987), p. 49.

20. Same as note 16.

21. "Mr. Winchester Orders a Pizza," *Fortune*, November 14, 1986, p. 134.

22. Same as note 15.

23. Same as note 3, p. 62.

24. Same as note 3.

25. Mary J. Rudie and H. B. Wansley, "The Merrill Lynch Quality Program," *Services Marketing in a Changing Environment* (Chicago: American Marketing Association, 1985), p. 9.

26. "Marriott Expands Frequent Travelers Program," *Hotel and Motel Management*, February 2, 1987, p. 93.

27. E. A. Locke, K. N. Shaw, L. M. Saari, and G. P. Latham, "Goal Setting and Task Performance, 1969–1980," *Psychological Bulletin*, no. 1 (1981): pp. 125–52.

28. Same as note 3.

29. Same as note 11, pp. 11–12.

30. Same as note 2.

31. Jeremy Main, "Toward Service Without a Snarl," *Fortune*, March 23, 1981, p. 61.

32. Same as note 3.

Chapter 6

GAP 3: THE SERVICE PERFORMANCE GAP

1. Daniel Yankelovich and John Immerwahr, *Putting the Work Ethic to Work* (New York: Public Agenda Foundation, 1983), p. 1.

2. As discussed in B. Katz and R. Kahn, *The Social Psychology of Organizations* (New York: John Wiley & Sons, 1978).

3. Same as note 2.

4. Bro Uttal, "Companies that Serve You Best," *Fortune*, December 7, 1987, p. 100.

5. "At Du Pont, Everybody Sells," *Sales & Marketing Management*, December 3, 1984, p. 33.

6. Leigh Bruce, "British Airways Jolts Staff with a Cultural Revolution," *International Management*, March 1987, p. 37.

7. J. Carey, J. Buckley, and J. Smith, "Hospital Hospitality," *Newsweek*, February 11, 1985, p. 78.

8. Lisa McGurrin, "Hillbilly Music in the Frozen Peas at Stew Leonard's," *New England Business*, February 17, 1986, pp. 38–41.

9. Same as note 7, p. 38.

10. "CS Close-Up," *Customer Service Management Bulletin*, March 25, 1987, p. 8.

11. Thomas J. Peters and Nancy Austin, *A Passion for Excellence* (New York: Random House, 1985), p. 15.

12. Orville C. Walker, Jr., Gilbert A. Churchill, Jr., and Neil M. Ford, "Motivation and Performance in Industrial Selling: Present Knowledge and Needed Research," *Journal of Marketing Research*, May 1977, pp. 156–68.

13. These issues are discussed in Charles Greene and D. W. Organ, "An Evaluation of Causal Models Linking Perceived Role and Job Satisfaction," *Administrative Science Quarterly*, March 1973, pp. 95–103; and R. L. Kahn, D. M. Wolfe, R. P. Quinn, J. D. Snock, and R. A. Rosenthal, *Organizational Stress* (New York: John Wiley & Sons, 1964).

14. As discussed in Arlie Russell Hochschild, *The Managed Heart: Commercialization of Human Feeling* (Berkeley: University of California Press, 1983).

15. Same as note 12.

16. "Service, Strategy Give Edge to Business Competitors," *Marketing News*, June 20, 1986, p. 5.

17. "Pul-eeze! Will Somebody Help Me?" *Time*, February 2, 1987, p. 49.

18. J. L. Heskett, "Lessons in the Service Sector," *Harvard Business Review*, March–April 1987, p. 118.

19. Same as note 18.

20. Same as note 4, p. 104.

21. Michael Kranish, "Somerville Lumber," *Boston Globe*, June 9, 1987, p. 47.

22. Same as note 4.

23. These issues are discussed in William G. Ouchi, "A Conceptual Framework for the Design of Organizational Control Mechanisms," *Management Science*, September 1979, pp. 833–48; and William G. Ouchi and Mary Ann McGuire, "Organizational Control: Two Functions," *Administrative Science Quarterly*, December 1975, pp. 559–69.

24. Same as note 23.

25. Leonard L. Berry, "Reconciling and Coordinating Selling and Service," *American Banker*, February 12, 1986, pp. 4–5.

26. Same as note 6.

27. R. H. Bork, "Call Him Old-Fashioned," *Forbes*, August 26, 1985, p./66.

28. Rosabeth M. Kanter, "From the Information Age to the Communication Age," *Management Review*, August 1987, p. 23.

29. Don Lee Bohl, ed., "Close to the Customer," *An American Management As-*

sociation Research Report on Consumer Affairs (New York: American Management Association, 1987), p. 47.

30. A. Parasuraman, "Customer-Oriented Corporate Cultures Are Crucial to Services Marketing Success," *Journal of Services Marketing*, Spring 1987, p. 13.

31. Same as note 11.

32. These issues are discussed in J. H. Geer and E. Maisel, "Evaluating the Effects of the Prediction-Control Confound," *Journal of Personality and Social Psychology*, no. 8 (1972): pp. 314–19; and D. C. Glass and J. E. Singer, *Urban Stress* (New York: Academic Press, 1972).

33. J. R. Averill, "Personal Control over Aversive Stimuli and Its Relationship to Stress," *Psychological Bulletin*, no. 4 (1973): pp. 286–303.

34. As quoted in speech by Larry Wilson, "Leadership Aspects and Reward Systems of Customer Satisfaction," at CTM Customer Satisfaction Conference, Los Angeles, California, March 17, 1989.

35. "McDonald's Tries to Keep Personal Touch," *Bryan-College Station Eagle*, May 28, 1985, p. 7A.

36. Thomas V. Bonoma, "Making Your Strategy Work," *Harvard Business Review*, March–April 1984, p. 76.

37. Same as note 29.

38. "Hot-Line!" The Forum Corporation, Boston, Mass., June 22, 1987.

39. "Management Autonomy Adds to Deli Success at Byerly's," *Progressive Grocer*, June 1984, p. 318.

40. George Russell, "Where the Customer Is Still King," *Time*, February 2, 1987, p. 56.

41. "May the Force Be with You," *Inc.*, July 1987, p. 75.

42. Scott McMurray, "Merrill Honors Quality Circles," *American Banker*, August 23, 1983, p. 23.

43. Same as note 42.

44. "How American Express Measures Quality of Its Customer Service," *AMA Forum*, March 1982, p. 30.

45. George H. Labovitz, "Keeping Your Internal Customers Satisfied," *Wall Street Journal*, July 6, 1987, p. 10.

46. As quoted in speech by David Bowen, "Leadership Aspects and Reward Systems of Customer Satisfaction," at CTM Customer Satisfaction Conference, Los Angeles, California, March 17, 1989.

Chapter 7
GAP 4: WHEN PROMISES DO NOT MATCH DELIVERY

1. William R. George and Leonard L. Berry, "Guidelines for the Advertising of Services," *Business Horizons*, May–June 1981, pp. 52–56.

2. As discussed in Leonard L. Berry, "The Employee as Customer," *Journal of Retail Banking*, March 1981, pp. 33–40; and Christian Gronroos, "Internal Marketing—Theory and Practice," *Services Marketing in a Changing Environment* (Chicago: American Marketing Association, 1985), pp. 41–47.

3. Same as note 1.

4. Leonard L. Berry, Valerie A. Zeithaml, A. Parasuraman, "Quality Counts in Services, Too," *Business Horizons*, May–June 1985, pp. 44–52.

5. Mike Burns, "Jiffy Lube International: Success Proves Too Slippery to Handle," working paper, Duke University, Durham, North Carolina, 1989.

6. Same as note 1.

7. As discussed in A. Parasuraman, Valarie A. Zeithaml, and Leonard L. Berry, "SERVQUAL: A Multiple-Item Scale for Measuring Consumer Perceptions of Service Quality," *Journal of Retailing*, Spring 1988, pp. 12–40; and A. Parasuraman, Leonard L. Berry, and Valarie A. Zeithaml, "An Empirical Test of the Gaps Model of Service Quality," working paper, Texas A&M University, College Station, Texas, 1989.

8. Valarie A. Zeithaml, "Consumer Perceptions of Price, Quality, and Value: A Means-End Model and Synthesis of Evidence," *Journal of Marketing*, July 1988, pp. 2–22.

9. Don Lee Bohl, ed., "Close to the Customer," *An American Management Association Research Report on Consumer Affairs* (New York: American Management Association, 1987), p. 80.

10. Same as note 9.

Chapter 8
GETTING STARTED ON THE SERVICE-QUALITY JOURNEY

1. A. Parasuraman, "Customer-Oriented Corporate Cultures Are Crucial to Services Marketing Success," *The Journal of Services Marketing*, Summer 1987, pp. 39–46.

2. Mimi Lieber, "Managing for Service Excellence in a Turbulent Environment," a speech to an American Marketing Association conference, Boston, Massachusetts, February 25, 1987.

3. As quoted in Leonard L. Berry, "Middle Managers Can Play a Key Role in Improving Service," *American Banker*, September 23, 1987, p. 4.

4. "The Chairman Doesn't Blink," *Quality Progress*, March 1987, p. 23.

5. Daniel Yankelovich and John Immerwahr, *Putting the Work Ethic to Work* (New York: Public Agenda Foundation, 1983), p. 1.

6. Same as note 4.

7. Benjamin Schneider, "Imperatives for the Design of Service Organizations," in *Add Value to Your Service*, proceedings of the American Marketing Association Services Marketing Conference, 1987, p. 97.

8. Leonard L. Berry, David R. Bennett, and Carter W. Brown, *Service Quality—A Profit Strategy for Financial Insttitutions* (Homewood, Ill.: Dow Jones-Irwin, 1989), pp. 122–23.

9. John J. Falzon, "Met Life's Quest for Quality," *Journal of Services Marketing*, Spring 1988, pp. 61–64.

10. Leonard L. Berry, Charles M. Futrell, and Michael R. Bowers, *Bankers Who Sell—Improving Selling Effectiveness in Banking* (Chicago: Bank Marketing Association and Homewood, Ill.: Dow Jones-Irwin, 1985), pp. 42–45.

11. Mortimer R. Feinberg and Aaron Levenstein, "It's Not My Job, Man," *Wall Street Journal*, November 11, 1985.

12. As paraphrased in Robert H. Waterman, Jr., *The Renewal Factor* (New York: Bantam Books, 1987), p. 225.

13. Howard Deutsch and Neil J. Metviner, "Quality in Banking: The Competitive Edge," *Bank Administration*, April 1987.

14. Same as note 13.

15. Chip R. Bell and Ron Zemke, "Do Service Procedures Tie Employees' Hands?" *Personnel Journal*, September 1988, p. 79.

16. Same as note 12, p. 73.

17. Same as note 12, p. 88.

18. As quoted in Bell and Zemke, "Do Services Procedures Tie Employees' Hands?," p. 81.

19. Same as note 13.

20. Peter F. Drucker, "Leadership: More Doing than Dash," *Wall Street Journal*, January 6, 1988.

Chapter 9
SERVICE-QUALITY CHALLENGES FOR THE 1990'S

1. G. Lynn Shostack and Jane Kingman-Brundage, "Service Design and Development," in *Handbook of Services Marketing*, ed. Carole A. Congram and Margaret L. Friedman (New York: ANACOM, in press).

2. G. Lynn Shostack, "Planning the Service Encounter," in *The Service Encounter*, ed. John A. Czepiel, Michael R. Solomon, and Carol F. Surprenant (Lexington, Mass.: Lexington Books, 1985), p. 246.

3. See G. Lynn Shostack, "Designing Services that Deliver," *Harvard Business Review*, January–February 1984, pp. 133–39.

4. William R. George and Barbara E. Gibson, "Blueprinting: A Tool for Managing Quality in Service," a presentation to the Symposium on Quality in Services, Karlstad, Sweden, August 1988.

5. Steve Bergsman, "Valley National Streamlines Loan Processes," *American Banker*, March 15, 1989, pp. 9–10.

6. Leonard L. Berry, "Big Ideas in Services Marketing," *The Journal of Consumer Marketing*, Spring 1986, p. 50.

7. Information supplied by Florida Power & Light company officials James Cartwright and Kathy Scott in telephone interviews on April 26 and 28, 1989.

8. Tom Peters, "Twenty Propositions about Service," a speech to the International Customer Service Association, Phoenix, Arizona, September 20, 1988.

9. "Among Restaurateurs, It's Dog Eat Dog," *Business Week*, January 9, 1989, p. 86.

10. "Where the Jobs Are Is Where the Skills Aren't," *Business Week*, September 19, 1988, p. 105.

11. "Help Wanted," *Business Week*, August 10, 1987, p. 49.

12. Louis S. Richman, "Tomorrow's Jobs: Plentiful, But . . . ," *Fortune*, April 11, 1988, p. 44.

13. Same as note 10, p. 104.

14. Roger Selbert, "The Educational Future," *FutureScan*, September 12, 1988, p. 1.

15. As quoted in "Tomorrow's Jobs," note 12, p. 48.

16. James Poisant, "Disney World's Happy-Employee Secrets," *Boardroom Reports*, October 15, 1987, p. 3.

17. Same as note 12, p. 52.

18. Same as note 11, p. 51.

19. Robin Clapp, "The Magic of Disney," unpublished paper.

20. Tom Peters, "Competitiveness Crusade Begins with Your Gripes," *Chicago Tribune*, March 6, 1989.

21. Adapted from Paul Hawkin, "You Are the Customer, You Are the Company," *Whole Earth Review*, 1986.

22. This paragraph is based on material appearing in note 8. The service-quality statistics appear in the *Deluxe Corporation 1988 Annual Report*.

23. This statistic was supplied by Jeff Jones of the product marketing department at Dunkin' Donuts in a telephone interview on April 28, 1989.

24. Donald K. Clifford, Jr., and Richard E. Cavanaugh, *The Winning Performance—How America's High-Growth Midsize Companies Succeed* (New York: Bantam Books, 1985), p. 66.

25. Leonard L. Berry, "Delivering Excellent Service in Retailing," *Arthur Andersen Retailing Issues Letter*, April 1988, p. 2.

26. Leonard L. Berry, A. Parasuraman, and Valarie A. Zeithaml, "The Service-Quality Puzzle," *Business Horizons*, September–October 1988, p. 43.

Appendix A
SERVQUAL AND ITS APPLICATIONS

1. Details about the procedure used in developing and testing SERVQUAL and empirical evidence of the instrument's reliability and validity can be found in A. Parasuraman, Valarie A. Zeithaml, and Leonard L. Berry, "SERVQUAL: A Multiple-Item Scale for Measuring Consumer Perceptions of Service Quality," *Journal of Retailing*, Spring 1988, pp. 12–40.

INDEX